AHM779
84

# Global
# AIDS
# Policy

# Global
# AIDS
# Policy_____

**EDITED BY**
**DOUGLAS A. FELDMAN**

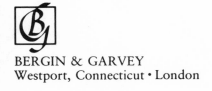

**BERGIN & GARVEY**
Westport, Connecticut • London

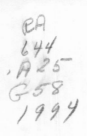

Library of Congress Cataloging-in-Publication Data

Global AIDS policy / edited by Douglas A. Feldman.
    p.  cm.
    Chiefly previously unpublished papers presented at the Mar. 1991
Society for Applied Anthropology Meeting in Charleston, S.C., and at
the Nov. 1990 American Anthropological Association Meeting in New
Orleans, La.
    Includes bibliographical references (p.   ) and index.
    ISBN 0–89789–282–8 (alk. paper).—ISBN 0–89789–412–X (pbk.)
    1. AIDS (Disease)—Government policy.  I. Feldman, Douglas A.
II. Society for Applied Anthropology. Meeting (1991 : Charleston,
S.C.)  III. American Anthropological Association. Meeting (1990 :
New Orleans, La.)
    RA644.A25G58   1994
    362.1'99792—dc20       94–2850

British Library Cataloguing in Publication Data is available.

Library of Congress Catalog Card Number: 94–2850
ISBN: 0–89789–282–8
     0–89789–412–X (pbk.)

First published in 1994

Bergin & Garvey, 88 Post Road West, Westport, CT 06881
An imprint of Greenwood Publishing Group, Inc.

Printed in the United States of America

The paper used in this book complies with the
Permanent Paper Standard issued by the National
Information Standards Organization (Z39.48–1984).

10  9  8  7  6  5  4  3  2  1

To my good friend
Steven Hersh
(1947–1992)
who died of AIDS

# Contents

# Preface

This volume of original, never previously published chapters grew in part out of two seminars that I chaired: "Issues in Planning and Evaluating AIDS-Related Interventions in Africa and Asia" at the March 1991 Society for Applied Anthropology meetings in Charleston, South Carolina, and "Global AIDS Policy" at the November 1990 American Anthropological Association meetings in New Orleans. Several of the chapters, however, were initially developed specifically for this volume.

All of the chapters were peer reviewed prior to acceptance, and I would like to cordially thank our distinguished panel of external reviewers: Dr. Ralph Bolton (Pomona College), Dr. Robert G. Carlson (Wright State University), Dr. Michael C. Clatts (Narcotic and Drug Research Inc.), Dr. Francis P. Conant (Hunter College, CUNY), Dr. Stephen L. Eyre (University of California, San Francisco), Dr. Vincent E. Gil (Southern California College), Dr. Janis Hutchinson (University of Houston), Dr. Carl Kendall (Tulane University), Dr. Norris G. Lang (University of Houston), Dr. Susan McCombie (University of Pennsylvania), Dr. Michael Melody (Barry University), Dr. Robert Porter (Porter/Novelli), Dr. Michael D. Quam (Sangamon State University), and Dr. Priscilla Reining (University of Florida). I would also like to thank Jean Dingee, Jonathan Bellman, Armando Castro, and Dieter Fredericks for editorial assistance, and Donna Rayburn and Maggie Dominguez for secretarial assistance.

The reader should keep in mind that AIDS-related events and circumstances change rapidly, and that the contributors to this volume maintain perspectives valid at the time their chapters were written. It is not the intention of this volume to be comprehensive on the topic of global AIDS policy. Indeed, volumes have already been written on this subject. However, the viewpoints expressed here are primarily based upon empirical social science research and theory.

While it was not my original intention necessarily to edit a volume that emphasized strong critiques of existing global AIDS policy, most of the chapters turned out this way. It is now clear that this development was not by chance. Rather, the overall direction of global AIDS policy through the 1980s and early 1990s has been essentially misguided, and serious rethinking of AIDS as a public health and social issue is now necessary. It has become obvious to most of the contributors of this volume, and to myself, that a restructuring of AIDS/HIV prevention programs, services for persons living with AIDS/HIV, and social institutions relating to all aspects of health is crucial on an international scale if there is to be any chance for success in our global struggle against AIDS. It is my hope that this volume will assist in showing us the way.

# 1

# Introduction

*Douglas A. Feldman*

As we look back at the social, cultural, and political dimensions of AIDS in the 1980s and early 1990s, it seems as though we have come so far in so short a time. From a virtually unknown disease in 1981, AIDS has become undoubtedly the most discussed, most thought-about, and most feared pandemic of our time. Few human activities generate as much concern and ambivalence as do sex and death, and AIDS links sex and death in our consciousness as has no other disease in the modern era. AIDS has had a profound influence in numerous aspects of our lives, especially in many developed nations. From the media to the workplace to health care to our educational systems, AIDS discourse has increasingly grown in importance in recent years.

AIDS has become a major concern in many aspects of public policy. Whether or not to have sex education and AIDS education in the classroom is no longer the issue in much of North America and Europe. The question has become to what extent abstinence or safer sex practices should be emphasized. The enormous economic impact of AIDS upon the health care system in the United States has forced us to begin seriously to plan for a fundamental restructuring of this previously intransigent social institution. Human resource managers are increasingly becoming more experienced in handling employment-related issues of their employees with HIV-spectrum disease. Major newspapers, newsmagazines, and television networks have devoted substantial resources and staff to cover various issues and perspectives of AIDS. For a virus that had infected only an estimated 13 million people by 1992, or a mere 0.25 percent of the world's 5.3 billion people, HIV has had a more pivotal effect on health research, health education, and the global biomedical infrastructure than any other single disease in this century.

Yet when we look at what has actually changed, at what behaviors have been fundamentally altered, and at what social institutions have been restructured as a consequence of AIDS, it is striking how little has been accomplished in terms of getting the pandemic under control through effective prevention programs and of ameliorating the social, cultural, political, and personal impacts of AIDS. In most of the developing countries where HIV is already rampant, while sexually active teenagers and adults may be very worried about getting AIDS, there is usually little or nothing that they are doing to change their sexual behavior to prevent HIV infection. In those African cities where one of every four sexually active adults is currently HIV seropositive, the alarming reality remains that only a tiny minority of the population uses condoms properly and regularly during sexual intercourse. The vast majority do not use condoms at all. Few individuals utilize other forms of safer sex, such as interfemoral sex, to reduce HIV risk. In those same African cities where funerals for persons who have died of AIDS have become commonplace, where the managerial sector of key industries has been especially hard hit by personnel losses due to AIDS, and where the number of AIDS-related orphaned children continues to climb more rapidly than the resources of either society or government to cope with the needs, AIDS is still viewed much as it was a decade ago. It remains a highly stigmatized disease that few care to talk about in public.

Policy decisions are being made throughout the world on how to best handle the AIDS crisis. Areas of policy formulation include such issues as mandatory or voluntary HIV reporting, mandatory or voluntary HIV testing, priorities in AIDS health and social services funding, quarantining and immigration restrictions, screening blood supplies in developing nations, effective strategies for HIV prevention, and HIV-related discrimination and neglect.

In general, politicians and biomedical administrators have set the direction for global AIDS policy until now. By and large, this policy has failed, and failed miserably. It is the premise of this book that to effectively accomplish the control of HIV on a global scale, it will be necessary to replace political considerations and a biomedical approach with a public health and social science approach. Needle exchange programs are a good example of the need to reformulate policy. Political considerations in the United States and elsewhere have prevented needle exchange programs from being implemented. Conservative politicians and some religious and African-American leaders have opposed needle exchange programs, asserting that they promote drug use. Those who favor a biomedical approach have been reluctant to support any program that will facilitate the use of a harmful narcotic. However, public health and social science research has demonstrated that such programs reduce HIV seroprevalence in an injecting drug-using population and do not promote greater drug use.

Vincent E. Gil's chapter ("Behind the Wall of China: AIDS Profile, AIDS

Policy") looks at AIDS in the world's most populous nation. HIV is spreading rapidly through injecting drug use in China's rural southern Yunnan Province and is also showing signs of nascent growth through sexual transmission in major urban centers. Restrictive attitudes toward sexuality and antidemocratic policies may hinder HIV prevention and control in China during the 1990s. Certainly, Asia is the continent to watch during the next few years. It has been projected that the number of new HIV infections in Asia will overtake the total number of persons with HIV in Africa by the year 2000. HIV transmission is increasing rapidly in India and Thailand, and it is likely that this pattern will soon occur in other neighboring countries as well.

Richard G. Parker ("Public Policy, Political Activism, and AIDS in Brazil") points to the dismal lack of achievement by the Brazilian government in handling its AIDS crisis. Poor planning, lack of governmental coordination, inadequate funding, and disinterest on the part of most Brazilian politicians concerning HIV prevention and AIDS services have led to the current disastrous situation in Brazil. Conditions that have contributed to the spread of HIV in Brazil include a large but politically unorganized gay community, rampant poverty where countless street children often turn to prostitution, a vast bisexually active population of married men who do not see themselves at risk, and poor sanitation in the *favelas* (slums) that promotes the proliferation of cofactor pathogens.

The problem of governmental neglect or incompetence is certainly not restricted to Brazil. Indeed, most of the governments in Latin America, the Caribbean, Asia, the Middle East, and Africa have performed poorly in their handling of the AIDS crisis. There are exceptions, Costa Rica and the Commonwealth of Puerto Rico in Latin America and the Caribbean, Uganda and Senegal in Africa, and Thailand and Australia in Asia and the Pacific, for example, where governments have made a sincere attempt to work against the epidemic through the provision of HIV prevention and AIDS health and social services within their borders. But even in these few countries where stigma, shame, fear, denial, corruption, and inaction do not shape AIDS/HIV policy, severe budgetary limitations in developing nations often delimit what such governments can do. It is interesting, though unfortunate, that the one developing country that spends the most funds on persons living with HIV on a per capita basis, Cuba, has developed the most draconian measures of incarceration of all HIV-positive citizens in several quarantine camps. Allocation and availability of resources by a government clearly do not necessarily mean that prudent choices will be made in the struggle against HIV.

Pamela Hartigan ("The Response of Nongovernmental Organizations in Latin America to HIV Infection and AIDS: A Vehicle for Grasping the Contribution NGOs Make to Health and Development") looks at the role that NGOs, national AIDS programs, and donor organizations have in working together to strengthen broad-based HIV prevention and AIDS care programs. Hartigan shows us some of the difficulties encountered by various kinds of NGOs in Latin America, which have led to inefficiencies and inadequacies of HIV-related services and prevention.

Norris G. Lang ("HIV, Immigration Policy, and Latinos/as: Public Health Safety versus Hidden Agendas") discusses the history and inequities of U.S. immigration policy as it relates to HIV and Latin America. It is peculiar that the United States, a nation that contributed heavily to global HIV transmission during the 1980s through international tourism and that has such a large population with HIV, is so restrictive against immigration by persons testing HIV positive. If this model of exclusion were adapted universally, no one with HIV would be permitted to migrate to any other nation. Since most HIV transmission is preventable, policies based on exclusion of infected persons, rather than behavioral change, are unnecessary and unfair. By the early 1990s this policy of exclusion led to the virtual stranding at a U.S. military base camp next to Cuba of HIV-positive Haitians who were otherwise eligible to come to the United States. It took a court decision, ruling this policy to be inhumane, to permit some of the Haitians to be brought over to a detention center in Miami.

Sub-Saharan Africa has so far been the region most deeply impacted by the AIDS pandemic. In spite of the imminent threat to their lives, most Africans remain wary of using condoms. Charles B. Rwabukwali and colleagues ("Culture, Sexual Behavior, and Attitudes toward Condom Use among Baganda Women") conducted a study among Baganda women in Uganda to find out how they feel about using condoms. Among the findings, quite remarkably, is that most of the women who have extremely negative feelings toward condoms have never even seen a condom, let alone used one. Successful behavioral change requires more than education. Fundamentally, long-term behavioral change may inevitably be dependent on much-needed structural changes in the political economy of developing nations in order to reduce relentless poverty, dichotomous income inequality, and the second-class status of women. In the short term, however, skills building, role playing, desensitization to discussing sex and handling condoms, and personal empowerment counseling are necessary tools for promoting safer sex behavior.

The lessened value of women in contemporary African societies may explain why female prostitutes in Ghana were seen as the source of the HIV problem in that country. Robert W. Porter ("AIDS in Ghana: Priorities and Policies") shows us the cultural biases of epidemiologic data and demonstrates how the HIV prevention priorities for this nation were wrongly constructed based upon a false foundation.

In South Africa political conservatives have mobilized antigay and antiblack bigotry to support an intentionally lethargic AIDS agenda. Virginia van der Vliet ("Apartheid and the Politics of AIDS") analyzes the political processes at work in that nation. The potential impact of AIDS in South Africa cannot be overstated, and van der Vliet is correct in stating that "AIDS will become one of the most important factors shaping [that nation] within the next ten years."

Dana Raphael ("The Politics of International Health: Breastfeeding and HIV") addresses the risk of breastfeeding among HIV-positive mothers in developing nations. She points to what she sees as the hypocrisy of international organizations that have one standard for developed nations and another riskier standard for developing nations. The question of HIV and breastfeeding raises some essential ethical dilemmas that need further examination.

This volume attempts to be truly global by including public policy concerns within the United States, where much of the work on HIV by social and behavioral researchers has been conducted. Michael D. Quam ("AIDS Policy and the United States Political Economy") assesses the status of HIV in relation to socioeconomic factors within the United States at the close of the Bush administration. Writing prior to Clinton's national health program, he is on target when he indicates, "We have no national health policy and we have no national strategy for funding such a policy. The AIDS crisis has exposed the brutal failure of the current health establishment."

In the United States millions of gay and bisexual men, both those who are HIV positive and those who are HIV negative, have been irrevocably affected by the pandemic. The gay community of the 1990s has been transformed quite dramatically since the advent of AIDS. With hundreds of thousands of gay men ill (or dead), the scourge has not only been devastating on a personal level, but has had a profound influence on the social and economic infrastructure and cultural norms of the gay community itself. In many respects, however, AIDS has strengthened the gay community. Political coalitions and demonstrations, gay economic development, and cultural activities have markedly grown. M. E. Melody ("Acting Up Academically: AIDS and the Politics of Disempowerment") describes some of the growing pangs of the gay community. Melody takes us from the reaction of the Reagan conservatives to the rise of ACT UP, an activist organization that has had a pivotal influence upon HIV public policy.

Robert G. Carlson, Harvey A. Siegal, and Russel S. Falck ("Ethnography, Epidemiology, and Public Policy: Needle-Use Practices and HIV-1 Risk Reduction among Injecting Drug Users in the Midwest") look at the cultural ecology of injecting drug use in two Ohio cities. They observe that the term *needle sharing* is a misnomer, since the process of needle transfer from one user to the other does not involve a communal sense of, or desire for, social sharing. When needle transfer does occur, it is out of necessity, rather than as a function of social solidarity within the injecting drug-using population. Indeed, the general availability of clean needles and syringes in Ohio has resulted in a very low rate of HIV seroprevalence among users.

Michael C. Clatts and colleagues ("AIDS Risk Behavior among Drug Injectors in New York City: Critical Gaps in Prevention Policy") review the findings from several studies conducted among drug injectors in New York City where needle transfer is common due to the scarcity of available unused needles. The authors conclude that knowledge about risk does not result in behavioral change among many of those involved in drug injection, and that condom use appears to be determined by a host of social and economic factors that compete with concerns about risk for HIV.

The struggle over AIDS policy is a microcosm of the essential political and social struggles currently raging within societies on a global level. Broadly speaking, AIDS spotlights the dysfunctional inadequacies and anachronisms of our times. AIDS forces us to revive our commitment to social, political, and economic change throughout the world. In responding to the challenge of AIDS, we undoubtedly will continue to encounter change-resistant forces that may seem formidable. Our role must first be to develop AIDS policy that is sound, reasoned, based upon research and evaluation, and not compromised by the omnipresent change-resistant forces, and then to implement well-financed, effective programs that will convert policy into action. It is urgent that we not waver from this approach. AIDS is giving us the opportunity to correct the structural and attitudinal discontinuities of modern social life and to guide the direction of rapid social and cultural change in virtually every nation. Equally as important, there are simply too many lives at stake. We cannot let them, and indeed ourselves, down. The new AIDS policy makers need to remain firm and uncompromising. History will judge us harshly if we fail.

# 2

# Behind the Wall of China:
# AIDS Profile, AIDS Policy

*Vincent E. Gil*

China has both fascinated and alarmed the West for centuries. Called the Middle Kingdom—Zhongguo in Mandarin—China has had the ability to remain enigmatic to most of the world, seeping out self-perceptions with measured restraint and as global opinion has required (Mosher 1990). Yet the universal human condition of our era cannot be divorced from the experiences of China's more than 1.16 billion people, nearly a quarter of the human population.[1]

As China has emerged from isolation and attained for itself a more comfortable global platform, it has been pressed to address issues that come from openness and reform. Such issues are no longer simply ideological or technological; they are also epidemiologic and medical. China's nascent HIV infection is already moving the country from being a poorly understood nation to one deserving once more a center position on the global stage.

Sadly, news of China's HIV infection has crept out slowly and cautiously. Initially given little press by official news agencies, it was later overshadowed by the more pressing economic reforms of 1988 and by the dramatic political events of 1989. The emerging pattern of infection led to China's classification by the World Health Organization (WHO) as a "Pattern III" country (Chin and Mann 1988), where infection rates are low and predominantly heterosexual or of unspecified origin. Viewing China's infection through the WHO taxonomy has also worked against understanding any unique dimensions of China's own HIV epidemic.[2] As will be discussed later, there are relevant differences in the Chinese case that merit specific attention.

This chapter is the result of fieldwork in China by the author, undertaken as part of a collaborative technical exchange and at the invitation of the

Chinese Medical Association. Fieldwork presented a rare opportunity to go "behind the Wall" and openly assess HIV/AIDS in most of its complexity. In developing countries such as China, multifactorial issues hinder prevention efforts and complicate epidemiologic forecasting (Alexander, Gabelnick & Spieler 1990; Feldman 1990:46). In this chapter I elaborate those cultural, social, and political elements involved in China's attempts to manage its growing HIV epidemic. Epidemiologic data from field visits conducted in Beijing, Chengdu, and Kunming summarize the status of the epidemic to date. Select data from the First Sino-American Management of HIV Disease Symposium (held in Beijing during 1990), to which I was a delegate, are also blended with the ethnographic material to further clarify present conditions.[3]

Particular attention is being devoted to understanding China's emerging HIV/AIDS policies. Attempts to clarify these policies and the issues they pose for Chinese socialism are framed within the tensions of prevention. HIV prevention in China cannot be easily divorced from political philosophy or from human rights issues. Containment of HIV thus poses an unrelenting challenge for China to transform its traditional treatment of sexual expression and—consequently—of people.

A report such as this is both necessary and timely, because China's HIV record should be kept distinct from the HIV/AIDS phenomenon in other countries totally unlike China. Today, with its ideology in flux, with its commitment to halting HIV formed under unique traditions and a socialist philosophy that is quintessentially Chinese, China is rapidly developing its own prevention system. Any effort to delineate just what that system is—or what it may become—must be to some degree hesitant, preliminary, and limited. This chapter is a first step toward understanding China's HIV problem and its unfolding policies and procedures to halt infection.

## CHINA'S HIV/AIDS HISTORY

Growth in international contacts eventually enabled the transmission of HIV to within China's borders. In 1984 an American foreigner was identified as being seropositive and was quickly deported (Zeng 1988). Shortly thereafter, the government commissioned seroepidemiologic studies on a wide scale. In 1985 Factor VIII sera produced in the United States were found to have infected four Chinese persons with hemophilia (Zeng 1990). There was now sufficient reason for the government to begin coordinated screening of potentially at-risk populations. In April 1986 several hospitals in Beijing and the Institute of Virology, Chinese Academy of Preventive Medicine, began screening sexually transmitted disease (STD) and other select outpatients.

Sexual transmission was discovered in January 1988 in a Chinese male who presented with penile erythema and atrophic lesions. Western blot and ELISA tests confirmed that the patient was HIV seropositive (Quin et al. 1990). The patient acknowledged that during the previous September he had had homosexual contacts with foreigners.

By September 1990 China had identified 446 HIV-positive individuals after an extraordinary effort to test over 300,000 in the population (Chen 1990). The emerging pattern, however, did not forecast HIV transmission through heterosexual contacts as much as it revealed its association with drug use in the southwestern provinces (Dai 1990). Then "Pattern III" characteristics began to weaken. It was obvious to the Chinese, even in 1988, that the Indochinese epidemic was spreading up through Thailand, a consequence of drug traffic in the Golden Triangle.

Most severely affected since 1988 has been Yunnan Province, a predominantly agricultural region bordering Myanmar (formerly Burma), Laos, and Vietnam. Through this region—and inevitably through southern China as well—passes the "opium express," a trafficking complex that since the late 1970s has produced the world's largest tonnage of opium and its derivatives (Inciardi 1986). Since the 1980s drug use has steadily increased in Yunnan and adjoining provinces (Guanxi, Guizhou, Guangdong). For centuries there has been a tradition of smoking opiates in this region, but the recent trend has been toward intravenous use of drugs, particularly heroin (He 1990). Estimates vary, but official reports put the region's intravenous drug users at above 100,000 (Dai 1991). Heroin availability masks the low availability of drug-injecting equipment, and thus promotes the onerous practice of communal use of syringes.

By 1990 Yunnan's HIV-infected accounted for 87.2 percent ($n=389$) of China's total HIV prevalence.[4] Ruili (county) had the strongest concentration of seropositives; 305 (of the then 389) cases living in its Dehong prefecture. This cluster was considered yet another recognizable but rare HIV nidus in a rural region (Peabody 1990). Lushui (county), in Jadi Prefecture, and Gejiu (county), again in Dehong, followed, with 11.4 percent and 4.3 percent of the nation's infected. (Mercifully, the rest of China enjoyed at that time a very low HIV rate, with only Beijing surfacing above the 1–2 percent proportion infected in the samples tested.)

Yunnan's topography and the particular lifestyle of the many minority groups in this region encouraged the consolidation of the epidemic early on. Rugged mountains and deep agricultural valleys dot the countryside. Agrarian populations in Yunnan, consequently, do not travel much or relocate unnecessarily. Even for those addicted, it is often easier to get drugs locally or cross into Myanmar than to travel extensively to cities in the province itself.

Moreover, this region of China is populated by "minority peoples," as the dominant Han Chinese refer to non-Han and related populations. Each ethnic minority group has sufficient lifestyle and historical distinctives to keep it from readily assimilating. Yunnan's Provincial Health and Anti-Epidemic Center was able to amass enough demographic information early, to clarify local conditions. The Dai, in the county of Ruili, Dehong Prefecture, accounted for 68.6 percent of those infected locally in 1990. Since they were ancestrally related to Thai farmers across the border, most did not even speak Mandarin. The Dai showed the strongest pattern of infection and also drug use (*China Daily* 1991a). However, learning to inject drugs is not part of the cultural legacy of these farmers (87 percent do agricultural work) and this requires needles: needles come from areas where other addicts live—cities and lives well beyond their imagination. The Jingpo, another ethnic minority, accounted for 17.7 percent of those infected in the province in 1990.

In sum, the overwhelming majority of seropositives to 1990 were ethnic minorities (372 of 389) who were occupationally tied to the land, male, young (between the ages of 20 and 39), and involved in parenteral drug use.

Yunnan women presented a low incidence rate at the 1990 juncture. The ratio of men to women infected was 76:1. Only two spouses of HIV seropositive males were identified as seropositive, and they were both Chinese. There were nineteen women of Myanmar origin living in this region identified as HIV seropositives. It was unclear from available data whether these Myanmar female cases were drug-use related. In 1990 it was also too early in China's epidemic to know whether women who were tested, and found seronegative, would seroconvert later on. The exact number of infected women in Yunnan is still not knowable, and is presumed by all forecasts to be higher than the 1990 statistics represent (Zhao 1990).

A significant difference emerged in the ensuing three years of the epidemic, between 1990 and 1993. Growth in seropositive cases between 1990 and 1992 more than doubled to 932 cases, making the growth rate for the period 206.5 percent. AIDS cases also grew from 2 to 11 in the same period (Ministry of Public Health 1992).

In 1990, those non-Han minority groups delineated above and residing in Yunnan, farmers and manual laborers who also drug injected, comprised the bulk of cases. By 1992 the distribution includes expatriate Chinese, prostitutes and their clients, hotel attendants, spouses and relatives of former HIV seropositives, persons with hemophilia, prisoners, those with other sexually transmitted diseases, homosexual men, and populations in the border regions with Tibet and southeast Asia. Drug injection users continue to be well represented (677) but now comprise 72.6 percent of the infected total. Eighty-four percent of medical and epidemiology personnel I interviewed in 1992 ($n=69/82$) agreed that most new HIV cases are discovered in residents that are not from the province where they were tested and found seropositive. Interviews also confirmed that increases in travel, especially foreign travel, and exposure to HIV through sexual contact abroad were implicated in the increase ($n=80/82$, or 97 percent of those interviewed were in agreement).

I also collected ethnographic data in 1993 through convenience interviews ($n=147$) of medical doctors, provincial epidemiology station personnel, family planning and STD clinic personnel, and local subjects in five provincial urban centers. All confirmed the effects of mass movements of persons in China during the past three years on HIV transmission and the widening sociogeographic distribution that the virus now shows. This point is worth elaborating.

Since 1989, China increasingly liberalized its policies on employment and thus on where people could relocate. A liberal policy enabled mass movements of peasants, especially from the southwest countryside (from provinces like Yunnan) to come to the burgeoning metropolises of China. The appeal to seek new fortunes in "open cities" like Guangzhou, Shanghai, and in Special Economic Zones (SEZs) like Shenzhen, Zhuhai, became irresistible (Morrison and Dernberger 1989). These are exactly the places where new HIV prevalences have been documented between 1990 and 1992. Moreover, expatriate Chinese during these years continued to travel freely between Hong Kong, Malaysia, Thailand, Macao, and the mainland. Thus, businessmen and wealthy overseas Chinese entrepreneurs are over-represented in the 1992 HIV positive expatriate population. Many expatriates combine business with pleasure, as evidenced by their engagement of call girls and occasional male homosexuals at hotels and exclusive discos in the mainland (Gil 1991). It is not surprising, then, that the number of expatriate Chinese who have been found to be HIV positive is also high in developing and SEZ cities: Yunnan (Sichuan), Beijing, Guangzhou (Guangdong), and Shanghai. Similarly, mainland Chinese who travel abroad are over-represented among the HIV positive cases ("Foreign Exposure" category of Table 2), confirming that their source of infection stemmed from sexual contacts abroad.

Small but visible numbers of the HIV infected in some populations in China now presage the global trend of association among STDs, sex industry workers, clients, and HIV infection (Lewis, Kenney, Dor, & Dughe 1989). In 1990 there were no reported HIV cases among sex industry workers or their clients, nor was a connection between STD patients and HIV seen in the case records (Gil 1991). By the close of 1992 all three groups (prostitutes, clients, and STD patients) show some HIV infectivity. Furthermore, HIV infections also show up among prisoners, as well as among male homosexuals screened for blood in Beijing.

By November 1993, 1,140 HIV seropositive cases were being reported in China, and nineteen patients with AIDS (Zeng 1993). Yunnan Province maintained the highest caseload of HIV/AIDS with 879 infections.

## THE GOVERNMENT'S RESPONSE TO HIV

The Chinese perspective on HIV and prevention is best understood within the emic context of China's social, political, and ideologic history. A view from many angles is thus required; only some of these can be fully addressed in this section.

Faced with a small but nonetheless fulminating and deadly epidemic on its soil, the Chinese government has acted quickly and in keeping with its ideological traditions. Essentially, HIV/AIDS required swift political action: new measures to insure that no repudiation of revolutionary ideals would occur while dealing with a crisis that could challenge the fiber of party social thinking.[5] Because HIV was linked early to homosexuality, and later to drug use, laws were enacted by the People's Congress to insure that control measures were framed within appropriate ideologies. The 1982 constitution had already shifted much of the authority for lawmaking and approving to the National People's Congress (Wu et al. 1988:47), enabling the passage of new laws within record time.

Two primary goals have thus surfaced in response to the threat of HIV/AIDS in China: (1) to tackle the social contexts in which HIV infectivity is possible; and (2) to generate the appropriate medical-epidemiologic infrastructure needed to prevent its spread. The former goal has required a comprehensive linkage of civil measures with legal and political ones. The latter goal has involved massive and coordinated expansion efforts in education and medicine.

### Sociolegal Actions

On January 14, 1988, regulations concerning the monitoring and control of HIV/AIDS were issued by the Ministry of Public Health and seven other ministries, with the approval of the State Council (He 1990). By February 1989 the Law of Preventing Infectious Diseases of the People's Republic of China was passed by the People's Congress (He 1990). Not only does this law require that non-Chinese foreigners coming to stay in China for more than one year bear proof of being HIV negative, but the same regulations are also made to apply to Chinese expatriates returning to China. Thirty-three articles also established a monitoring and control system for "relevant persons" (i.e., those HIV seropositive) and a reporting system that identifies them to the proper authorities. Moreover, under these articles, anyone infected who knowingly transmits the virus to another person could be criminally prosecuted, if identified.

The articles also furnish provinces with the right to restrict the movement of seropositive individuals, enabling local "quarantine" measures for the "provision of medical care to infected persons" (China Daily 1990; He 1990). In Yunnan, for example, individual "registration cards" are now issued to HIV-positive persons in order to trace their movements. No one so identified and tagged can travel without appropriate notification and release from the local epidemiology station (*China Daily* 1990).

These measures are consistent with China's historical restrictions on individual interests in light of the superseding priorities of the state.[6] Freedom of movement, for example, has been restricted by law since 1958, and mobility is premised principally on the allocation of human resources as the state sees fit. As an HIV control measure, restricting movement of seropositive individuals simply reinforces the argument of selfless sacrifice for the common good (Han and Go 1986). Furthermore, due to its present low level of HIV infection, China has not yet determined the relative risks associated with its infected populations. There are no epidemiologic models that would provide a probabilistic basis from which to predict infectivity and transmission potentialities. HIV transmission remains predominantly rural at this time. Yunnan's villages are the focal points of infection. Restricting movement of those infected from their rural villages is China's hedge against the possibility of HIV transmission beyond the known geographic boundaries of infection.

A high rate of HIV infection among injecting drug users aroused great attention from the Chinese government early on. Laws introduced in 1988 were aimed at strengthening those already in existence to insure that drug dealers, traffickers, and users were swiftly prosecuted (He 1990; Wu *et al.* 1988:46). Not only is drug dealing illegal in China, but so is drug taking. Regulations such as "Strongly Cracking Down on Prostitution, Whoring and Drug Abuse," and "Strengthening the Management of the Public Social Order" (He 1990) express the sentiment that the government will not tolerate what it perceives to be a threat to the society. To this end, the Departments of Social Security, Customs, and Public Security work together with epidemiology surveillance stations and medical establishments as a network. For drug users, rehabilitation centers exist and are operative. These combine detoxification programs with measures for social restoration using work programs.[7]

At other levels, the government has moved to identify at-risk groups beyond drug injecting ethnic minorities. The Asian Games held in 1990 are a good example of what has been happening. Beijing's municipal government intensified surveillance and preventive education in an effort to "encourage people to refuse to be contaminated by evil influence, not to have sexual contacts with [potentially HIV-positive individuals,] and not to engage in needle sharing" (Foreign Broadcasting Information Services [FBIS] 1990b; bracket my translation). Six categories of persons were targeted for special attention: "street prostitutes, upstarts or recently wealthy/aspiring industrialists/businessmen, young women longing for study abroad, teenage [women] who have been raped and thus are indifferent to further sex, young women with [a] vengeance toward men, and persons who are indifferent to [the risks of] venereal diseases" (*ibid.*; brackets my translations). All of these were presumed risk groups for the spread of HIV.

Categorically, the targets appear predominantly female (at least four of six). Most important in this illustration, however, is the continuation of a socialist ideology about classes of people. That ideology is applied to the HIV/AIDS social metaphor without alteration. Both Sabatier (1988) and Farmer (1990) have illustrated the effects of categorizing individuals believed to be at high risk, resulting often in the accusation of groups because of their presumed potential for transmitting the virus. Here, Chinese socialists evidence their use of "associative logic," a framework that regards classes of people as essentially sharing the same characteristics (Wu *et al.* 1988). Such associations, in turn, promote a particular treatment of the group as a whole.

### Epidemiologic and Medical Actions

Stepped up prevention and education activities now underscore China's desire for early precautions. In 1986 the Chinese Ministry of Public Health added HIV/AIDS to the list of diseases requiring notification to health authorities (Zhu and Deng 1988). Monitoring stations were set up in Beijing, Shanghai, Guangzhou, Fuzhou, Hangzhou, Xian, Shengyang, and Nanning. In 1988 Chengdu and Kunming epidemiology prevention stations were added to the list (making them the closest monitoring sites to the sources of infection) and now operate ongoing serosurveillances for HIV (Dai 1990).

The relationship between HIV and other STDs is known and is taken into consideration (Dai 1990; He 1990; Xu and Fan 1990). From 1980 to 1989, 220,222 STD cases were reported in the country, after a previous decade of extremely low incidence (Xu and Fan 1990). In early 1991 the cumulative figure stood at 370,000 (*China Daily* 1991b). Modernization and reforms have had liberalizing consequences, most significantly on the sexual mores of the younger generation (Link, Madsen, and Pickowicz 1989). Premarital intercourse is now known to be higher than ever in China's socialist history (Pan 1989, 1990). Sociologists estimate that between half and two-thirds of all STD cases occur in unmarried individuals. In this population the incidence of STDs has more than doubled since 1989 (FBIS 1990b). Coupled with low levels of contraceptive use by unmarried, sexually active persons, STD infections pose a serious potential route for enhancing HIV transmission in China. Aware of this threat, the National Institute of Virology now coordinates the monitoring of STDs. Screening of groups with high rates of STDs is routine in tourist areas, coastal "special economic zones," and the twelve provinces with epidemiology surveillance stations (Xu and Fan 1990).

At the medical level, seroepidemiologic, virologic, and clinical research studies are under way (Ji and Su 1990; Wang, Shao, and Zeng 1990; Zeng 1990). Studies have also been undertaken using traditional Chinese medicinal herbs (Su 1990; Wu 1990) and even *qigong* (breathing exercises) (Cui 1990). Some herbal remedies have shown *in vitro* antiviral action against HIV-1, although the scope of this work is very limited at present (Guan 1990; Jin 1990).

China has recently requested assistance from abroad in managing HIV. In March 1990 WHO was asked to help formulate a three-year national program for HIV/AIDS control. The program's aim is to strengthen local efforts while attempting to bring these into conformity with global HIV/AIDS policies and strategies (FBIS 1990a; Peabody 1990). The plan calls for perfecting epidemiologic assays and surveillance work, coordinating established medical resources at the provincial and municipal levels, training health personnel, and targeting populations perceived to be at risk (Zhang 1990). In November 1990 the First Sino-American Symposium on the Management of HIV Disease took place in Beijing. Hosted by the Chinese Medical Association, the symposium brought 148 American delegates with wide-ranging expertise to China for technical exchanges with Chinese counterparts.

Travel throughout China by the author made field assessments of medical facilities and interventions possible. HIV-infected individuals are treated with a regimen of traditional Chinese medicine (TCM) and Western medicine, but this is mediated by a patient's locale, access to medical clinics, and access to available technology. In outlying prefectures little medical intervention is possible. In the West zidovudine/azidothymidine (AZT) treatment is an accessible alternative when a patient is in progressive T4 cell immunosuppression, and clinical programs of ddI, recombinant CD4, and interferon are at least trial options for some. HIV-positive Chinese, however, have none of these. In the clinic as well as the laboratory in China, TCM is increasingly relied on as a feasible therapeutic alternative.[8]

Presently, Chinese medical facilities are not able to provide ongoing interventional medical therapy—in the Western tradition—for HIV/AIDS. Should viral infection grow to any significant extent in the population, resulting in the development of a large AIDS caseload, the medical infrastructure would be hard pressed to deliver medical care by any Western standard. Health care expenditures in China provide an average of only eight dollars per person annually. Hospitals in general suffer from lack of funds, and in some provinces up to one-third are already "bankrupt" (*China Daily* 1991c). The cost of azidothymidine (AZT) and pentamidine alone can average three hundred dollars a month. Moreover, the lack of the medical technology required for the application of aerosol pentamidine for *Pneumocystis carinii* pneumonia and for the administration of various therapies would be compounded by shortages in equipment, laboratories, and even sterilization methods (Chi 1990; He 1990). Overall, such a short-age of funds, necessary facilities, and testing laboratories, and the lack of experienced public health personnel would severely impede medical inter-ventions.

Inevitably, questions also arise as to how this anomaly of two distinct medical traditions—TCM and Western medicines—can jointly prevail against HIV/AIDS. Policy concerns come clearly into view if one considers the inherent worldview differences these systems represent. Western science underscores empirically tested clinical interventions: technically the goal of Western science is to continually test and modernize, and ideologically to be open to modifications, following the tradition of empiricism. Chinese traditionalism emphasizes subjective therapies and standardization of in-terventions based on an epistemology of disease that is in harmony with conceptions of the universe, conceptions that are themselves rooted in Chi-nese mythology. In an herbally rich but technologically and monetarily deficient context, the final outcome of the clash between these two medical systems will only be determined by the pressures that HIV/AIDS itself will impose. Nevertheless, tradition-based thinking is likely to complicate Chi-na's ability to move beyond prevention and into effective long-term medical interventions.

## PROPAGANDA AS PREVENTION POLICY

Often ignored in studies of HIV-infected societies are ideological differ-ences that exist between Western nations and those professing various forms of socialism. Epidemiology attempts to maintain political neutrality. However, political differences do impose themselves on, and influence, any methodology used to prevent HIV in a population (Mann 1987, 1988; Sabatier 1989). This section deals with prevention education and its com-plications in Chinese culture, where sexual mores are tied to an "official" and socialist ideology of sex. China's growing modernization has de-manded that the vocabulary of Chinese politics be informed by the norms of its evolving popular culture. However, in the arena of sexuality and in light of the exigencies that HIV imposes, dialogue between official percep-tions and modern sexual realities is a difficult undertaking.

The government is convinced that appropriate sexual education ("prop-aganda," as it is nonchalantly called by the Chinese health authorities) is the cornerstone of preventive sexual behavior, and that it will also change behaviors oriented toward high HIV risk (FBIS 1990b; Dai 1990; Tong and Fang 1990). To understand this view of change, one must consider how the state views sexuality and people, and how these perceptions were formulated over time. Such views become critical factors in determining the success of any HIV prevention effort in the Republic of China.

China's epistemology of sexuality is not "scientific" by Western standards, but it is well developed nonetheless, rooted in historical conceptions about the body and in appropriate expressions of "sexual satisfaction," and based on Confucian moral principles (Ng and Lau 1990). Confucianism provided a set of well-understood rules of conduct, rules that dictated how human comportment should be carried out, and that also taught people to accept the consequences of their actions, whatever these were (Bond 1986). Nearly two millennia of medical involvement with the human body promoted certain ideas and beliefs about its functions. Among these, sexual expression was ultimately seen as predominantly utilitarian. Socialism provided the parameters by which to interpret appropriate sexual expressions, ones that would build the collective while underscoring those proprieties of time, place, and person that Confucianism had already delineated (Butterfield 1983).

HIV/AIDS has now raised onerous questions about whether these official understandings are correct, and whether the government's posturings about human nature and sexual behavior are indeed accurate. Being challenged, most fundamentally, is the party-line belief that what composes the guiding force of sexual expression is "sexual knowledge." The underlying assumption is that people act according to how much they know, with "knowledge" being viewed as the regulator of sexual behavior and morals. From these views emerges a conception that if one wants to produce sexual behavior change, one then has to change the level of "sexual knowledge" a person has (Dai 1990). The government has pursued this line of thinking with vigor.

Since mid-1988 the National Health Education Institute in Beijing has been prompted to establish a Division of AIDS Health Education and to undertake limited KAPB (knowledge, attitudes, practices, and beliefs) surveys. The institute has also begun publishing AIDS prevention materials in the form of pamphlets and brochures explaining HIV and routes of infection. Similarly, there has been a flood of sex education stemming from other official sources that has nearly caused a "sexual [i.e., educational] revolution" of unprecedented scope and strength.[9] Sadly, the capacity of this flood to alter behavior has been questionable and appears limited, despite official studies to corroborate that all this effort is working (C[h]ui 1990).

Part of the problem China faces lies in its use of sexual terminology. As a "culture contact" disease (Bateson 1988), HIV/AIDS has often forced a culture clash of sexual terms (Abramson and Herdt 1990). In China issues of meaning and assessment are surfacing from within the very infrastructure commanded to combat the epidemic (Gil 1990). Sexuality has heretofore been explained by using officially sanctioned sexual rhetoric: traditional and quasi-feudal, culturally moral and appropriate, but always vague in its terms. Now, the need to be explicit in dealing with how one gets infected with HIV creates an unrelenting pressure within the system itself. The government is continually asked to clarify exactly how far bureaus should go in explaining sexual acts and those practices implicated in transmission. In a culture where sex is scarcely talked about, this is difficult and confusing work. Also, some bureaus commissioned to fight HIV/AIDS have never dealt with "sexual matters" before. As a case in point, the Department of Tobacco Control and Disease Prevention of the National Health Education Institute of China is now commissioned to undertake local (Beijing) sex surveys and publish pamphlets on "AIDS avoidance."

Such tensions between a reliance on traditional rhetoric and the use of more explicit language readily manifest themselves. Official declarations regarding HIV/AIDS cautiously proclaim: "The government calls to the attention of its citizens whether their words and deeds conform to the standards of the Chinese nation," and whether they "know what to do and what not to do when making sexual decisions and avoiding unnecessary agony" (FBIS 1990b). In this format "education" and "information" take on old, propagandistic, and vague overtones. In contrast, the more progressive language and efforts were in evidence at a Beijing exhibit prepared by doctors from the Municipal Health Education Institute and aimed at educating the public about STDs, sexual physiology, and sexual morality. Attracting more than 200,000 visitors, the exhibit explicitly laid out sexual reproduction and sexuality information ("sex sense") in living-color illustrations and blush-candid language (C[h]ui 1990; Tian 1990).

Even such liberal experiments, vesting people with sexuality information, do not alter or negate the pervasive undercurrent that from the government's view, sexuality always embraces a social and moral referent. Intended to be socially constructive, sexual expression must be based on a shared set of understandings and guided by the collective norms of society. Young adults, particularly unmarried adults, are specially targeted with these messages. Thus the "sex" part of HIV, that is, its modes of sexual transmission, are never mentioned without a moral background in official statements.

Certain sexual behaviors in Chinese sexual philosophy clearly fall beyond the boundaries of social approval. From a policy perspective, these are openly decried as a means of HIV prevention education. Chinese presenters at the First Sino-American Management of HIV Disease Symposium (Beijing, November 1990) often made reference to sexual immorality and openly denounced nonmarital sexual intercourse:

Wrong behavior which violates the biological and sociological laws has to incur the double punishment of nature and society. . . . The wild spread of AIDS is the most severe penalization. . . . In China, health education for the prevention of AIDS never includes the use of condoms, and our guiding principle is mainly . . . [to advocate] against non-marital sexual relations and . . . [in favor of] sexual morality (Zhu 1990:2–3).

Education's role is to enable sexual decisions along approved, traditional lines of thought. Its main goal is to ward off "the consequences of sexual libertinage, the bane of modern society, economics and politics" (Jiang 1990:3).

Corroborated by my own fieldwork (Gil 1991), I note, nevertheless, that there is an active undercurrent of sexual expression in China that does not comply with those parameters set by tradition, morality, or social grouping (see also Butterfield 1983; Pan 1990; Schell 1988). Ten years of reforms, allowing more open policies to emerge and, consequently, a growing adulation of Western forms, have inevitably influenced the population. The Chinese people are diversifying in sexual practices, as in almost all other areas of life, and neither socialist categorization of groups nor manipulations through propaganda are now easy undertakings.

Given the new parameters of Chinese sexual behavior, will infusions of "sex knowledge" and overreliance on educational approaches serve the state well in light of its desire to curb the spread of HIV? Moreover, can sex education also halt—if not reverse—any present tidal wave of liberal sexual mores in the popular culture? Rhetorical as these questions are in the present, they presage the widening gulf between public practices and public policy. Moving, as it were, among the "fault lines" of a society (Bateson 1988), HIV/AIDS is making the cracks between official understandings about sex and social realities as apparent in China as they are elsewhere.

Targeting education as China has done generates a narrow prevention strategy, one that unequivocally leaves out other epidemiologically relevant avenues. I was told repeatedly, as answers to my questions on how the government would deal with divergent sexual practices and at-risk populations, that "we will just provide more propaganda [education]".[10] More education, alone, will probably not solve the inherently complex and diverse problems of prevention.

## CONCLUSION: THE SPECTER OF HIV/AIDS

> Drugs and sex speak louder than the Buddha and the State.
> Buddhist monk, Yunnan Province

A predominantly localized HIV epidemic is now a reality in China. It has demanded and received sober attention. Yet, as elsewhere, the incidence rate has continued to climb. What makes HIV so troubling to prevention strategists is that its transmission occurs in the context of the most intimate social behaviors—contexts that have proven gravely resistant to controls. Even in a culture like China's, whose political system dictates the major dimensions of human life, the private nature of common transmission

routes—sex acts and parenteral drug use—makes these practically imper-
meable to broad regulation.

The Chinese government is convinced, however, that its other successes
at indoctrination and using propaganda prove that such an approach will
work equally well with HIV. This viewpoint interprets the dynamics of
human sexuality and the strength of addictive behaviors from the basis of
scientific socialism (Wu *et al.* 1988:3–5). In this paradigm, historical necessity requires the state to govern human relationships and set limits to
what individuals can and cannot do. In turn, the individual (when obligated
by conscience and the social good) will conform. Today, even with China's
modernization in full swing, individual compliance is still sought through
persuasion.

As regards HIV, any required changes in sexual behavior must be linked
to deep psychological motivations and desires. Such changes demand great
acts of restraint and deprivation of drives on the part of the person as well
as alteration of meaning systems and these cannot be encouraged by dictum
or education alone.

For the rural populations who remain true to socialist customs and ideology, the government's approach may well serve as an inroad to HIV
prevention. But here the strong association of drug injecting with HIV
among the infected may require more than education or legal restraints to
be effective. China's response to this association has underscored its view
of the injecting drug user as a social criminal and thus aims at medical
treatment blended together with social rehabilitation. Such an approach
leaves unaddressed those tacit, important other dimensions of HIV transmission among drug users. For the more than one billion others who do
not inject drugs, HIV poses a certain and future concern. Globally, HIV
has proven that it does not remain confined to any specific group.

Where does this leave China? For a nation faced with a fatal epidemic
that has the potential for grave social disruption, the temptation to resort
to more coercive policies has been seductive. Mercifully, this approach has
been avoided. Nevertheless, a society constructed of powerful hierarchical
bonds can be expected to look to individual needs only from a special
perspective. In short, if hierarchical allegiances dominate an official ideology, then individual needs will be secondary and possibly only subservient
to the needs of the majority (Hofstede 1984). Whatever the determinants,
it is clear that the "decision" to restrict HIV-infected persons from movement is consistent with the priorities of a vertical and collectivist society.
In this regard, China's decision separates its treatment of HIV-seropositive
individuals from those practices in virtually all other infected societies.

Remaining politically unaddressed is the great disparity between sexual
practices as these actually occur in the population and the state's views on
sexuality. Seriously recognizing any present sexual expressions that vary
from the party's norms will only come about if there is a paradigmatic shift

in the way China thinks about sex. The government must first modify its epistemological basis of beliefs about human sexual expression and its guiding forces: it must come to view sexual behavior as more than an outcome of knowledge and physiology. At present, the government's instrumental view of sexuality as primarily procreative, as well as its socialist policies toward sexual expression, can only generate a guarded approach to embracing these difficulties. For all its good efforts to date, China's posturings fall far short of what is needed to work through the issues and toward a resolution.

Confronted with the enigma of how to proceed, the state has embraced education. Here the risk is that the politically attractive will become confused with the socially effective. Growing reification of education as the most comprehensive prevention method can shield one from noting the difficulties inherent in this approach. Sex education and HIV prevention information are already taking on the uniformity that reflects China's socialist preference. For instance, generalizations about sexual behaviors in men and women abound in the sex education literature. Information made uniform cannot be expected to embrace individual differences nor, for that matter, be able to transcend China's subcultural diversity and effect cogent HIV prevention.

From a policy perspective, China must acknowledge and inform itself about the great rift that exists within its walls: national minorities; regional and linguistic groups with broad divergencies in sexual customs, not to mention cognitive differences in worldview; and socioeconomic segments with diverse sexual appetites. China must attend to further studies of its populations and their sexual practices and attitudes. Any homogenous thinking about sexuality in the Republic is certain to insure failures in HIV prevention. Finally, education alone, without the support of other interventions, both medical and social, offers little in the way of actual behavior change (U.S. GAO 1988; U.S. OTA 1988). China will need to realize what the fundamental limits are to its education policy and creatively combine education with other measures that will work in the culture.

HIV has imposed upon Chinese medicine, sexual philosophy, and political culture new and possibly transforming challenges: to syncretize effective disease prevention efforts, to realistically appraise sexual expression, to modify traditional sexual language and symbols, and to revamp those avenues by which China presently addresses sexual matters. The real question before us is whether China will be able to meet these challenges with timely reason and compassion. The specter of AIDS demands nothing less.

## NOTES

I would like to thank Constance B. Wofsy, M.D. (University of California, San Francisco, and San Francisco General Hospital) for the invitation to join the *Man-*

*agement of HIV Disease Delegation* to the People's Republic of China; the many delegates and now friends in attendance, who encouraged my later ethnographic overtures; and Douglas A. Feldman (D. A. Feldman & Associates) for continuing to encourage global AIDS dialogue. Special thanks go to Allen F. Anderson (University of South Alabama) for helpful suggestions and support, and to Donna Zeigler for extraordinary library help. Segments of this chapter appeared in an earlier version in "An Ethnography of HIV/AIDS and Sexuality in the People's Republic of China," *Journal of Sex Research* 28, no. 4 (Fall 1991).

1. The size of China accentuates the dimensions of the Chinese experience. So does the fact that Chinese culture continues to be unique and influential in human affairs. Successes or failures with HIV/AIDS will affect not only China, but all of Asia and the global community.

2. While "patterns" are useful as broad categorizations, they have a tendency to obscure culture-specific cofactors to HIV transmission (Sabatier 1989). Flam and Stein (1986) alluded early on to the complications inherent in simple epidemiologic modeling (cf. Anderson and May 1988).

3. The symposium was hosted by the Chinese Medical Association and co-led by the director of the *Management of HIV Disease Delegation* to the People's Republic of China, Constance B. Wofsy, M.D. Dr. Wofsy is associated with the University of California, San Francisco, and San Francisco General Hospital, where she codirects the AIDS Activities Programs. Chinese delegates representing both the political and medical establishments and U.S. delegates from a broad range of fields jointly presented papers and engaged in technical exchanges during November 8–9, 1990.

4. Serosurveillance figures as of September 1990 were provided by the Yunnan Provincial Health and Anti-Epidemic Center, Kunming, Yunnan Province, People's Republic of China. More recent reports (May 1991) from Beijing's Ministry of Public Health, Epidemic Department, placed the number of discovered HIV seropositive persons at 493, with 397 of them in Yunnan.

5. Chinese political culture does not regard sexual expression outside of stated norms very favorably. Individualism and individual sexual expression must always be subsumed under what is best for the majority. Left unchecked, the "AIDS issue" could unlock related issues of party control over the private lives of citizens. This the government could not allow.

6. Rights in China differ from rights in the United States in conception, in scope, in content, and in essential significance. The view in the United States begins with the individual, and the individual remains central, with a person's well-being the primary purpose of society. China begins with the society, the collectivity, and concentrates on general (not individual) welfare (Anderson 1991).

7. Some distinctions clarifying how the Chinese differentiate between types of infractions might be helpful here. There is a strong "rehabilitative" component in Chinese sociolegal thinking, a tradition that seems to predate communism by centuries (Allen 1987: 101–110). The "internal" mechanism of Chinese law is a rehabilitative/reformist-oriented philosophy and is the driving force behind the success of the "external" law (the written code). It is to the internal agent, or human conscience, that the external law appeals. When there is an infraction, the entrenched ideal by which the offender is dealt with is thus rehabilitative and reformist in essence. Hence drug users, while "criminals," are dealt reformist punishments

that aim at rehabilitation through social restitution, not just detoxification. Some distinction must also be made here between these types of offenders and what one would call "political" offenders. Political criminals seek to change the status quo of political balance and are therefore dealt more severe punishments. General criminals, however, not being a threat to the political order, receive the more traditional punishments of rehabilitation/reformation (Anderson 1991).

8. At the First Sino-American Management of HIV Disease Symposium a session was devoted to diagnosis and treatment of HIV-infected patients. All five of the Chinese medical presentations on treatment involved uses of traditional medicines or techniques. None mentioned Western medical regimens or antiviral compounds. Treatment regimens using TCM are scheduled for patients in light of such factors as how the individual was infected, the clinical symptoms, if any, and present pathology. Diagnosis is undertaken from the point of view of a "consumptive disease," often within the theoretical premises of "febrile diseases" (both belong to diagnostic categories in TCM). Deficiencies of *qi* (vital energy) and of *yin* (earth energy) are seen as resultant from the infection itself and amenable to intervention using herbal medicines identified to date. Fourteen compounds are presently being tested and used in varying combinations on some HIV-positive patients (Su 1990).

9. China has been slowly liberalizing its stance on sexual information. Since 1985 Chinese government officials have been increasingly persuaded to authorize sex education classes and to allow publication of sexuality-related education materials and the address of such concerns in the public press (Ruan and Bullough 1989). The present impetus under the threat of HIV has swept aside many remaining restrictions, but not without escalating political nervousness and generating bureaucratic confusion.

10. Conversations with Zhang Jiapen, M.D., Vice-Director, Yunnan Provincial Health and Anti-Epidemic Center, Kunming, Yunnan; Zhao Shangde, M.D., Director, Yunnan Provincial Health and Anti-Epidemic Center; and Zhu Xi-Ying, M.D., Director, Division of Health Education, Training Center for Health Management, Beijing Medical University, Beijing.

## REFERENCES

Abramson, P. R., and G. Herdt. 1990. The Assessment of Sexual Practices Relevant to the Transmission of AIDS: A Global Perspective. *Journal of Sex Research* 27(2): 215–232.

Alexander, N. J., H. L. Gabelnick, and J. M. Spieler. 1990. *Heterosexual Transmission of AIDS*. New York: Wiley-Liss.

Allen, G. Frederick. 1987. Where Are We Going in Criminal Justice? Some Insights from the Chinese Criminal Justice System. *International Journal of Offender Therapy and Comparative Criminology* 31:101–110.

Anderson, Allen F. 1991. China Report: AIDS, Law, and Social Control. *International Journal of Offender Therapy and Comparative Criminology* 35:303–309.

Anderson, R. M., and R. M. May. 1988. Epidemiological Parameters of HIV Transmission. *Nature* 333:514–519.

Bateson, M. C., and Richard Goldsby. 1988. *Thinking AIDS*. Reading, MA: Addison-Wesley Publishing Co.

Bond, M. H., ed. 1986. *The Psychology of the Chinese People.* Hong Kong: Oxford University Press.

Butterfield, Fox. 1983. *China: Alive in the Bitter Sea.* New York: Bantam Books.

Chen, M. 1990. Opening Speech. Plenary session, First Sino-American Symposium on Management of HIV Disease, November 8–9, Beijing, People's Republic of China.

Chi, B. 1990. China's Health Service System and Disease Control. Plenary session address, First Sino-American Symposium on Management of HIV Disease, November 8–9, Beijing, People's Republic of China.

Chin J., and J. M. Mann. 1988. The Global Patterns and Prevalence of AIDS and HIV Infections. *AIDS* 2 (suppl. 1): S247–S252.

*China Daily.* 1990. Yunnan Steps up Fight against AIDS. Beijing, May 31.

———. 1991a. Dehong Cracks Down on Drugs. Beijing, April 6, p. 3.

———. 1991b. A Warning That the AIDS Threat Is Real. Beijing, March 15, p. 1.

———. 1991c. Hospitals Suffer from Lack of Funds. Beijing, April 18, p. 4.

C[h]ui, Y. 1990. An Investigation on Sex Knowledge and Sex Sense of 200 University Students. Paper presented at the First Sino-American Symposium on Management of HIV Disease, November 8–9, Beijing, People's Republic of China.

Cui, J. 1990. Research for Curing AIDS by Qigong. Paper presented at the First Sino-American Symposium on Management of HIV Disease, November 8–9, Beijing, People's Republic of China.

Dai, Z. 1990. Prevention and Control of HIV Disease in China. Paper presented at the First Sino-American Symposium on Management of HIV Disease, November 8–9, Beijing, People's Republic of China.

———. 1991. Opening Address, International Conference on the Prevention and Control of AIDS in China. (A report of the conference and Dr. Dai's address appeared in *China Daily,* A Warning That the AIDS Threat Is Real, Beijing, March 15, 1991, p. 1.)

Farmer, Paul. 1990. AIDS and Accusation: Haiti, Haitians, and the Geography of Blame. In *Culture and AIDS,* ed. Douglas A. Feldman, 67–92. New York: Praeger.

Feldman, Douglas A. 1990. Assessing the Viral, Parasitic, and Sociocultural Cofactors in AIDS Transmission in Rwanda. *Culture and AIDS,* ed. Douglas A. Feldman, 45–54. New York: Praeger.

First Sino-American Symposium on the Management of HIV Disease. 1990. Organized by the Chinese Medical Association and People to People International, Citizen's Ambassador Program. Constance B. Wofsy, M.D., Delegation Leader. November 8–9, Beijing, People's Republic of China.

Flam, R., and Z. Stein, 1986. Behavior, Infection, and Immune Response: An Epidemiological Approach. In *The Social Dimensions of AIDS: Method and Theory,* ed. Douglas A. Feldman and Thomas M. Johnson, 61–71. New York: Praeger.

Foreign Broadcasting Information Services Reports. Arlington, VA: FBIS (CIA), Electronic Communications. 1990a. (FBIS-CHI-90-043). Three Year Plan to Fight AIDS Drafted (March 2, 1990). Reported by B. Zhu for *China Daily.*

———. 1990b. (FBIS-CHI-90-135). Beijing Intensifies Surveillance and Education among Six Categories of People, and Is Strictly on Guard against the Coming

On of AIDS during the Period of the Asian Games (July 13, 1990). Reuters.

Gil, V. 1990. Prevention Issues in the Sexual Transmission of HIV/AIDS: The Assessment of Sexual Practice as Behavioral Co-factors. Paper presented at the Meeting of the HIV Disease Management Delegation and Faculty, West Sichuan University School of Medicine, November 12, Chengdu, People's Republic of China.

————. 1991. An Ethnography of HIV/AIDS and Sexuality in the People's Republic of China. *Journal of Sex Research* 28(4): 521–538.

Guan, C. 1990. Screening of Anti-HIV Drugs from Natural Products of Chinese Medicinal Herbs. Paper presented at the First Sino-American Symposium on the Management of HIV Disease, November 8–9, Beijing, People's Republic of China.

Han, Mingli, and Yuzhao Go. 1986. Democracy Is a State System; Also Discussing Its Relationship with Legality. *Faxue Yanjui*, no. 3, June 23. (Translation quoted in R. R. Edwards, L. Henkin & A. J. Nathan et al. 1986. *Human Rights in Contemporary China*. New York: Columbia University Press, p. 141.)

He, J. 1990. Management of HIV Disease in China. Plenary session address, First Sino-American Symposium on the Management of HIV Disease, November 8–9, Beijing, People's Republic of China.

Hofstede, G. 1984. The Cultural Relativity of the Quality of Life Concept. *Academy of Management Review* 9(3): 389–398.

Inciardi, J. A. 1986. *The War on Drugs*. Palo Alto, CA: Mayfield Publishing Co.

Ji, C., and C. Su. 1990. Detection of Human Immunodeficiency Virus Type-1 Gag Gene by Polymerase Chain Reaction. Paper presented at the First Sino-American Symposium on the Management of HIV Disease, November 8–9, Beijing, People's Republic of China.

Jiang, F. 1990. Role of Education in Prevention and Treatment of AIDS. Paper presented at the First Sino-American Symposium on the Management of HIV Disease, November 8–9, Beijing, People's Republic of China.

Jin, E. 1990. Screening Investigations of 14 Kinds of Chinese Traditional Herbs against HIV in Vitro. Paper presented at the First Sino-American Symposium on the Management of HIV Disease, November 8–9, Beijing, People's Republic of China.

Lewis, M. A., G. M. Kenney, A. Dor, & R. Dighe. 1989. *AIDS in Developing Countries*. Washington, DC: The Urban Institute Press (UI Report 89-5).

Link, P., R. Madsen, and P. G. Pickowicz. 1989. *Unofficial China: Popular Culture and Thought in the People's Republic*. Boulder, CO: Westview Press.

Mann, J. 1987. The World Health Organization's Global Strategy for the Prevention and Control of AIDS. *Western Journal of Medicine* 147 (December): 732–734.

————. 1988. The Global Picture of AIDS. *Journal of Acquired Immune Deficiency Syndromes* 1:209–216.

Ministry of Public Health. 1992. *AIDS Surveillance Reports*. Beijing: Chinese Academy of Preventive Medicine, Center for AIDS Surveillance.

Morrison, C., and R. F. Dernberger. 1989. *Asia-Pacific Report 1989*. Focus: China in the Reform Era. Honolulu, HI: East-West Center Publications.

Mosher, Steven W. 1990. *China Misperceived*. New York: Basic Books.

Ng, M. L., and M. P. Lau. 1990. Sexual Attitudes in the Chinese. *Archives of Sexual Behavior* 19(4):373–388.

Pan, Sui-ming. 1989. On the Sexual Revolution: A Comparative Study between China and the West since 1919. Beijing: China Women's Publishing House. [In Mandarin.]

———. 1990. Manual, Oral, Anal, and Homosexual Behavior Today in Chinese Civil People: Analysis of Their Interrelationships with Sexual Knowledge, Attitude, Practices, and Response. Paper presented at the First Sino-American Symposium on the Management of HIV Disease, November 8–9, Beijing, People's Republic of China.

Peabody, J. 1990. Conversations held during meeting with Management of HIV Delegation to the People's Republic of China, November 14, Kunming, People's Republic of China. (Dr. Peabody is the World Health Organization's delegate to the PRC regarding HIV/AIDS.)

Quin, S., A. Wang, J. Fan, D. Chen, S. Li, and X. Li. 1990. First Case of Sexual Transmission of HIV in Mainland China. Paper presented at the First Sino-American Symposium on the Management of HIV Disease, November 8–9, Beijing, People's Republic of China.

Ruan, Fang-fu, and Vern L. Bullough. 1989. Sex in China. *Medical Aspects of Human Sexuality.* 2(2) (July), pp. 59–62.

Sabatier, Renee. 1988. *Blaming Others: Prejudice, Race, and Worldwide AIDS.* Philadelphia: New Society Publishers.

———, ed. 1989. *AIDS and the Third World.* Philadelphia: Panos Institute/New Society Publishers.

Schell, O. 1988. *Discos and Democracy.* New York: Pantheon Books.

Su, C. 1990. Treatment of AIDS by TCM. Paper presented at the First Sino-American Symposium on the Management of HIV Disease, November 8–9, Beijing, People's Republic of China.

Tian, X. 1990. Evaluation of the Importance of STD Exhibition: Dissemination of STD Knowledge. Paper presented at the First Sino-American Symposium on the Management of HIV Disease, November 8–9, Beijing, People's Republic of China.

Tong, W., and J. Fang. 1990. The Role of Education in Prevention and Treatment of AIDS. Paper presented at the First Sino-American Symposium on the Management of HIV Disease, November 8–9, Beijing, People's Republic of China.

U.S. General Accounting Office (U.S. GAO). 1988. *AIDS Education: Reaching Populations at Higher Risk.* Report to the Chairman, Committee on Governmental Affairs, U.S. Senate (September). Washington, DC: General Accounting Office, GAO-PEMD-88-35.

U.S. Office of Technology Assessment (U.S. OTA). 1988. *How Effective Is AIDS Education?* OTA Staff Paper no. 3. Prepared for the U.S. Congress (June). Washington, DC: Office of Technology Assessment.

Wang, Z., Y. Shao, and Y. Zeng. 1990. Research on HIV Test Reagents in China. Paper presented at the First Sino-American Symposium on the Management of HIV Disease, November 8–9, Beijing, People's Republic of China.

Wu, B. 1990. Countermeasure Role Played by TCM against AIDS. Paper presented at the First Sino-American Symposium on the Management of HIV Disease, November 8–9, Beijing, People's Republic of China.

Wu, Yuan-li, Ta-ling Lee, F. Michael, M. S. Chang, J. F. Cooper, and A. J. Gregor. 1988. *Human Rights in the People's Republic of China.* Boulder, CO: Westview Press.

Xu, Wenyan, and Jiang Fan. 1990. Prevention and Control of HIV Infection through Sexual Transmission in China. Paper presented at the First Sino-American Symposium on the Management of HIV Disease, November 8–9, Beijing, People's Republic of China.

Zeng, Y. 1988. Isolation of Human Immunodeficiency Virus from AIDS Patient. *Chinese Journal of Epidemiology* 9(3): 135–137.

———. 1990. Seroepidemiological Studies on HIV-1 Antibody in China. Paper presented at the First Sino-American Symposium on the Management of HIV Disease, November 8–9, Beijing, People's Republic of China.

———. 1993. *HIV infection and AIDS in China.* Paper presented at the First Symposium on Sexology—East and West, Beijing, People's Republic of China (October 15–16). Sponsored by the Chinese Medical Association and People to People, International.

Zhang, Aiguo. 1990. Strategies of AIDS Prevention and Control in Shangdon Province. Paper presented at the First Sino-American Symposium on the Management of HIV Disease, November 8–9. Beijing, People's Republic of China.

Zhao, S. (Director, Yunnan Provincial Health and Anti-Epidemic Center.) 1990. Data presented during meeting with Management of HIV Delegation to the People's Republic of China, November 16, Kunming, Yunnan Province, People's Republic of China.

Zhu, Jia, and Shulin Deng. 1988. AIDS: Prevention and Control. *China Reconstructs,* April, pp. 13–14.

Zhu, Q. 1990. HIV Is Nothing, Health Behaviour Is Everything: An Oriental View on AIDS. Paper presented at the First Sino-American Symposium on the Management of HIV Disease, November 8–9, Beijing, People's Republic of China.

# 3

# Public Policy, Political Activism, and AIDS in Brazil

*Richard G. Parker*

By mid-1991 the Brazilian Ministry of Health had recorded nearly 20,000 cases of AIDS—the highest number of cases reported in Latin America and among the highest number anywhere in the world. Since its emergence precisely a decade earlier, the AIDS epidemic had taken shape as one of the most serious public health problems in the country, and official estimates that more than 700,000 Brazilians are already infected with HIV suggest that the impact of the epidemic will continue to grow dramatically in the foreseeable future. Yet in spite of these facts, the history of the epidemic in Brazil has been marked by the relative failure of government authorities to develop coherent policies and programs in response to AIDS and by the current lack of anything even remotely resembling a coordinated plan of action for responding to the epidemic in the coming decade.

In the absence of a more effective governmental response, AIDS activism and political mobilization have been especially important in drawing public attention to the developing crisis, as well as in offering an alternative vision of how Brazilian society might respond to it. Yet even AIDS activists have been unable to effectively shape the policy agenda in ways that would lead to more effective programmatic development, and the growing tension between activists and authorities has left little room for constructive dialogue. As Brazil moves ever deeper into a rapidly expanding epidemic, the prospects for the future would seem to offer little reason for optimism.

This chapter examines the politics of AIDS in Brazilian society. Following a brief overview of the epidemiology of AIDS in Brazil, it describes the development of AIDS programs and policies from the early 1980s to the early 1990s, as well as the emergence of AIDS activism in response to the ineffectiveness of governmental programs. On the basis of this review, it seeks to identify the key policy issues currently facing Brazil as the AIDS epidemic moves into its second decade.

## THE CHANGING EPIDEMIOLOGY OF AIDS IN BRAZIL

Before turning to a more detailed discussion of AIDS-related policy, it is worthwhile to situate these issues within the wider social and epidemiologic context of AIDS in Brazil. What is most immediately striking is the country's remarkable diversity, and, perhaps not surprisingly, the complexity that has emerged in the epidemiology of AIDS within this context. Brazil is an immense country with an area of approximately 8,500,000 square kilometers and a population estimated at more than 150 million people. It is marked by a range of important regional differences, as well as by highly varied processes of modernization and social change in different parts of the country and among different sectors of the society. It was perhaps best described some years ago by Roger Bastide as a "land of contrasts" in which the divisions of class, race, and gender are constantly apparent.

The many contradictions that seem to characterize Brazilian life have become even more apparent in recent decades as the result of a series of social and political changes. Rapid growth and urbanization have transformed the once largely rural society, creating a range of new social and economic divisions that has stretched the fabric of Brazilian life. The political economy of debt and dependence has produced a series of severe economic crises, resulting in a deeply rooted and apparently long-term recession by the late 1980s and early 1990s. Perhaps most important, twenty years of authoritarian military rule between 1964 and 1984, followed by a gradual return to democratic government in the mid- to-late 1980s, have largely undermined the legitimacy of many political institutions. Together, these developments have resulted in the extensive deterioration of both the public health and social welfare systems, limiting Brazilian society's capacity to address its many already existing health problems and conditioning the ways in which it might respond to the emergence of a new socially, culturally, and epidemiologically explosive infectious disease (Daniel and Parker 1991).

It is within this context that the HIV/AIDS epidemic began to take shape in Brazil during the early 1980s, and the ways in which this epidemic has developed, as well as the ways in which Brazilian society has responded to it over the course of its first decade, have been affected by this particular set of circumstances. Like Brazilian society itself, AIDS in Brazil has been marked, perhaps above all else, by its complexity and diversity. By June 1991, with 19,361 reported cases and 9,484 known deaths (see table 3.1), AIDS had clearly emerged as one of the most serious problems in contemporary Brazilian life. While the vast majority of these cases have been in

Table 3.1
Number of AIDS Cases and Deaths in Brazil by Year of Diagnosis, 1980–1991

| Year | Cases | Deaths |
|------|-------|--------|
| 1980 | 1 | 1 |
| 1981 | – | – |
| 1982 | 7 | 5 |
| 1983 | 31 | 26 |
| 1984 | 122 | 102 |
| 1985 | 469 | 338 |
| 1986 | 952 | 652 |
| 1987 | 2,200 | 1,300 |
| 1988 | 2,984 | 1,973 |
| 1989 | 4,654 | 2,203 |
| 1990 | 5,498 | 2,265 |
| 1991 | 1,800 | 619 |
| **TOTAL** | **19,361** | **9,484** |

*Source:* Ministério de Saúde, Divisão Nacional de DST/AIDS.
ªData through June 1, 1991.

large urban centers such as São Paulo (7,946, or 41 percent of the national total) and Rio de Janeiro (2,415, or 12 percent), AIDS cases have now been reported from every state and region of the country (see Parker 1990).

Even greater diversity emerges in turning from its regional distribution to the specific modes of HIV transmission that have characterized the AIDS epidemic in Brazil. Whether we look at sexuality, the exchange of blood and blood products, or the use of injected drugs, the complexity that characterizes Brazilian life can be found in almost all of the specific contexts in which HIV infection has become significant. While homosexual contacts have been important in the spread of HIV, for example, the social and cultural organization of such contacts in Brazil seems to be especially complex, and multiple subcultures or sexual communities have developed over the course of recent years, at least in urban Brazil, in which same-sex sexual behaviors are linked to the construction of sexual identities in a variety of diverse ways (Parker 1987, 1990). Same-sex interactions do not always translate into the conscious elaboration of homosexual or even bisexual identities, and the links between specific sexual practices and perceptions of risk are mediated by diverse social structures and cultural representations (Daniel and Parker 1991; Parker 1987, 1988, 1990). Perhaps not surprisingly, then, although homosexual contacts had accounted for 34 percent of the cases of AIDS reported in Brazil as a whole by June 1991, bisexual contacts had accounted for another 16 percent, while cases linked to heterosexual interactions had risen to 13 percent of the national total (see table 3.2).

Much the same complexity can be found, as well, in the exchange of blood and blood products in Brazil, where humanitarian values have always been less important than commercial interests. Blood has traditionally circulated from the poorest sectors of Brazilian society, with the least access to adequate medical care, to the more well-to-do, and the commercialization of blood has long resulted in high incidences of diseases such as Chagas' disease. Not surprisingly, 7 percent of the reported cases of AIDS in Brazil have been linked to receipt of blood and blood products on the part of persons with hemophilia and blood transfusion recipients (see table 3.2). Even though important attempts have been made recently to regulate the blood industry, these efforts have often been resisted and, in some parts of the country, have resulted both in the creation of a kind of underground or parallel blood market and in widespread uncertainty concerning the possible risks involved in both blood donation and the receipt of blood products (ABIA 1988; Parker 1990).

Finally, although injection drug use lagged behind other modes of transmission during the early years of the AIDS epidemic in Brazil, it has recently become the most rapidly expanding mode of transmission, accounting for 18 percent of the cases reported in the country as a whole (see table 3.2). In some areas, such as parts of the state of São Paulo, where drug-traffic routes have traditionally functioned (and have become even more frequently used, probably in large part as the result of changing drug-control policies in other parts of South America), this percentage is significantly higher and has been especially difficult to confront. When compared to the situation in at least some other nations, injection drug use in Brazil is perhaps less clearly defined as the focus for a unique, sharply bounded or defined underworld, yet it seems to be characterized by a number of factors (such as the widespread injection of cocaine as opposed to heroin) that may contribute in significant ways to the rapid spread of HIV. That clearly will continue to pose a growing problem in the foreseeable future.

As a result of these different factors, the shape of the AIDS epidemic in Brazil has continued to change in a number of significant ways over the

Table 3.2
Number and Percentage of Cases of AIDS in Brazil According to Category of Transmission and Sex, 1980–1991

| Category of transmission | Males | | Females | | Total | |
|---|---|---|---|---|---|---|
| | Number | (%) | Number | (%) | Number | (%) |
| **Sexual transmission** | **11,382** | **(67)** | **754** | **(35)** | **12,136** | **(63)** |
| Homosexual contact | 6,475 | (38) | -- | -- | 6,475 | (34) |
| Bisexual contact | 3,122 | (19) | 11 | (0) | 3,133 | (16) |
| Heterosexual contact | 1,785 | (10) | 743 | (35) | 2,528 | (13) |
| **Blood transmission** | **3,935** | **(22)** | **1,031** | **(49)** | **4,966** | **(25)** |
| IV drug use | 2,971 | (17) | 666 | (32) | 3,637 | (18) |
| Transfusion | 557 | (3) | 365 | (17) | 922 | (5) |
| Hemophilia | 407 | (2) | -- | -- | 407 | (2) |
| **Perinatal transmission** | **174** | **(1)** | **174** | **(8)** | **348** | **(2)** |
| **Undefined or other** | **1,742** | **(10)** | **169** | **(8)** | **1,911** | **(10)** |
| **Total** | **17,233** | **(89)** * | **2,128** | **(11)** * | **19,361** | **(100)** |

*Source:* Ministério de Saúde, Divisão Nacional de DST/AIDS; data through June 1, 1991.
[a]Proportional distribution by sex. Male/female ratio: 8/1.

course of the past decade. Perhaps most dramatically, what once appeared to be a disease primarily of homosexual men has rapidly come to impact upon a much larger population: the male/female ratio in reported cases of 121/1 in 1984 had fallen to 8/1 by 1991 (see table 3.3). At the same time, the social and economic profile of the epidemic has rapidly changed, increasingly affecting the poorer sectors of Brazilian society—clearly the greatest mass of what is an overwhelmingly poor nation. Taken together, these developments have intensified the impact of AIDS on Brazilian society as a whole, posing one of the most serious crises currently facing the public health system and severely stretching the limits of a range of already problematic legal and social services (ABIA 1988; Daniel and Parker 1991).

## PUBLIC POLICY AND PLANNING

Given the seriousness of the situation, the obvious urgency of an effective and coordinated policy response can hardly be overestimated. Yet the possibilities for such a response have also been conditioned by a range of factors. The emergence of the epidemic in the early 1980s coincided with the development of a severe social, political, and economic crisis. Cases of AIDS were first reported in 1982, near the end of the authoritarian military regime that had ruled the country since 1964, and the continued development of the epidemic has taken shape within the context of Brazil's gradual return to democracy during the late 1980s (ABIA 1988; Daniel and Parker 1991; Parker 1990).

Within this context, and at least in part as a result of the legacy of authoritarianism, it is perhaps not surprising that the Brazilian government failed to offer any significant response to the emerging epidemic during the early 1980s. Attention focused instead on a range of other public health problems and political processes that seemed more salient as part of the transition to democracy. AIDS was largely dismissed as a disease limited to homosexual men—a relatively small and already marginalized segment of Brazilian society. By the mid-1980s such popular prejudices had become deeply ingrained, and the level of official denial had become almost absolute. Successive ministers of health described AIDS as an epidemic of the elite—privileged, well traveled, and able to pay for their own health care needs—rather than a serious public health concern for the wider Brazilian population (ABIA 1988; Daniel and Parker 1991; Parker 1990).

Even by the mid-1980s, after AIDS had begun to become statistically significant, the Brazilian government, like so many others, was slow to take action. Only in 1985, in the wake of mounting international pressure, was a government *Portaria* or executive order issued calling for the establishment of a Programa Nacional da AIDS (National AIDS Program) to be elaborated by a new Divisão Nacional de Controle de DST-AIDS (National Division for the Control of STD-AIDS) within the Ministry of Health. It

Table 3.3
Number of AIDS Cases, According to Sex, by Year of Diagnosis, 1980–1990

| Year | No. of cases | | Ratio |
|------|------|------|------|
|      | Male | Female | M/F |
| 1980 | 1 | – | 1/– |
| 1981 | – | – | – |
| 1982 | 7 | – | 7/– |
| 1983 | 30 | 1 | 30/1 |
| 1984 | 121 | 1 | 121/1 |
| 1985 | 452 | 17 | 27/1 |
| 1986 | 900 | 52 | 16/1 |
| 1987 | 1996 | 204 | 10/1 |
| 1988 | 3175 | 452 | 7/1 |
| 1989 | 4128 | 526 | 8/1 |
| 1990 | 4869 | 629 | 8/1 |
| TOTAL | 15679 | 1882 | 8/1 |

*Source:* Ministério de Saúde, Divisão Nacional de DST/AIDS.

was only in 1986 that this new division actually began to function, at first in a relatively limited and marginal way, and began to work on the development of an initial five-year plan intended to guide the Ministry of Health's response to the epidemic between 1988 and 1991 (Ministério de Saúde 1987; Rodrigues 1988).

From 1986 to 1990, throughout the remainder of the conservative Sarney administration, the indirectly elected regime that had replaced the military dictatorship in 1985, this newly created National AIDS Program was directed by Dr. Lair Guerra de Macedo Rodrigues, a medical doctor who had worked briefly at the Centers for Disease Control (CDC) in the United States, and who was particularly well connected politically thanks to her influential brother, Carlyle Macedo, the director of the Pan American Health Organization (PAHO). In large part due to these political connections, as well as her own undeniable political skill, in spite of occupying an appointed position that would normally be expected to change with ministerial substitutions, Rodrigues went on to survive four different ministers of health. She left her post only after the entry of the Collor administration in March 1990. Over this period, she succeeded in building AIDS into the largest and most controversial program within the Ministry of Health, with an annual budget of more than thirty million dollars and more than thirty staff members by the time of her departure (Parker 1990; Rodrigues 1988; *Jornal do Brasil* 1988, 1990b).

In spite of its director's political astuteness, the National AIDS Program constructed under the Sarney administration was generally marked by inconsistencies and questionable successes. While much attention was directed toward controlling the quality of the blood supply, which was seen as the one area where the federal government could immediately exercise a positive effect to control the epidemic, the record of the National AIDS Program was a dismal failure. For example, it was only in May 1987 that the Ministry of Health ordered the screening of blood donations. In 1988 a law passed by the Brazilian Congress and signed by the president required the registration of all blood donors and the testing of all blood donations for HIV. Later that year the new Brazilian constitution was passed, prohibiting the commercialization of blood and blood products. Throughout this period, however, the lack of enforcement of legal sanctions at the local level, together with the failure to implement any kind of official regulatory apparatus, made it impossible to guarantee effective screening procedures. While relatively thorough control of the blood supply seems to have been achieved in some parts of the country, such as the state of São Paulo, in other areas, such as the state of Rio de Janeiro, the late 1980s and early 1990s have been characterized by the rapid rise of an extensive black market of clandestine blood banks, often linked to organized crime, that have completely escaped official control (Parker 1990).[1]

The contradictions and difficulties that marked attempts to control the blood supply were no less apparent in the AIDS education and health promotion strategies developed by the Ministry of Health. While education and information were quickly identified as the key to reducing the spread of the epidemic, it was only in 1987 and 1988 that a large-scale educational program began to be implemented—and, even then, only inconsistently and at times incoherently. As the communication medium that most clearly cuts across the major divisions of Brazilian society and unites the country's diverse geographical regions, television quickly emerged as the natural focus for AIDS education campaigns developed on a national level. Although a range of other materials (such as posters, pamphlets, and advertising billboards) were developed for use in conjunction with television, the major focus of AIDS education activities was a series of nationally broadcast public health announcements developed for the Ministry of Health by commercial advertising agencies (Parker 1992).

The earliest materials developed for these national campaigns focused on the presentation of very basic information concerning how HIV is (and is not) transmitted, the role of sexual relations, injecting drug use, blood transfusions, and related issues. As the national campaigns developed, a strategy emerged in which new television spots were periodically introduced, successively shifting the message. A campaign focusing on the risk of HIV transmission due to multiple sexual partners would be followed some time later, for example, by a new campaign directed at drug injection. Yet the underlying messages of such campaigns were often highly contradictory, ranging from the early slogan, "Love Doesn't Kill," to the later "Don't Die from Love." Although the campaigns appear to have had an important role in raising public knowledge and concern about HIV/AIDS, limited behavioral research carried out at the end of the 1980s suggested that they may have been considerably less effective in leading to measurable behavioral change in response to the epidemic (Parker 1992a, 1992b, 1993).

Although attempts to reduce the conditions facilitating the transmission of HIV seem to have largely failed during this first phase of the National AIDS Program, some progress was made in attempting to overcome the especially chaotic nature of the Brazilian public health system and to build bridges between a number of different sectors whose collaboration was correctly seen as crucial. At least to a certain extent, it was possible to unify federal, state, and local services in relation to AIDS more effectively than in relation to almost any other health concerns. Such unification was always far from perfect, but nonetheless did create conditions in which some degree of cooperation was possible. The establishment of a National AIDS Commission involving representatives from the public health system as well as the scientific community, and concerned civic groups also provided a forum for bringing together diverse sectors of Brazilian society. In spite of their differences, they opened up a debate concerning the development of effective policy responses to the epidemic.

In spite of the mixed record of success and failure that seems to have characterized the development of AIDS-related policy and the National AIDS Program during the Sarney administration, it is hard to deny that accomplishments of the period seem more impressive today than they did at the time. In 1989 Brazil's first direct presidential election in more than twenty years pitted a leftist coalition built up around the candidacy of Luís Inácio (Lula) da Silva against the conservative populist Fernando Collor de Melo. Following Collor's narrow victory and his inauguration in March 1990, a series of mistakes on the part of the inexperienced administration threw the country into an ever-deepening cycle of recession combined with uncontrolled inflation, and the general deterioration of social services continued hand in hand with the lack of definition and direction in economic policy. Collor's appointment of Alceni Guerra, a medical doctor turned conservative politician, accentuated the impact of these factors on the public health system, particularly given the new minister's commitment to privatized medical care. Alceni Guerra's unceremonious dismissal of Lair Rodrigues and appointment of Eduardo Côrtes, a young epidemiologist trained at UCLA, but with no previous administrative or political experience, to head the National AIDS Program under the new administration marked a major change in the federal government's response to the epidemic.

In appointing Côrtes, Alceni Guerra called for a new, more aggressive response to the AIDS epidemic (*Jornal do Brasil* 1990a). At the same time, however, preoccupied with what he saw as the unwieldy growth of the National AIDS Program into the largest unit within the Ministry of Health during the previous administration, he slashed both its budget and its staff, leaving its inexperienced director with the unpleasant task of fighting to create a place for his program within the complicated structure of the Ministry of Health. It is perhaps hardly surprising, then, that for much of the next year, without experience, without staff, and without a significant budget, the National AIDS Program lapsed into an almost absolute silence, notable not so much for what it did as for what it failed to do.

During the first year of the Collor administration, the Ministry of Health discontinued the most significant aspects of the AIDS program that had been initiated under the previous regime. One of the major accomplishments of the mid-1980s had been partial improvements in epidemiologic surveillance, together with the monthly publication and relatively widespread distribution of an epidemiologic bulletin listing cases reported to the National Division of STD/AIDS. By mid-1990 this bulletin had been discontinued, replaced by a photocopied report that could not always be obtained even on request, and whose new format was explained as a cost-cutting measure. An ambitious, but sometimes not well-coordinated, program of educational activities had been initiated under the previous administration, but these educational programs, like the epidemiologic bulletins, were largely discontinued under the new government. The National AIDS Commission that had been established to work with the National Division of STD/AIDS in elaborating a plan of action in response to AIDS faded into disuse. At the same time that the new administration failed to develop meaningful new initiatives in response to the epidemic, it also dismantled much of the program that had been initiated under the previous administration.

This situation grew increasingly worse by the end of 1990, when the Collor government's first major AIDS prevention program, a national educational campaign, was finally unveiled. Not surprisingly, given its high visibility, this educational campaign was seen, at least in the eyes of the general public, as the clearest example of the government's response to the epidemic. Yet when it was finally initiated, the result of this new campaign could hardly have been worse. Produced by a private advertising agency working together with the National AIDS Program, and financed through donations from large corporations, the campaign was intended as a concrete example of Alceni Guerra's promise for a more "aggressive" AIDS prevention program and included a moderately integrated set of visual materials such as posters and billboards together with a series of public service announcements on Brazilian television. The graphic materials featured line drawings of a male and a female, each in black and white, with red and white targets over the genital area, apparently implying the danger of sexual relations. Even more astounding, the program of television announcements was initiated with a series of four talking heads—the first three claiming to have suffered different diseases (such as tuberculosis and cancer) that had fortunately been successfully treated, while the fourth dolefully identified himself as an AIDS patient and reminded the public that his disease has no cure. The spot ended with a disconcerting jingle: "Se você não se cuidar, a AIDS vai te pegar" (if you don't take care of yourself, AIDS will get you).

Not surprisingly, in spite of the government's repeated claims to have conducted evaluation research proving the remarkable effectiveness of its new educational program, the campaign was widely decried by AIDS activists, public health officials, and even its corporate sponsors. For much of 1991 debate about AIDS-related policies in Brazil focused on this campaign, held up as perhaps the clearest example of the government's reactionary and irresponsible policies (see Daniel 1991). Yet the campaign itself was simply the most visible example of a range of growing problems. Less than a week after implementing a new round of wage controls as part of its economic stabilization program, the federal government authorized increases in the prices of all medicines used in the treatment of AIDS-related infections. Shortly after the government announced federal financing for the purchase of AZT, its distribution to hospitals around the country was initiated, only to be discontinued when it was realized that the expiration date of the medication had already passed. In short, in the wake of its ill-fated educational campaign, one new questionable policy decision after another was announced, yet with no sense of a more all-encompassing or comprehensive plan of action guiding any kind of effective decision-making process.

By the end of 1991, as both the AIDS epidemic and the Brazilian economy seemed to teeter on the brink of hyperinflation, the legitimacy of the National AIDS Program had all but vanished. Eduardo Côrtes, the director of the National Program since the beginning of the Collor administration, had come under increasingly heavy criticism from a range of different fronts. While some hope could still be found in the government's renewed efforts to purchase and distribute AZT within the public hospital system, the commitment of extensive resources to this potentially important program seemed also to have immobilized a range of other activities. The possibility, announced by the World Health Organization, that Brazil might serve as a site in the developing world for testing vaccines against HIV/ AIDS had created both interest and unease, particularly after the director of the National AIDS Program announced at a public meeting that he was unaware of the reasons behind such a choice or how this proposed program was to be implemented. As the AIDS epidemic in Brazil continued its rapid advance, the governmental response to the epidemic seemed almost paralyzed, in a state of general disarray, and without any clear long-term plan of action.[2]

## AIDS ACTIVISM

Precisely because the development of a coherent, consistent, and effective government program aimed at responding to the AIDS epidemic in Brazil has been so problematic, the role of nongovernmental organizations (NGOs) has been especially important (Daniel and Parker 1991). This is perhaps not entirely surprising, given the historical context of the emerging epidemic. The end of the military dictatorship and the return to civilian rule in the early 1980s was marked by a major increase in the formation of nongovernmental organizations of various types, focusing on issues as diverse as land reform, racial equality, women's health, and ecology. These otherwise apparently diverse organizations were united, above all else, by their shared concern with the role of civil society in defending the democratic process, the values of citizenship, and the preservation of basic human rights that had so often been violated during the authoritarian period.

By the mid-1980s, even before the formation of a National AIDS Program, AIDS had begun to emerge as a focus of attention on the part of a number of different types of organizations. On the one hand, preexisting organizations, in particular, gay organizations such as the Grupo Gay de Bahia (Gay Group of Bahia) in Salvador and Atobá in Rio de Janeiro, began to become active in a range of prevention and education activities aimed at responding to the perceived risk facing their clienteles. At the same time, however, following the much wider trend in the rapid formation of NGOs in Brazil, an increasing number of new organizations focusing specifically on AIDS as their exclusive concern began to take shape. These new AIDS service organizations ranged from organizations such as GAPA, the Grupo de Apoio à Prevenção à AIDS (Support Group for AIDS Prevention), formed in more than a dozen major urban centers by diverse groups of health professionals, social workers, gay activists, and individuals concerned with providing social and psychological support for people with AIDS, to institutions such as ABIA, the Associação Brasileira Interdisciplinar de AIDS (Brazilian Interdisciplinary AIDS Association), formed by influential intellectuals and scientists, or ARCA, the Apoio Religioso Contra AIDS (Religious Support Group against AIDS), an ecumenical group formed by liberal religious leaders (see Daniel and Parker 1991; Parker 1990).

Between 1985 and 1989 more than fifty nongovernmental AIDS service organizations (ASOs) had emerged, playing an increasingly important role not only in AIDS education, but in defending the civil liberties of people with AIDS and in providing basic care and treatment services for AIDS patients. As the first critics of government policy, these organizations provided the key focus for an emerging AIDS activism in Brazil, yet were sharply divided by a range of differences in strategies and goals. While some organizations, such as ABIA, focused heavily on critically monitoring public policy as the key task of nongovernmental organizations, the majority of the new NGOs/ASOs were involved in providing a range of services to people with AIDS, as well as in developing educational programs aimed at preventing the spread of the epidemic (Daniel and Parker 1991).

These differences, together with the important distinctions characterizing the populations served by many organizations (ranging from gay organizations and prostitutes' associations to ASOs directed to a more amorphous or general public), led to a series of difficulties in the development of collaborative initiatives on the part of the wider NGO/ASO movement. In 1989, at least in part as the result of discussions initiated at the international NGO meeting sponsored in conjunction with the International Conference on AIDS in Montreal, a serious attempt to form a national network of NGOs and ASOs in Brazil was launched, only to be abandoned more than six months and two national meetings later, after it had become clear that ideological differences between the now nearly seventy organizations involved in community-based AIDS prevention activities were too severe to permit a more formal association. While a range of important differences existed, perhaps more than anything else it was the split between organizations linked to specific constituencies (such as gay groups or prostitutes associations), formed before or independent of the AIDS epidemic, and between ASOs formed exclusively in response to AIDS-related concerns that was fundamentally important. The limitation of dialogue between such different organizations had become intense by the beginning of 1990 (see Vallinoto 1991).

While the profile of different organizations seems to have been especially important in defining the terms of this split and in limiting the possibilities of collective action among different organizations, it was the way in which these divisions translated into relations between nongovernmental organizations and the Brazilian government that was perhaps fundamental to the ideological split between different organizations. Ironically, although many of the organizations, formed not in response to AIDS but in order to defend the rights of minority populations such as homosexual men, had suffered severe oppression on the part of the state in the past, they were now better able to work together with policy makers and planners in the development of a range of different activities. Particularly during the National AIDS Program initiated under the Sarney administration, but continuing on even into the Collor government, a kind of coalition politics was practiced by the Ministry of Health that counted heavily for its success on its ability to involve such groups as representatives of communities at risk and to make them the key focal points for AIDS education activities.

Such an approach was far more difficult, however, in relation to the more recently formed AIDS service organizations, many of which had been created in fact as a response to government inertia and inactivity. Concerned not simply with preventing HIV infection among one or another group, but with mobilizing Brazilian society more generally in response to the epidemic and with developing a more all-encompassing view of AIDS prevention, these newer AIDS service organizations (even if they often lacked any clearly defined community base of support) tended to be far more critical of government policy and to reject, sometimes out of hand, any kind of coalition with government authorities. Such tendencies were aggravated even further by the long-standing and profoundly important political differences between members of the newly formed AIDS organizations, many of whom were political leaders with long-term commitments to leftist and resistance politics more generally, and the dominant figures in the conservative Sarney and Collor governments, who were the representatives, in many ways, of the continued legacy of the authoritarian military dictatorship.

Particularly given this important split between different nongovernmental organizations and the kind of political inertia that it seemed to have created by the end of the 1980s, among the most important developments within this context in the early 1990s has been the formation of the Grupo Pela VIDDA (the Group for Life, signified in Portuguese with an acronym representing the valorization, integrity, and dignity of people with AIDS) in Rio de Janeiro. Formed initially by Herbert Daniel, a leading AIDS activist and one of the coordinators of ABIA, the Grupo Pela VIDDA was the first organization in Brazil formed principally by people with HIV and AIDS along with their families and friends. While the majority of the organizations formed in response to AIDS had sought to provide some form of assistance to people with AIDS and to speak for them and represent their needs and demands in relation to the wider society, the Grupo Pela VIDDA consciously rejected what it described as an "assistance model," seeking to give people with AIDS their own voice and to develop a range of activities aimed at defending their human and civil rights (Vallinoto 1991).

Coinciding, not incidentally, with a series of transformations taking place internationally in the perception of HIV infection and AIDS, the Grupo Pela VIDDA focused its attention on fighting against what Herbert Daniel described as the "morte civil" (civic death) of individuals infected by HIV (Daniel 1989). It established a groundbreaking legal assistance program to combat discrimination within the justice system, as well as a series of support groups (including the first women's support group in Brazil) and AIDS education services such as an AIDS information hotline staffed by volunteers from the group. Perhaps above all else, it was of crucial importance in introducing the notion of "living with AIDS" (as opposed to dying from it) as a key to responding to the epidemic in the 1990s—publicizing this view through activities ranging from public demonstrations to the organization of the first national meeting of people living with HIV and AIDS in Brazil (Vallinoto 1991).

By 1991 loosely linked chapters of the Grupo Pela VIDDA had emerged in São Paulo, Curitiba, and Victória, and similar organizations had taken shape in smaller cities around the country. While the development of Grupo Pela VIDDA has certainly not been without difficulties (see Vallinoto 1991), it is perhaps characteristic of a number of important changes taking place in the AIDS NGO movement more generally. While problems of sustainability and instability have been common among virtually all of the organizations formed in response to the epidemic, a growing sense of political commitment and political criticism vis-à-vis the insensitivity of the Brazilian government has become increasingly important in the self-perceived role of the majority of the NGOs that have emerged in response to AIDS. No doubt in large part because of the almost complete absence of any kind of coherent national strategy in response to the epidemic, the notion of AIDS activism as central to the activities of even those organizations otherwise focusing on the provision of services or assistance has become increasingly widespread.

It would appear, in turn, that this increasing emphasis on AIDS activism, while still not clearly articulated or directed in terms of effective collective action, has been important in helping to overcome at least some of the differences and divergences that have characterized the interaction of many organizations in the past. By late 1991, for example, a meeting organized by GAPA–São Paulo had brought together representatives of nearly fifty organizations and had provided an opportunity not only for an exchange of ideas and experience between organizations, but also for discussion and interchange with the director of the Ministry of Health's National AIDS Program. As a result of this meeting, a range of collective activities, such as an organized response to WHO proposals for vaccine testing, had been initiated, and the possibilities for interaction and collaboration between organizations seemed more promising than at any time since the beginning of the epidemic. How such collaborative initiatives will develop in the future remains an open question, but a new sense of the possibilities for cooperation clearly had begun to emerge by the end of 1991, offering some hope for more effective interactions between at least some organizations in the future. These possibilities have increasingly come to fruition in 1992 and 1993, following the return of Lair Guerra and the reorganization of the National AIDS Program. New collaborative interactions between activists and government officials have continued to be tense and sometimes strained, but a growing awareness of a range of common interests and goals has made possible a new dialogue across sectorial boundaries that was largely absent during the first decade of the epidemic.

## CONCLUSION

By the early 1990s a range of issues had clearly emerged as fundamental to the future politics of AIDS in Brazil. The inadequacy of what had developed as a National AIDS Program by the end of 1991 and the pressing need for its thorough reformulation had become apparent. While a bureaucratic and administrative structure necessary to respond to the epidemic clearly exists, without the elaboration of a coherent plan for responding to AIDS in a coordinated way, along with both the necessary technical expertise and political will, it is apparent that little can be expected from the Brazilian Ministry of Health. Ultimately, form must be accompanied by content.

In the absence of meaningful action on the part of the Brazilian government, it is tempting to view nongovernmental AIDS service organizations as the only real alternative at the present moment—and to hope that they will in some way be able to bridge the gap and take up many of the actions that the Brazilian authorities have failed to carry out. Yet such expectations are themselves unfair, implicitly asking minimal and often highly fragile organizations to provide services that they are in no way adequately equipped to offer. On the contrary, a more realistic hope might be that such organizations will in some way be able to exert sufficient pressure to demand that the state take action and develop a coherent policy response in ways that it has thus far failed to do. Yet this, in turn, will require collective initiatives and forms of influencing the political process that have thus far failed to emerge, and that have never been well developed in the Brazilian political system more generally.

Indeed, among the most important points that must be emphasized in thinking about the development of AIDS-related policy in Brazil is the extent to which it is in many ways a prisoner to a broader political process. It is impossible to understand the development of policy initiatives on the part of the Brazilian government, for example, without recognizing the broader historical and political context within which the epidemic emerged—the heritage of the authoritarian period, the tentative return to democracy, and the disruption caused by the transition from one administration to another. In much the same way, the development of AIDS activism in Brazil must be situated and contextualized, understood in relation to leftist politics more generally. The difficulties faced by activists in seeking to influence the seemingly monolithic government bureaucracy are themselves a function of the Brazilian political process, with its inability to incorporate a more meaningful approximation between the state apparatus and a range of diverse interest groups.

These questions, of course, are not unrelated to the much larger stage of world events. It is not without reason that transformations in the Brazilian National AIDS Program should take place at precisely the same moment that similar transformations were under way in the development of the World Health Organization's Global Program on AIDS—that the Ministry of Health's concern with bringing the question of AIDS more effectively into its traditional structures, and thus controlling what was perceived as the unwieldy growth of the National AIDS Program and, consequently, its almost dangerous political power, should in many ways mirror similar trends at an international level. Again, it is no surprise that attempts to build a national network of NGOs and ASOs should follow on the heels of similar attempts at an international level, or that a movement of people living with AIDS should emerge as perhaps the most creative and powerful collective response to the epidemic.

The particularities of HIV/AIDS, not simply as an international biological pandemic, but as a global social phenomenon at this historical moment, have meant that the emerging events and the formulation of public policy decisions in any specific context are necessarily linked to the world system more broadly. It is this tension between the particularities of specific context, such as the Brazilian case, and the more general patterns of a much broader world system, within which global AIDS policy initiatives are shaped and formulated, that we must ultimately seek to understand as we move into the second decade of the epidemic. As the case of Brazil clearly shows, progress over the course of the past years has been inconsistent and problematic at best, and the challenges that must be confronted are immense. While much has been accomplished in mounting an initial response to the epidemic on a variety of fronts, much more remains to be done. Success or failure may depend, in large part, on an ability to realize that the most pressing questions that must be confronted may be less technical than, fundamentally, political, shaped by the complicated forces that determine the political landscape in different settings and dependent upon a renewed commitment to the political process.

## NOTES

Research on the social dimensions of AIDS in Brazil has been made possible by grants from the Wenner-Gren Foundation for Anthropological Research; the Joint Committee on Latin American Studies of the Social Science Research Council and the American Council of Learned Societies, with funds provided by the National

Endowment for the Humanities and the Ford Foundation; and the Foundation for the Support of Research in the State of Rio de Janeiro (FAPERJ).

1. Important differences existing in the quality and effectiveness of the public health systems of different states have been especially influential in shaping the extent to which AIDS-related policies, such as blood testing, have been effectively implemented.

2. In 1992, the Ministry of Health underwent a number of major changes that have had an important impact on the development of AIDS policy. Following a series of scandals involving accusations of fraud within the Ministry of Health, Alceni Guerra was forced to resign as Minister in early 1992, and was replaced by the highly respected heart surgeon and former Secretary of Health for the State of São Paulo, Abid Jatene. In March 1992, Eduardo Côrtes was dismissed as director of the National AIDS Program, and the reappointment of the Program's ex-director, Lair Guerra de Macedo, was announced (*Jornal do Brasil* 1992). Lair Guerra's return was marked by a new attempt to create partnership's and alliances across traditional boundaries—particularly between government services, researchers, and community-based organizations. While the results of these initiatives remain to be seen, a new willingness to work more effectively with other sectors of Brazilian society nonetheless offers important promise for a more effective response during the second decade of the epidemic.

## REFERENCES

ABIA. 1988. The Face of AIDS in Brazil. Paper presented at the IV International Conference on AIDS, Stockholm, Sweden, June.

Bastide, Roger. 1978. *Brasil, Terra de Contrastes*. Rio de Janeiro and São Paulo: Difel.

Daniel, Herbert. 1989. *Vida Antes da Morte/Life before Death*. Rio de Janeiro: Jaboti.

———. 1991. AIDS: Alvos Equivocados. *Políticas Governamentais* 65 (January/February): 20–23.

Daniel, Herbert, and Richard Parker. 1991. *AIDS: A Terceira Epidemia*. São Paulo: Iglu Editora.

*Jornal do Brasil*. 1988. Programa da AIDS perde Cz$ 900 milhões. September 9.

———. 1990a. Demissão de Lair da DST causa saída de 12 técnicos da Saúde. April 23.

———. 1990b. Salários baixos impedem Saúde de preencher cargos. March 29.

———. 1992. Demissão no programma anti-AIDS. March 6. Ministério de Saúde (Divisão Nacional de DST-AIDS). 1987. *Estrutura e Proposta de Intervenção*. Brasília: Ministério de Saúde.

Parker, Richard G. 1987. Acquired Immunodeficiency Syndrome in Urban Brazil. *Medical Anthropology Quarterly* 1(2): 155–175.

———. 1988. Sexual Culture and AIDS Education in Urban Brazil. In *AIDS 1988: AAAS Symposia Papers*, ed. Ruth Kulstad, pp. 169–173. Washington, DC: American Association for the Advancement of Science.

———. 1990. Responding to AIDS in Brazil. In *Action on AIDS: National Policies in Comparative Perspective*, ed. Barbara Misztal and David Moss, pp. 51–77. Westport, CT: Greenwood Press.

————. 1992a. Sexual Diversity, Cultural Analysis, and AIDS Education in Brazil. In *The Time of AIDS: Social Analysis, Theory, and Method,* ed. Gilbert Herdt and Shirley Lindenbaum, pp. 225–242. Newbury Park, CA: Sage Publications.

————. 1992b. AIDS Education and Health Promotion in Brazil: Lessons from the Past and Prospects for the Future. In *AIDS Prevention Through Education: A World View,* ed. Jonathan Mann, Harvey Fineberg, and Jaime Sepulveda. Oxford: Oxford University Press.

————. 1993. After AIDS: Changes in (Homo)sexual Behavior. In *Sexuality, Politics and AIDS in Brazil,* ed. Herbert Daniel and Richard Parker. pp. 97–114. London: The Falmer Press.

Rodrigues, Lair Guerra de Macedo. 1988. Brazil's Educational Programme on AIDS Prevention. In *AIDS Prevention and Control,* pp. 37–40. Geneva: World Health Organization/Oxford: Pergamon Press.

Vallinoto, Tereza Christina. 1991. A Construção da Solidariedade: Um Estudo sobre a Resposta Colletiva à AIDS. Master's thesis, National School of Public Health, Rio de Janeiro.

# 4

# The Response of Nongovernmental Organizations in Latin America to HIV Infection and AIDS: A Vehicle for Grasping the Contribution NGOs Make to Health and Development

*Pamela Hartigan*

The winds of democratization and decentralization appear to be sweeping through Latin America and the Caribbean, making the 1990s a decade of new approaches and exciting possibilities. This mood upswing paradoxically coexists with continuing economic and social problems: debt that strangles the economies of most of the hemisphere, stifling poverty, illiteracy, and a shortage of health care and other services. At least one-third of the people in Latin America are still without adequate health care.

On the positive side, the spread of democracy nurtures opportunities for the poor to have a say in the development programs that affect them. Fiscal constraints help to sway bureaucrats into admitting that illiteracy is not synonymous with ignorance and that the poor can and must be allowed to do formally what they have often had to do informally for years: play an active role in serving their own basic needs.

Throughout Latin America, civil society is being enriched by a web of nongovernmental organizations (NGOs) with visions of a different, more equitable world. The AIDS epidemic provides an opportunity to more closely examine the dynamics and motivations of many NGOs working in areas of health and development. This analysis of the NGOs' response to AIDS provides insights into the features of different types of organizations that comprise the NGO universe and helps us to understand the types of NGOs that might best accomplish a specific health goal: AIDS prevention and care. It also examines the influence and responsibilities that donor organizations have in shaping the NGO response to identified needs in developing countries.

This chapter initially presents an overall view of the dynamics that motivate NGOs to do development work and subsequently seeks to specifically apply this framework to NGOs engaged in AIDS prevention, education, and care activities. By grasping the dynamics that motivate NGOs to engage in health and development activities, one can achieve a better understanding of their unique role as development entities and as effective partners with public and other private-sector organizations in preventing AIDS and caring for those who live with HIV infection.

## NGOs: PROBLEMS WITH DEFINITION

Many institutions have provided taxonomies or classifications of NGOs in order to describe their activities (World Bank 1988; World Health Organization 1985). The "nongovernmental" label tells us more about what these organizations are not (Brown and Korten 1989) than what they are. In addition, the term has been imported from the North, where NGO activities and functions differ from those in the Third World. But the very vacuousness of the term may be useful, as was pointed out by a Brazilian observer of NGO evolution (Landim 1987).[1]

The lack of definitional boundaries is revealed when one solicits a definition of NGOs from professionals in public or private organizations. It is then that one is reminded of the well-known tale of the five blind men who were each asked to describe the whole of an elephant from knowledge of the configuration of one of its parts. However, unlike the elephant, which can be perceived as a whole, the key to understanding the vast universe of organizations that fall under the NGO rubric is not to look at the whole, but rather to focus on the specific dynamics and forces underlying these entities.

## GENERAL DISTINCTIONS BETWEEN PUBLIC, PRIVATE FOR-PROFIT, AND NONGOVERNMENTAL ORGANIZATIONS

Organizations in the governmental or public sector are primarily motivated by the need to stimulate progress and maintain social order. Thus government programs and priorities are geared toward achieving national economic and social objectives supported by consensus and stability. At times, governments participate directly in the production or delivery of goods and services where it is felt for some reason that private initiative cannot be relied upon to do this satisfactorily. Increasingly, however, government interventions are being curtailed and confined to indirect means such as rules and regulations, designed to help ensure the achievement of social and economic objectives. In the exercise of these roles, government is accountable to its citizens.

Commercial or private-sector organizations, meanwhile, are motivated almost exclusively by profit and other economic goals. They contribute to the development of society mainly through the efficient use and production of goods and services. Mechanisms for resource mobilization are based on negotiated exchanges in market systems, which, in turn, are enforced through mechanisms of reciprocity and contracts (Olson 1971).

In examining the distinctions between NGOs, Brown and Korten (1989) differentiated voluntary organizations (VOs) from other NGOs. Organizations in the voluntary sector can be distinguished by two general characteristics: Voluntaryism and non-profit-making status. Primarily motivated by a vision of a better future, members of these organizations share some core value, be it political, religious, or interpersonal, that is so strongly entrenched within their ranks that the pursuit of this value or vision channels all behavior, even in the most hostile circumstances.

The priority of these voluntary organizations is organizing people around the shared core value; economic incentives are secondary (Cernea 1988:7–8). Consequently, the organizational capacity that springs to life through voluntary organizations and becomes engaged in development activities represents the fundamental strategic resource and the most important contribution of these voluntary organizations.

Given these characteristics, it becomes apparent that not all NGOs are voluntary organizations. The degree of voluntaryism varies, as does the extent of the links to specific communities. This is important because donor organizations often assume that legally, not-for-profit, nongovernmental organizations are all voluntary and have direct access to grassroots communities.

Special characteristics of voluntary organizations include their low cost, elusiveness, and escalating impact (Brown and Korten 1989). Their low cost, however, does not imply that voluntary organizations can operate without financial backing. On the contrary, they must depend on external contributions from donors who recognize that their greatest asset is their ability to unite people in the pursuit of collectively shared goals.

Moreover, the contributions made by voluntary organizations are not easily assessed. As a practical matter, they are not easy to control. There is a mystique surrounding the value-based motivations of these entities that transcends simple economic and social considerations. Voluntary organizations often draw into their ranks idealistic individuals who may later emerge as charismatic leaders who tap into the social consciences and wider values of citizens, mobilizing voluntary energies from all sectors. The interaction of shared values, innovative ideas as to how to achieve common goals, and the new alliances that may result often produce self-reinforcing escalation of social energies with wide impact (Uphoff 1988). Among voluntary organizations themselves, there are important distinctions that will be outlined later.

Brown (1990) made an important contribution to the analysis of the three sectors (public, private for-profit, and voluntary) by observing that the prevailing classifications of NGOs have been derived by political scientists or economists. He noted that through the "lens of economic analysis," NGOs emerge as a result of various forms of market failure. This type of analysis focuses on what need can be met by the nonprofit organization that is not met by the for-profit sector. Because market vulnerability is particularly acute in developing countries where large segments of the population lack the financial resources to participate, alternative forms of organization (i.e., NGOs) spring up in response to these market failures (Jorgensen, Hafsi, and Kiggundu 1986).

But if the economist analyzes the existence of NGOs from the market-failure perspective, the political analyst focuses on NGOs as indicative of government failure. For political analysts, NGOs provide public goods (e.g., health services) for relatively small groups of people. This focus on small groups sparks special interest in the role of NGOs in local development. Thus the political analyst attributes the existence of NGOs to social diversity and specific unmet social needs (Cernea 1988).

It is important to keep in mind that all three sectors (public, private, and voluntary) share these motivations to some degree, although each is guided by specific and distinct primary motivations (i.e., shared values and volunteerism for the NGOs, progress and maintenance of social order for the governmental organizations, and production of goods and services for private-sector organizations). One can easily find examples of shared values and volunteerism in both governmental and private-sector organizations. Likewise, voluntary organizations, as well as governments, are also motivated to some degree by the production of goods and services and the maintenance of social order. Through intersectoral collaboration, these three sectors can achieve more far-reaching and sustainable results in such endeavors as AIDS prevention and care than they could independently.

## A CLOSER LOOK WITHIN THE NGO UNIVERSE

The previous discussion highlights some general distinctions between public, private, and voluntary NGO sectors. But there are also distinctions within the voluntary sector itself. The following discussion attempts to provide insights into the dynamics of voluntary and other NGOs. It is important to keep in mind that characteristics highlighted for each type are not mutually exclusive, and many NGOs combine several aspects. Figure 4.1 clarifies these distinctions.

1. Voluntary service delivery organizations are motivated by shared values, usually stemming from religious tradition (Beckman 1985). Their objectives revolve around relieving the immediate symptoms of a problem. These organizations are usually funded by a donor in the developed world, and services are delivered by a satellite member within the developing country. Because of the nature of their work, voluntary organizations of this type have little accountability to beneficiaries and may create a counter-

# Figure 4.1
## Types of Nongovernmental Organizations

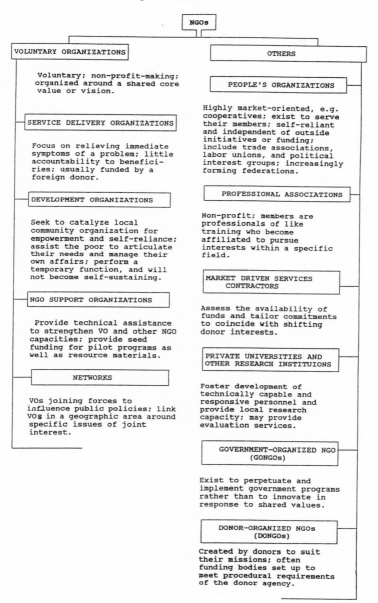

*Source:* Based on distinctions made by David L. Brown and D. Korten, *The Role of Voluntary Organizations in Development* (Boston: Institute for Development Research, 1989).

*Note:* Characteristics highlighted for each type are not mutually exclusive, and many NGOs combine several aspects.

developmental dependency that perpetuates the need for foreign charity rather than building local systems that can respond to similar future problems (Yudelman 1989).

2. Developmental catalyst organizations (Brown and Korten 1989) are also motivated by shared values and visions of a better world.[2] However, their objective is to catalyze local community organizations for empowerment and self-reliance. They seek to establish arrangements that will be accountable to the community itself and remain in place without continuous need of its presence. The more effective developmental catalysts are promoting the development capacity of sectors of civil society by assisting the poor or disenfranchised in articulating their needs and managing their own affairs.

This type of voluntary organization depends on a continuing flow of external contributions from donors willing to let the organization remain autonomous so that it can execute its catalytic role. Problems can often arise from pressures by donors for it to move into service delivery roles so that donor resources can be matched clearly with measurable outputs. In addition, because the developmental catalyst performs a temporary function, it will not itself become self-sustaining (Calavan 1984).

With the growth of the voluntary NGO sector, certain voluntary organizations have become specialized service providers to other voluntary or nongovernmental organizations. In addition, there has been a growth of networking among these organizations. Thus two more types of organizations can be identified within the realm of voluntary organizations: sector support organizations and networks.

3. Sector support organizations are voluntary organizations that provide technical assistance through training in management skills and related expertise to strengthen capacities of other NGOs. In the area of AIDS, the Confederación de Mexicanos Contra el SIDA is rapidly emerging as a sector support organization that provides technical assistance and resource materials to other Mexican voluntary organizations working in AIDS prevention, education, and care.

4. Networks in Latin America and the Caribbean are a rapidly growing phenomenon as voluntary organizations join forces with one another in order to influence public policies that provide greater access to opportunities and resources that distribute benefits more equitably (Yudelman 1989). The motivation has been a conscious one, prompted by the realization that greater leadership is needed if the sources of underdevelopment, rather than just the effects of it, are to be significantly altered. In the area of AIDS, regional and subregional networks are rapidly being formed by NGOs in order to pool scarce organizational know-how and share experiences and knowledge.[3]

There are three other types of social-action NGOs that bear special mention because of their relevance to health objectives, but that are not necessarily voluntary organizations. The latter two are of particular relevance to AIDS.

5. People's organizations are NGOs that are highly market oriented in their external exchange transactions (e.g., cooperatives and unions). Unlike the developmental catalysts, people's organizations are expected to be self-sustaining and independent of outside initiatives or funding. These NGOs are formed to mutually benefit their members, and in so doing they can create demands for greater responsiveness to grassroots concerns and provide the collective bargaining power that enables the poor to negotiate with representatives of government or private corporations. Others are composed of individuals with similar professional orientations who join together to pursue selected health-related goals, such as the American Medical Association, the American Psychological Association, or the Latin American Confederation of Clinical Biosciences. The key difference between people's organizations and other voluntary organizations is that the former exist primarily to serve their members, while the latter are committed primarily to values that transcend the immediate interests of their members.

6. Public service contractors (Brown and Korten 1989) are a special type of NGO that are often what multilateral, bilateral, and other donor organizations are seeking when they contract with NGOs for advisory services and implementation of projects. It is often difficult to distinguish between other voluntary organizations and public service contractors, but it is important to be aware of their differences since the end result is dependent upon what motivates each one. The influx of funding in any field of development (e.g., environment, child survival, AIDS) gives rise to public service contractors that act like businesses in the "development racket." AIDS is no exception. Unlike the mission-oriented voluntary organization that is primarily motivated to work in AIDS for humanitarian reasons, these market-driven service contractors, although legally identified as not-for-profit, sell health services that the donor market wants. One year their focus may be child survival; the next year, the environment; the next year, AIDS.

A voluntary organization defines its program based on its social mission and then seeks the funding required to implement it. The market-driven public service contractor assesses the availability of funds and tailors its commitments to coincide with shifting donor interests. Thus track record is critical in distinguishing between the two, and the success of an AIDS intervention, for example, may depend on the dynamics that motivate the mission-oriented as opposed to the market-driven NGO.

7. Private universities and other research institutions are nonprofit, nongovernmental organizations of particular relevance for AIDS work. They foster the development of technically capable and responsive health care personnel who will strengthen the ability of the health care system to respond to the needs in Latin America and the Caribbean. They also provide

local research capacity to search for local solutions to health concerns, such as AIDS.

## PSEUDO-NGOs

Some NGOs are created by governments. Government-organized NGOs (GONGOs) have proliferated in Latin America due to two interrelated factors: the desire to perpetuate and implement government programs rather than innovate in response to shared values (Brown and Korten 1989), along with the influx of foreign funding to NGOs from donors more willing to donate to NGOs where they feel their monies will more directly benefit the poor than to the Latin American governments, whom they view as inept and corrupt.

Likewise, donors create NGOs to suit their missions. These donor-organized NGOs (DONGOs) are often funding bodies that are set up to meet philosophies or procedural requirements of the donor agency. While the creation of DONGOs does not present a problem in itself, difficulties can arise if a number of donors decide to channel funds through a single DONGO. In this case, the DONGO can exercise inordinate power over the indigenous NGO community (van der Heijden 1987).

## THE AIDS EPIDEMIC AND NGOs

AIDS is a relatively new phenomenon in Latin America and the Caribbean, with the first cases emerging in the early 1980s. Almost immediately, however, community-based responses to the disease surfaced, beginning in Brazil, where the epidemic spread rapidly. Most of these responses were initiated by individuals who had lost loved ones to AIDS. Initially, most of these groups were formed by individuals who themselves felt marginalized by societal norms that stigmatized their personal sexual orientations and behaviors. Many of these newly formed groups voiced frustration with non-existent or top-down governmental programs, expensive and ineffective AIDS education campaigns, and continued ostracism by the very national programs that were created by governments to respond to the epidemic (Hartigan 1991).

At first, these groups were few in number and were motivated, like other developmental catalyst NGOs, by shared values and visions of a world without discrimination toward sexual orientation. But since the late 1980s the world has witnessed a mushrooming of NGO responses to AIDS. Among countries in Latin America and the Caribbean, for example, Mexico reports a total of ninety-two NGOs working in AIDS education, prevention, and care (Figueroa 1991). A rough estimate for the region as a whole puts the count currently at about five hundred (Pan American Health Organization 1991).

In Latin America and the Caribbean, NGOs working in AIDS are engaged in one or more of the following functions: (1) education for prevention; (2) advocacy in support of specific AIDS-related policies or changes in institutions that are responsible for the provision of health care services; (3) provision of services for persons with HIV infection and AIDS and their families; and (4) networking for mutual exchange of experiences and joint formulation of policies and programs. In addition, many NGOs working in AIDS address specific groups (e.g., gay men, lesbians, heterosexual men and/or women, teenagers, street children, persons with HIV infection and AIDS, prisoners, injecting substance users, and factory workers).

The premise underlying the need to work closely with NGOs in formulating and implementing AIDS prevention and care programs is the same premise that underlies the incorporation of NGOs into health care activities in general. That is, if health promotion programs are to emphasize the maintenance or modification of particular behaviors, these behaviors can be affected only when the pressure to change comes from within the individual or community and is not perceived to be imposed from without. This pressure from within is often generated by key individuals at the helm of NGOs who galvanize members to action.

However, NGOs are only part of the answer. They are community-based responses to specific situations, although when they come together, they can and do exert considerable political pressure. But NGOs have limited access to funds, needed technologies, research, and other support. Their activities are initiated by leaders committed to a cause, but not necessarily interested in replicating their efforts nationally. This task falls to governments. It is the responsibility of donors who mobilize resources to the developing regions to understand the importance of fostering partnerships between NGOs and their respective governments. This, unfortunately, has yet to happen in AIDS.

## THE DONOR RESPONSE TO NGOs WORKING IN AIDS

Much has been written about the donor/NGO relationship, often termed a North-South dialectic (Brodhead 1987; Brown and Korten 1989; Spoerer 1990).[4] Analysis of the donor response to AIDS in Latin America and the Caribbean provides a springboard from which to more closely examine donor influence on NGO activities in other areas of health and development. Moreover, it underlines the need to reconsider the donor/NGO equation in light of political changes throughout the region, and to consider in particular the urgency of fostering the inclusion of NGOs as important actors in new but still-fragile democracies.

There is little doubt that donors may exercise inordinate influence on NGOs, and AIDS is no exception. Donors have their own institutional philosophies and administrative requirements. The problem arises when donors direct support to certain activities, but not to others that may be more consistent with the mission envisaged by a given NGO. In AIDS this donor-driven NGO response has been reflected in two ways: (1) an emphasis on prevention/education over care and (2) an emphasis on "seed money" for start-up activities over funds for NGO medium- and longer-term programmatic needs.

NGOs often act as barometers of community needs. That is, because they operate at the grassroots level, they are the first to be aware of changing patterns and accompanying needs. For example, a number of NGOs are attempting to respond to the increasing demand for care for AIDS patients. However, they have found that few donors are willing to consider proposals to fund home-based care and/or hospice services. NGOs that wish to respond to this need find themselves pushing education and prevention proposals instead, thus compromising their desire to respond to the growing demand for care of HIV-seropositive individuals and people with AIDS.

In addition, almost all donor initiatives to date that provide funds to NGOs working in AIDS have stipulated that they will consider supporting only proposals for "seed funds" to help groups initiate prevention and education activities. There are no donor initiatives in Latin America and the Caribbean aimed at helping successful NGOs continue effective activities. Having monies only for start-up programs prevents NGOs from formulating medium- and longer-term objectives. Instead, they live from project to project. Ironically, donors often criticize NGOs for lack of planning.

The emphasis on seed funds has another effect as well. As previously pointed out, funding availability in specific areas invariably gives rise to a variety of "market-driven NGOs," among which can be included public service contractors and GONGOs. Donor emphasis on including NGOs in development projects can backfire as governments, seeking to tap funds directed to the not-for-profit entities, create GONGOs that compete for funding with the mission-oriented NGOs.

Perhaps a more fundamental concern is the proclivity for donors to view NGOs as alternatives to government in the provision of health care. This industrialized-country bias is understandable given the role of the private sector in health care delivery in the wealthier countries. But in Latin America the scenario is different. Mesa-Lago (1992) reported that in twenty out of twenty-eight countries in Latin America and the Caribbean, most health services are supplied by the public sector, mainly by the Ministry of Health. The poorest sector of the population usually has access only to the services provided by the Ministry of Health since they are not eligible for social insurance and cannot afford private medicine. The author also made reference to a study by the Economic Commission for Latin America and the Caribbean (ECLAC) showing the magnitude, trends, and incidence of absolute poverty levels in Latin America in 1970, 1980, and 1986 and projected figures for 1989. When total population figures were used, national poverty incidence steadily increased in 1970–86 from 40 percent to 43 percent. Thus even if current efforts to privatize health care were to be successful, the poor would continue to seek free health care provided by the public health sector. However, public coffers are critically stretched, and this is particularly true in the area of health. Ministries of health throughout the region are traditionally the weakest of the ministries and have been generally unsuccessful in convincing their respective ministries of finance that investment in health is synonymous with their country's development.

The public health sector has viewed the emergence of myriad NGOs into the region as a mixed blessing. Democratic Latin American governments have yet to throw off the vestiges of authoritarian rule, and many still tend to view the advocacy role of NGOs as dangerous to their political hegemony, rather than as necessary to the health of a pluralistic society.

Governments are also conscious of the considerable transfer of resources flowing directly to NGOs from external donors (GONGOs are evidence of this awareness). In fact, many administrators of successful NGOs make salaries several times larger than those of public health officials. Thus rather than foster the strengthening of the relationship between NGOs and their respective governments in the service of the poor, donor funding to NGOs alone can serve to polarize government and NGO sectors, decreasing the chances of building trust and ensuring important intersectoral linkages between the organized community and fledgling democratic governments.

There are several donor-driven initiatives that seek to direct financial support to NGO efforts against AIDS in developing countries. Some of these initiatives call for approval of the national AIDS programs (NAPs) in the country where the project will be executed, such as the Partnership Program of the Global Program on AIDS (GPA/WHO). Others, such as the initiative spurred in 1991 by the Rockefeller Foundation and taken up by certain bilateral donors, appear to bypass the NAPs and siphon monies directly to NGOs, under the assumption that the NAPs, like other government agencies in Latin America, seek to control NGO activities.

While the latter assumption has been based on well-grounded experience, the current evidence is that NAPs and NGOs are beginning to collaborate and pool their efforts, albeit sometimes reluctantly.[5] In addition, because NGOs that are working together in the area of AIDS are becoming conscious of the need to join together in networks in order to influence policy and priorities, GONGOs are more easily identified, as are public service contractors whose motives are more market-oriented than vision-oriented.

Donors must be prepared to review internally (1) whether their financial support should go toward providing an enabling environment in which governments and NGOs work in partnership in the attainment of specific health goals, or (2) whether this idea of partnerships is simply an unattainable ideal, and donors are better off ignoring the political context in which these NGOs function in order to carry out a specific necessary action in AIDS prevention. The second option is easier than the first. It is much more difficult to fund processes and ensuing activities than activities alone. However, in development work, and more specifically in AIDS work, it is the process of eliminating fears and stigmas and of building trust and understanding that is critical to raising awareness of the threat AIDS presents in developing countries. Donor money will be ill spent if it has only served to support the implementation of activity X in AIDS prevention by one or more NGOs. While it is critical to support NGOs that work in AIDS, it is also especially critical to ensure the gradual construction of health systems that are responsive to and responsible for marginalized groups. This will only occur if the barriers of unfamiliarity and ensuing suspicion are worn down.

In practical terms this means setting up a funding mechanism that supports NGOs directly in AIDS prevention, education, and care within the context of the broader medium-term plan for AIDS designed by each country. Thus it necessitates previous consultation and planning with NAPs. "Consultation" is a key concept that can be interpreted in various ways. In this context it means identifying needs by the NGO, joint brainstorming with the NAP and other NGOs to discuss the most efficient use of human and financial resources necessary to address the problem, and subsequent proposal writing if it is deemed that outside funding is required to support the intervention.

Such a consultative approach must be free from all manipulation or control by the NAP; for the NGO it means envisioning its efforts as part of the broader national plan to fight AIDS. The only way to achieve this seemingly utopian situation is by fostering joint identification and planning between NGOs and their respective NAPs. Thus NAPs, NGOs, and donors have a large role to play in strengthening broad-based AIDS interventions.

## NOTES

1. Many NGOs in the Latin American/Caribbean region make the distinction of refusing to call themselves NGOs and instead call themselves OPDs (organizaciones para el desarrollo, or organizations for development).

2. Developmental catalyst organizations are also termed nongovernmental development organizations (NGDOs) by Mario Padrón, founder of DESCO (Centro de Estudios y Promoción del Desarrollo, Lima, Perú).

3. Two examples in Latin America include the Latin American Network of AIDS Service Organizations and the Pan American Association for People Living with AIDS and HIV Infection.

4. The term *donor* in this chapter refers to foreign donors in industrialized countries, including bilateral agencies, international NGOs, and foundations. The term

*NGO* in this section will refer specifically to indigenous, community-based NGOs, referred to as "developmental catalyst" volunteer organizations.

5. This gradual shift may be due to donor pressure of NAPs to include NGOs in their medium-term plans if they wish to access continued donor support.

## REFERENCES

Beckman, David. 1985. *Religious and Humanitarian Groups in the U.S. and Third World Development*. Washington, DC: International Relations Department of the World Bank.

Brodhead, Tim. 1987. NGOs: In One Year, Out the Other? In *Development Alternatives: The Challenge for NGOs*, ed. A. G. Drabek, pp. 1–5. Oxford: Pergamon Press.

Brown, David L. 1990. Lecture delivered at the World Bank, April 6, 1990.

Brown, David L., and D. Korten. 1989. *The Role of Voluntary Organizations in Development*. Boston: Institute for Development Research.

Calavan, Michael. 1984. Appropriate Administration: Creating "Space" Where Local Initiative and Voluntarism Can Grow. In *Private Voluntary Organizations as Agents of Development*, ed. R. Gorman, Boulder, CO: Westview Press.

Cernea, Michael M. 1988. *Non-governmental Organizations and Local Development*. World Bank Discussion Papers no. 40. Washington, DC: World Bank.

Figueroa, Adrian. 1991. *Participación Civil en la Lucha Contra el SIDA en México*. Mexico City: Ford Foundation.

Hartigan, Pamela. 1991. NGOs Working in Latin America and the Caribbean: An Overview. *AIDS and Society Bulletin* (Hanover: African-Caribbean Institute) 3(1): 6–7.

Jorgensen, J., Taieb Hafsi, and Moses Kiggundu. 1986. Towards a Market Imperfection Theory of Organizational Structure in Developing Countries. *Journal of Management Studies* 23(4): 417–442.

Landim, Leilah. 1987. Non-governmental Organizations in Latin America. In *Development Alternatives: The Challenge for NGOs*, ed. A. G. Drabek, pp. 29–38. Oxford: Pergamon Press.

Mesa-Lago, Carmelo. 1992. *Atención de Salud Para los Pobres en America Latina y el Caribe*. InterAmerican Foundation and PAHO 1992 Scientific Publication #539.

Olson, Mancur. 1971. *The Logic of Collective Action: Public Goods and the Theory of Groups*. Cambridge: Harvard University Press.

Pan American Health Organization, 1991. Office of External Relations Coordination. Data Base on NGOs working in health and development in the Latin American and Caribbean Region.

Spoerer, Sergio. 1990. Las ONGDs latinoamericanas: Democracia y cooperación internacional. In *Gestión y Políticas Institucionales en Organismos No Gubernamentales de Desarrollo*, ed. Carlos Salazar, pp. 63–92. Lima: DESCO e IRED.

Uphoff, Norman. 1988. Assisted Self-Reliance: Working with Rather Than for the Poor. In *Strengthening the Poor: What Have We Learned?* ed. John P. Lewis. New Brunswick: Transaction Books for Overseas Development Council.

van der Heijden, H. 1987. The Reconciliation of NGO Autonomy, Program Integrity, and Operational Effectiveness with Accountability to Donors. In *Development Alternatives: The Challenge for NGOs,* ed. A. G. Drabek. Oxford: Pergamon Press.

World Bank. 1988. *Operational Manual Statement: Collaboration with NGOs.* No. 5.30. Washington, DC: World Bank.

World Health Organization. 1985. *Collaboration with NGOs in Implementing the Global Strategy for Health for All.* A/38/Technical Discussions (4).

Yudelman, Sally. 1989. NGOs and Social Change in Central America. Prepared for Off-the-Record Workshop on Peace, Development, and Security in Central America. Oaxaca, Mexico: Center for the Study of the Americas.

# 5

# HIV, Immigration Policy, and Latinos/as: Public Health Safety versus Hidden Agendas

*Norris G. Lang*

Immigration law can often provoke strong controversy. When immigration law and AIDS are juxtaposed, the subsequent conflicts between opposing value systems and ideologies are made more evident. International skirmishes gave rise to moving the 1992 International Conference on AIDS from Boston to Amsterdam, where there are no restrictions on HIV-positive migrants or visitors. Such public policy debates have occurred repeatedly in recent years, evoking public outrage by members of HIV activist groups (*Houston Post* 1990; Siegworth 1990; Somerville 1989). Beginning in 1989, the Bush administration vacillated on its relaxation of restrictions for foreigners infected with HIV who want to attend certain conferences in the United States, a move aimed at defusing protests against U.S. immigration policy.

There is another side to this debate, however, that is not as public and where the social rights of the individuals involved are disregarded with impunity because they are, for the most part, politically disenfranchised. Internationally, countless individuals face discrimination, deportation, and social injustice due to immigration laws and HIV infection, bringing to mind the warning by Bateson and Goldsby (1988:2) of the propensity of HIV to "reveal the fault lines of a society and to become a metaphor for understanding that society." This situation is hardly in line with the humanitarian concerns that Congress and the U.S. Immigration and Naturalization Service (INS) have maintained are behind their tempering of the enforcement of immigration laws designed to exclude categories of people who are potential carriers of contagious diseases.

Immigration is as old as wars, famines, and droughts. Any natural or human-made disaster has often caused mass movements of people. AIDS raises the specter of yet another series of legal discussions over social policies and their ethical implications. However, in this instance the persons involved have no one to speak for them. These are the "illegal aliens," the "undocumented workers," made unwelcome in the United States by the increasing economic pressures of the last decade, the Reagan years. "Braceros" and others were once welcomed in the United States because they filled an economic need. With the growing awareness of the extent of the permanency of their illegal residency and with their increasingly greater claims on social services, they became targeted as economic liabilities and perceived as politically expendable.

Covello and Johnson (1987:viii) stated that each society has its own distinctive set of risks. In this view, risk is not a matter of objective reality but a social process. They write that "each society highlights some risks and downplays others; and each society institutionalizes means for controlling some risks and not others." They added that what societies choose to call risky is largely determined by social and cultural factors, not nature.

Douglas and Wildavsky (1982:6) also argued that people do not focus on particular risks simply in order to protect health, safety, or the environment; the "choice also reflects their beliefs about values, social institutions, nature, and moral behavior." They pointed out that people's concerns and fears about different types of risks can often be more accurately portrayed as ways of maintaining social solidarity than as reflecting health or environmental concerns. The cultural construction of risk involves the embedding of hidden agendas where conflicts emerge from the tension between hidden value systems and agendas of social institutions and their public presentations. Restrictive immigration laws and health concerns, in this era of AIDS, are yet another form of the cultural construction of risk.

This chapter includes a brief overview of the history of immigration laws in the United States that have excluded undocumented migrants on the basis of health concerns, implications of this public health policy for Latino/a populations in the United States, a review of relevant characteristics of Latino/a communities in Houston, Texas, and a summary discussion of these factors and their implications for decision making in the future.

## A BRIEF HISTORICAL OVERVIEW

According to Druhot (1986:86):

> The history of United States immigration law is a "tale of accommodation between the humanitarian goal of accepting into this country those immigrants who seek to build a new life here and a variety of reasons for restricting immigration." Exclusion, referring to the process by which a sovereign nation prohibits aliens from entering its territory, is one method of restricting immigration.

Druhot (1986:87) pointed out that before 1875 different American states, and colonies before them, regulated immigration in a piecemeal fashion that virtually guaranteed immigrants unrestricted entry into the United States. Until 1879 the regulations restricting immigration had to do with protection of the labor market and of the character of immigrants. The earliest restrictions specified convicts and prostitutes for exclusion. The subsequent legislation had to do with the increasing medicalization of immigration—succeeding refinements of laws concerning the prevention and control of the spread of contagious disease—and with the appropriate establishment of officers and boards to implement and enforce such legislation.

Druhot (1986:110) argued that the U.S. Public Health Service should add AIDS to its list of "dangerous contagious diseases" and should incorporate the HIV test into the medical examination of immigrants. With such an addition, immigration authorities could exclude immigrants infected with HIV from entering the United States and thereby attempt to control the growth of the disease. However, problems would then arise. One such controversy stems from the assertion that use of the blood test is merely an instrument for reinstating past discriminatory immigration practices against gay and bisexual men.

Druhot (1986:111–112) concluded that the U.S. government has the authority to exclude immigrants who might endanger the health of the people of the United States. This would require a reassessment of U.S. immigration policy in relation to AIDS. She admonished, however, that the way in which the United States and other countries deal with AIDS "may measure the extent to which such nations have the right to call themselves civilized."

Druhot (1986) apparently wrote her article just before the immigration laws were indeed changed to include AIDS as a "contagious disease" that must be regulated to protect the health and safety of U.S. citizens. In June 1987 the U.S. Public Health Service (PHS) added AIDS to the list of "dangerous contagious diseases." At the same time, Congress passed the Supplemental Appropriations Act of 1987, in which section 518 added HIV infection to the list of "dangerous contagious diseases" (Wolchok 1989: 129).

The U.S. Department of Health and Human Services issued new rules substituting HIV for AIDS on the list of "dangerous contagious diseases" making an immigrant inadmissible to the United States and requiring HIV serological testing of all applicants for permanent residence, including applicants for legalization under the amnesty law and refugees (*ibid.*). The INS has taken an even more restrictive approach than was intended by Congress in the Immigration Reform and Control Act of 1986. Wolchok (1989:127) wrote:

In the face of the worldwide AIDS health crisis, the rights of aliens to enter and remain in the United States have become even more complicated and controversial, implicating foreign policy and international health concerns as well as domestic health issues. Seeking to secure our border against an invasion of AIDS, the United States now requires HIV-antibody testing of 500,000 immigrants, nonimmigrants, and refugees annually. In addition, in what may be the most massive use of HIV testing in this country, more than 2.5 million aliens living in the United States must be tested in order to qualify for legal residence.

## IMPLICATIONS: AIDS IMMIGRATION HEALTH POLICY AND LATINOS/AS

The focus of this chapter concerns a group of people who have little political clout, who are openly discriminated against by American immigration law, who do not arouse the passion of more highly placed activists because they are an underclass with no spokesperson to articulate their social needs, and who are significantly impacted by the AIDS epidemic. Latino/a immigrants to Houston, Texas, who have requested political asylum or who have entered the amnesty process under the Immigration Reform and Control Act of 1986 are required to undergo HIV testing (Wolchok 1989:131). At-risk behaviors for HIV transmission (e.g., injecting drug use, bisexuality, and breastfeeding) are increasingly identified as commonplace for many Latino/a immigrants, based upon preliminary ethnographic data obtained by this author. Given the stigma that attaches to HIV and the precarious nature of the basis for their U.S. residency that most applicants for naturalization and refugees have been accorded, it is unlikely that precise figures for the number of Latino/a illegal immigrants can ever be obtained.

Singer et al. (1990:74) found that because health status and health-related behavior are inexorably tied to social class, Latinos/as in the United States

suffer disproportionately high rates of infectious and parasitic diseases, higher infant mortality, lower life expectancy, and a higher prevalence of morbidity rates of all kinds than most other subgroups in this country. . . . Moreover, they often are poorly reached and badly served by existing health and prevention services.

By March 1990 there had been 795 cases of AIDS reported among Latinos/as in the Houston area (Houston Department of Health and Human Services 1992). There is no breakdown of this figure on whether the HIV-infected individual is an undocumented immigrant or a citizen.

A crucial policy issue that emerges concerns the lack of guidelines and procedures for handling the deportation process for immigrants who test positive for HIV, their grounds to claim an HIV waiver, and the subsequent events should they be forced to return to their community or country of origin. The case-by-case reality that has evolved results in uneven policy and unfair practice, enormous fear and distrust on the part of the immigrant, and the creation of an incipient underclass of immigrants who go underground, thereby denying themselves access to the health care system.

The immigrant seeking political asylum or amnesty is inevitably the last priority for those professionals whose duty it is to aid the applicant in completing the requirements for the naturalization process. This author has identified five patterns that have evolved so far and that interrelate with this policy issue, thwarting the original intention of the legislation.

First, exploitation with respect to the process of acquiring proper documentation and credentials to conform to the amnesty process is rampant. Many of the physicians, lawyers, and others who are contracted are widely perceived as overcharging immigrants and causing endless delays in meeting their obligations. Second, unbridled illicit dealing in black-market documents for Latinos/as is a readily familiar part of the immigration process in Houston. Third, testing HIV positive, or simply the fear of testing HIV positive, makes candidates for citizenship fearful and predisposes them to go underground rather than risk possible deportation if HIV waivers are denied.

Fourth, once they have returned to their community or country of origin, these HIV-positive immigrants fear discrimination by their former neighbors and even their relatives for having resided in the United States. AIDS is widely framed as a "gringo" disease, and once such former immigrants are identified as being ill, it is usually assumed that they have AIDS. Fifth, whether the immigrant remains in the United States and goes underground or whether he or she returns to the community of origin, he or she is denied access to the health care system. In the former case, once immigrants have gone underground, they cannot readily access the health care system from fear of reprisal by INS agents. In the latter case, the health care systems in their communities of origin do not have adequate technology, therapies, or resources to take care of HIV-infected individuals. The subsequent burden on these community health care systems expands the bases for discrimination that already exist.

Within five years this set of circumstances will undoubtedly create an underclass of Latino/a refugees in the United States who are badly in need of medical care and knowledge of HIV education, but are unable to access the appropriate systems. The denial of access will further increase HIV transmission unless a vaccine becomes available during the 1990s. This will further contribute to the expansion of a two-tier system, already emergent between persons with AIDS in industrialized nations and those in developing countries. Those immigrants who are forced to return to their country of origin add as well to the increase of HIV infection and suffering.

Former immigrants, who may be former political refugees, will become even more isolated and discriminated against by their own people.

## CHARACTERISTICS OF LATINO/A POPULATIONS IN HOUSTON

The political instability in Central America that accelerated during the late 1970s has generated large waves of migration: several hundred thousand "without papers" to the United States, especially to urban centers with large Latino/a populations (Rodriguez 1987). In Houston, a city with over 300,000 Latinos/as, including an undocumented Mexican population estimated at over 80,000 in the early 1980s, conservative estimates by observers familiar with Latino/a immigration of the number of undocumented Central Americans were placed at over 100,000 in 1986. This Central American population is composed principally of Salvadorans, Guatemalans, and Hondurans. This undocumented Central American population has drawn different attention and response from law-enforcement agencies of the U.S. government than have undocumented Mexican migrants:

> The surveillance and interrogations of undocumented Salvadorans in Houston, in 1985, by U.S. government agents demonstrate that the U.S. government perceives these migrants with a special political concern. . . . Prosecution of sanctuary movement workers by the U.S. is seen as another indication of the government's special political concern with undocumented Central American immigrants. (ibid.:5)

It would appear, from the perspective of a cultural construction of risk, that the enforcement of the HIV immigration laws against these individuals is publicly cloaked with the humanitarian concern for the migrant, on the one hand, and the concern with the public health of U.S. citizens, on the other, that rationalize immigration policy enforcement. There is lurking, however, a suggestion of a private, hidden agenda for these immigrants that would account for the varying handling of HIV waivers and the lack of established public guidelines to determine such issues.

Another contrast with undocumented Mexicans is the Central Americans' prior level of community organizational experience. This experience can be an important resource for the migrant's incorporation into the host society (ibid.). In addition, about half of all undocumented Central Americans reside in neighborhoods that form zones of Latino/a transition or of new Latino/a settlement (ibid.:6). The Central Americans also came at a time when Houston's economy experienced a severe downturn.

While the data are currently unavailable, it would be interesting to know the figures comparing the rate at which citizenship is denied in Houston for these Central American immigrants, on the basis that they cannot demonstrate that they would not go on public assistance, with the rate of denial for Mexican immigrants, on the basis of public health concerns. In the case of the undocumented Mexican immigrant, it is more likely that he or she contracted HIV while already in the United States. Deportation would also lead to the severing of kinship and friendship ties that have been established in the United States.

Whatever the U.S. government's motives might be, the practice of enforcing immigration laws puts undocumented immigrants in precarious situations over which they can exert little control. Ethical issues involve their right to confidentiality and their right to access health care. Many of the candidates for naturalization, when they are denied HIV waivers, are left to the vagaries of other governmental policies in countries that have even less knowledge about HIV. They are forced to return to communities under threat of political reprisal and with greatly diminished abilities to obtain employment and medical care. The amnesty candidates, already adapted to the United States and usually gainfully employed, are forced to return to communities with even fewer ties of kin and friends on whom they can rely.

The unfairness of INS policies both in the legalization of Central American undocumented migrants and of Mexican immigrants under the amnesty clause reveals a mixed agenda. On the one hand, foreign policy goals are being pursued internally in the United States that might possibly have grave consequences for international relations. On the other hand, the claim of public health urgency erodes the humanitarian facade that the government places on immigration policy.

## CONCLUSION

Gostin and Ziegler (1987:14), in their review of HIV-related legislative and regulatory policy in the United States, concluded that there is a fertile area of nonpunitive law that can significantly contribute to public health strategy:

> The law can be an effective means of setting a high standard of care in the professions, mobilizing resources, planning for education, designing outreach programs, offering treatment and services, and safeguarding persons with HIV infection against breaches of confidentiality and unfair treatment.

They challenged federal legislators to develop legal and regulatory policies that impede the spread of AIDS while protecting the privacy, rights, and dignity of vulnerable individuals.

These same attitudes would be equally appropriate in the area of immigration policy and HIV infection. The public presentation of government policy toward both legalization of political refugees and processing amnesty candidates would be better served by different public health strategies than are now the case. The present set of policies appears at best punitive and at worst inhumane. The social process that stems from the cultural construction of risk thus far has been to deny citizenship to HIV-infected individuals under the premise that it is necessary to protect the public health of citizens. Since the United States is already one of the countries most severely impacted by the AIDS epidemic, this argument appears ill advised.

Public health strategists would be better counseled to take a different approach and to invest their publicly announced concern for humanitarian treatment with greater integrity. If, as they state, their goal is to contain the spread of HIV, it would be more effective to provide treatment and education for Latinos/as who are HIV infected. Also, the knowledge that HIV infection is not a cause for deportation would encourage the immigrants to come to appropriate PHS officials for help.

With regard to cost-containment issues, education and treatment for the relatively few HIV-infected Latinos/as would be far less expensive than the testing of a half-million immigrants per year. Moreover, such a response is far more humane. Both the safety of U.S. citizens and the control of the spread of HIV are ends better served by this more humane approach.

In the cultural construction of risk, the stigma attached to AIDS and homosexuality/bisexuality, and discriminatory policy carried out against Latinos/as, far outweigh the public protestations of public health safety compared with humane tempering in the enforcement of immigration policy. The politically powerful segments of the United States disapprove of injecting drug use and homosexuality and do not wholeheartedly endorse the influx of Latino/a immigrants because they are perceived as economic liabilities. These latent attitudes and hidden agendas, cloaked in public health concerns and humanitarian ideals, are far more insidious in their contribution to the spread of this epidemic than the behaviors of the applicants for citizenship.

## REFERENCES

Bateson, M. C., and R. Goldsby. 1988. *Thinking AIDS*. Reading, MA: Addison-Wesley Publishing Co.

Covello, V. T., and B. B. Johnson. 1987. The Social and Cultural Construction of Risk: Issues, Methods, and Case Studies. In *The Social and Cultural Construction of Risk: Essays on Risk Selection and Perception,* ed. B. B. Johnson and V. T. Covello, pp. vii–xiii. Boston: D. Reidel Publishing Company.

Druhot, D. M. (1986). Immigration Laws Excluding Aliens on the Basis of Health: A Reassessment after AIDS. *Journal of Legal Medicine* 7(1): 85–112.

Douglas, M., and A. Wildavsky. 1982. *Risk and Culture: An Essay on Selection of Technical and Environmental Dangers.* Berkeley: University of California Press.

Gostin, L., and A. Ziegler. 1987. A Review of AIDS-related Legislative and Regulatory policy in the United States. *Law, Medicine, and Health Care* 15(1–2): 5–16.

Houston Department of Health and Human Services. 1992. *AIDS Surveillance Update.* Bureau of HIV Prevention, July.

*Houston Post.* 1990. U.S. Relaxes Restrictions of Foreigners with AIDS. *Houston Post,* April 14, p. A-3.

Rodriguez, N. 1987. Undocumented Central Americans in Houston: Diverse Populations. *International Migration Review* 21(1): 4–26.

Siegworth, Mark, ed. 1990. U.S. Policy on HIV Threatens International AIDS Conference. *Positively* (Houston: Body Positive/Houston) 3(4).

Singer, M., F. Flores, L. Davison, B. Burke, Z. Castillo, K. Scanlon, and M. Rivera. 1990. SIDA: The Economic, Social, and Cultural Context of AIDS among Latinos. *Medical Anthropology Quarterly* 4(1): 72–114.

Somerville, M. A. 1989. The Case against HIV Antibody Testing of Refugees and Immigrants. *Canadian Medical Association Journal* 141(9): 889–894.

Wolchok, C. L. 1989. AIDS at the Frontier: United States Immigration Policy. *Journal of Legal Medicine* 10(1): 127–142.

# 6

# Culture, Sexual Behavior, and Attitudes toward Condom Use among Baganda Women

*Charles B. Rwabukwali, Debra A. Schumann,*
*Janet W. McGrath, Cindie Carroll-Pankhurst,*
*Rebecca Mukasa, Sylvia Nakayiwa, Lucy Nakyobe,*
*and Barbara Namande*

## BACKGROUND

Through 1990 over 17,000 cases of AIDS had been reported in Uganda (WHO 1991), the second highest number of cases in the world during that period, after the United States. This figure clearly represents an undercounting because some AIDS patients, especially in remote rural areas, are never reported to hospitals or are not properly diagnosed and hence do not appear in the official statistics. As in most of East and Central Africa, HIV infection in Uganda is primarily transmitted through heterosexual intercourse ("pattern II transmission") (Ankrah 1989; Larson 1989; Mann *et al.* 1988). Several studies have found that the most important risk factors associated with infection in these populations include number of sexual partners, having a history of other sexually transmitted diseases, having received or given money for sex, having had sex with someone with an AIDS-like illness, and contact with contaminated blood through injections or blood transfusions. (Berkley, *et al.* 1989; Carswell 1987; Quinn, *et al.* 1986).

The male/female sex ratio for AIDS cases in Uganda is approximately 1/1 (48 percent males and 52 percent females) (Ministry of Health 1988), although recent data indicate that women have slightly higher HIV infection rates (1.4 times) than men (Berkley *et al.* 1990). The mean age for males with AIDS is thirty-two and for women with AIDS, twenty-seven (*ibid.*). The highest rates of infection and disease are in young women aged twenty to twenty-nine (Berkley *et al.* 1989), and up to 28 percent of women attending a prenatal clinic in Kampala are HIV infected (Hom *et al.* 1991).

These data suggest that young women are at particularly high risk of becoming HIV infected. This risk is of double concern because not only are these young women themselves at risk, but as a result of infection in young women, there is a growing number of cases of pediatric AIDS in Uganda. For example, Okware (1988) reported that in Uganda approximately 10 percent of the AIDS cases are infants and children under age five years. There is a clear and urgent need for well-designed programs for preventing further infection among women. Unfortunately, in the past the tendency has been to focus on the role of prostitutes (e.g., Carswell 1987; Carswell, Lloyd, and Howells 1989) in transmitting HIV infection, while the behavior of African women who are not prostitutes has been neglected or ignored. The epidemiologic data suggest that this view is shortsighted and that the widespread assumption that "promiscuous behavior," as defined in a Western cultural context, is at the root of the AIDS epidemic in East and Central Africa dangerously underplays the risk present for the entire population. Such assumptions have been challenged by social scientists (e.g., Brokensha 1988; Caldwell, Caldwell, and Quiggin 1989; De Zalduondo, Msamanga, and Chen, 1989; McGrath, Schumann, and Rwabukwali 1990; Schumann, Rwabukwali, and McGrath 1990). To achieve a concrete understanding of the cultural patterning of female sexual behavior that places women at risk of infection with HIV, it is necessary to document the range of tolerated sexual behavior. Understanding the context underlying female sexual behavior can help in the design and implementation of programs to control infection through behavior change.

This chapter presents data from an International Collaboration on AIDS Research (ICAR) project on the social organization of risk behaviors in HIV transmission in a population of HIV-infected and uninfected women drawn from the pediatric follow-up project at Mulago Hospital in Kampala, Uganda. This is one of four projects investigating clinical and behavioral aspects of HIV infection and AIDS being undertaken jointly by Makerere University and the Ministry of Health of the Republic of Uganda and Case Western Reserve University, Cleveland, Ohio, the United States, under the International Collaboration on AIDS Research Program of the National Institutes of Health. The primary objectives of the study were (1) to ascertain sexual behaviors of urban married women in Kampala, Uganda, that place them at risk of HIV infection; (2) to ascertain the "social organization" of risk behavior, that is, the cultural patterning of social relationships, particularly sexual relationships, that promote continuance of risk behaviors; and (3) to identify explanatory factors in the use or nonuse of barrier methods (such as condoms) to control the spread of HIV infection in the study population. This chapter will focus on objective 3: explication of the factors determining women's attitudes toward using condoms with their sexual partners. Although we speak of condom use with reference to women, this is done only as a convenient shorthand to refer to women's attitudes regarding the use of condoms by their male partners.

### Sexual Behavior and Condom Use

Since the AIDS epidemic shows no signs of retreating, and since neither a cure nor a vaccine has been found, most experts agree that prevention is the only viable option to stem the spread of the disease (e.g., Carswell 1987; Feldblum and Fortney 1988). This prevention can be in the form of sexual abstinence, monogamy, reduction in the number of sexual partners, non-penetrative forms of sex, and the use of barrier methods in general, and condoms in particular, during sexual intercourse (e.g., Feldblum and Fortney 1988; Larson 1989; Sullivan and Roskens 1991).

*In vitro* studies suggest that HIV cannot pass through latex condoms despite the use of higher virus titers than those found in human semen (Feldblum and Fortney 1988), although the efficacy of natural skin condoms is questioned. Studies in high-risk populations have confirmed the efficacy of condom use. For example, Ngugi *et al.* (1988) reported that none of the prostitutes who always used condoms were infected, compared to 5 percent of those using condoms less than half the time and 72 percent of the nonusers. Mann *et al.* (1987) reported similar findings in Zaire.

Despite evidence of the efficaciousness of condoms in preventing infection, acceptance of condom use among the people of Africa, including Ugandans, has been extremely low and quite problematic for a number of reasons. First, condoms are often associated with risky sexual encounters, especially sex with prostitutes, and therefore promotion of condoms for all sexual encounters is difficult because it must overcome this association of condoms with paid sex (Rwabukwali and Kirumira 1989). Second, condoms are often interpreted as an intrusion into a relationship. Therefore, while condoms may be used between a prostitute and a client, condom use during sex between lovers or long-standing girlfriends and boyfriends is generally unacceptable, because a suggestion to introduce a condom can be interpreted as an insult or a sign of mistrust (Day 1990; Larson 1989; Rwabukwali and Kirumira 1989; Worth 1989).

Furthermore, it has been pointed out that for women who have been taught that sex should be "natural," condom use implies a decision to have unnatural or undesirable sex (Worth 1989). In addition, the perception that condoms are unattractive and uncomfortable for men makes women reticent to suggest or insist on their use, particularly when they feel the need to protect their men (Worth 1989). Above all, condoms carry implications that go beyond a need for contraception or prevention of STDs. They suggest that one is sexually active and either "seeking sex" or "available" for sex (Worth 1989).

In Uganda the extent of condom use has been low, and attitudes toward condom use have been, by and large, negative. McCombie, Bukombi, and Rwakagini (1991) reported on 283 Ugandan women factory workers interviewed in March and November 1990. In March, 1.9 percent of the women reported always using condoms, 6.6 percent had used a condom within the preceding two months, and 17.9 percent had used one sometime in their lives. In November, 7 percent reported always using condoms, 15.1 percent had used them within the preceding two months, and 20.9 percent reported never having used a condom. Out of 1,099 men and women interviewed, a total of 78 percent of all respondents had heard of condoms, and 18 percent had used a condom previously. Of persons with more than one sexual partner in the previous two months, 8 percent had used a condom (McCombie et al. 1991). Forster and Furley (1988) surveyed Ugandans randomly approached on the streets of Kampala. They reported that 100 percent of the men in their sample and 79 percent of the women had heard of condoms, but only 9.4 percent of the men and 1 percent of the women used condoms regularly. For most men, nonuse of condoms was based on the belief that condoms are dangerous because they could easily break or come off inside the woman, and this would necessitate an operation to remove the condom that might result in death (Forster and Furley 1988). Overall, according to McCombie et al. (1991), men and women both reported the same reasons for failure to use condoms: that they were unfamiliar with condoms, they trusted their partner (and therefore did not need protection), or they found it difficult to ask a partner to use a condom. A substantial proportion of those asked also did not know where to obtain a condom.

In response to the low levels of condom use in Africa, some African countries have taken steps to introduce or increase condom use by the sexually active population, particularly those at high risk due to frequent partner changes (e.g., prostitutes and their clients). Ngugi et al. (1988) reported a striking increase in condom use among a cohort of Nairobi prostitutes after a program of AIDS and STD education and free distribution of condoms. It is too early to say whether such success can be replicated elsewhere since currently only limited data are available on condom promotion and distribution programs in non-high-risk groups. Clearly the issue of how to increase condom use and how to distribute condoms practically and prudently is of critical concern at this time.

## The Baganda

This study focuses on the Baganda of Kampala, Uganda. It is important to understand the cultural values regarding sexual relationships and sexual behavior in order to understand the variables that influence condom use in this population.

Extensive ethnographic material exists for the Baganda (see, for example, M. C. Fallers 1960; L. A. Fallers 1964; Kilbride 1979; Kilbride and Kilbride 1990; Kisekka 1972, 1973; Mair 1965; Obbo 1980; Roscoe 1966; Southall and Gutkind 1957; Southwold 1972, 1973, 1978). The Baganda are a

Bantu-speaking people who constitute the predominant ethnic group in Kampala and number around two million. They occupy the area around Lake Victoria that was formerly known as the Kingdom of Buganda and ruled by the kabaka (king) of Buganda. Traditionally, the Kingdom of Buganda was highly centralized and powerful (L. A. Fallers 1964; M. C. Fallers 1960; Roscoe 1966), and the Baganda themselves were, and still are, largely peasant cultivators. They grow green plantains, sweet potatoes, yams, and cassava. The colonial administration introduced cash crops such as coffee, tea, and cotton (Kilbride and Kilbride 1990). The Baganda descent system is patrilineal, so that they tend to be affiliated with the clan of their fathers, although individuals do not necessarily reside in the village of the clan (*ibid.*).

Traditionally, polygyny was the ideal among the Baganda, although few could actually afford to maintain multiple wives and their children (Southwold 1978). Today, polygyny among the Baganda is common but far from universal. Recent estimates suggest that 33 percent of all unions in Uganda, 31 percent of those in urban areas, and 33 percent of those in rural areas are polygynous (Kaijuka et al. 1989). Several studies have reported that marriage among the Baganda tends to be impermanent (Mandeville 1975; Parkin 1966). One factor that may contribute to marital dissolution is the high rate of infertility within the region, which has been linked to high levels of sexually transmitted diseases, especially gonorrhea (Griffith 1963). The area around Lake Victoria and including Kampala is reported to have the highest rate of infertility (21–40 percent) in Uganda and probably the highest rate in the whole of East Africa (Frank 1983). This, in conjunction with a strong desire to have children, may have contributed to the practice of multiple marriages and multiple sexual partners (M. C. Fallers 1960). This cultural pattern indicates how sexually active Baganda men and women may be at high risk for HIV infection in the absence of epidemiologically defined risks, such as prostitution and drug use.

Early marriage among Baganda girls is the norm, and studies indicate that most Baganda girls are sexually active before they marry (Kisekka 1972; Southwold 1973). It can therefore be assumed that many young Baganda girls are exposed to risk of infection with HIV at an early age.

Several other studies have directed their focus on sexual values and behavior of the Baganda (Kisekka 1972; McGrath, Schumann, and Rwabukwali 1990; McGrath et al. 1992). Their main conclusion has been that Baganda cultural values support multiple partnerships for men, but not for women. Baganda women do have extra-union sexual relationships, however, under certain conditions. For example, women report that extra-union partnerships may occur out of economic necessity, as revenge against their partner's extra-union sexual activities, and for sexual satisfaction if the current union partner is sexually incompetent (Kilbride 1979; Mandeville 1975; McGrath, Schumann, and Rwabukwali 1990; McGrath et al. 1992,

1993; Obbo 1980; Parkin 1966; Rwabukwali, Schumann, and McGrath 1990; Schumann *et al.* 1991; Schumann, Rwabukwali, and McGrath 1990; Southall and Gutkind 1957; Southwold 1973). These Baganda cultural values and expectations represent idealized behavior, and it can be assumed that they will be modified in response to structural changes in society, such as urbanization and mass education, for example, resulting from modernization. Harsher economic conditions may result in males having fewer wives and, coupled with raised expectations for children, may lead to smaller family sizes. Mass communication and exposure to "Western" media promoting nuclear families may change cultural values as well. Finally, the continued influence of modern religion may successfully encourage monogamous unions. For purposes of the present discussion, sociocultural values about sexual behavior influence the likelihood of taking preventive action and/or condition the type of preventive action taken.

## METHODOLOGY

A case-control design (Schlesselman 1982) using 65 HIV-infected and 65 HIV-uninfected Baganda women, matched for age (plus or minus two years) was utilized. Subjects were recruited through the Case Western Reserve University/Makerere University Collaborative Pediatric Follow-up Clinic at Mulago Hospital in Kampala. Subject selection was nonrandom, so that our sample may not be representative of the general population of women in Kampala. All women in the study were at least three months postpartum at the time of recruitment into the study. Serostatus data were provided by the clinic.[1] All participants were given the option to know their serostatus, but most women did not choose to be informed at the time of this study (Laura A. Guay, personal communication).[2]

All interviews were conducted in Luganda, the language of the Baganda, and the interviewers were blinded to the serostatus of the subjects. An initial demographic interview ascertaining maternal and paternal education, employment, and income status was undertaken at the time of the follow-up visit to the pediatric clinic or in the subject's home. Extensive follow-up interviews in the home addressed cultural rules regarding sex, rules regarding love and marriage, issues regarding fidelity and infidelity, attitudes toward sex, individual sexual behavior, contraceptive knowledge and use, self-reported history of STDs and AIDS, and preferences with respect to medication and disease treatment. Questions regarding condom use were included with discussions of both AIDS knowledge and prevention.

## RESULTS

Data analysis included qualitative analysis of interviews and bivariate (chi-square test) and nonparametric correlation analysis. The data pre-

Table 6.1
Descriptive Demographic Information

|  | Cases (N=65) | | Controls (N=65) | |
| --- | --- | --- | --- | --- |
| Mean age: | 20.985 | | 20.831 | |
| Range: | 17-30 | | 15-30 | |

Education: (p-value = 0.219)

|  | N | % | N | % |
| --- | --- | --- | --- | --- |
| None | 4 | 6.2 | 0 | 0.0 |
| Some primary | 27 | 41.5 | 24 | 36.9 |
| Primary completed | 11 | 16.9 | 18 | 27.7 |
| S3 completed | 21 | 32.3 | 22 | 33.8 |
| S4-S6 | 1 | 1.5 | 1 | 1.5 |
| Teacher's training /technical school | 1 | 1.5 | 0 | 0.0 |
| Literate: (p-value = 0.317) | 60 | 92.3 | 62 | 95.4 |

Woman's Reported Personal Income:  (p-value = 0.008)

| Ugandan Shillings per month | N | % | N | % |
| --- | --- | --- | --- | --- |
| None | 32 | 49.2 | 36 | 55.4 |
| 1-3000 | 5 | 7.7 | 5 | 7.7 |
| 3001-5000 | 9 | 13.8 | 3 | 4.6 |
| 5001-7000 | 10 | 15.4 | 4 | 6.2 |
| 7001-10000 | 2 | 3.1 | 12 | 18.5 |
| >10001 | 5 | 7.7 | 2 | 3.1 |
| Unknown | 2 | 3.1 | 3 | 4.6 |

Religion: (p-value = 0.067)

|  | N | % | N | % |
| --- | --- | --- | --- | --- |
| Muslim | 12 | 18.5 | 17 | 26.2 |
| Catholic | 21 | 32.3 | 30 | 46.2 |
| Protestant | 27 | 41.5 | 16 | 24.6 |
| Other | 5 | 7.7 | 2 | 3.1 |

sented here focus on the sociodemographic characteristics of the study population and an examination of the determinants of condom use for this group of women.

## Sociodemographic Summary of Data

The study population can be briefly summarized as follows (see table 6.1): the mean age for both cases and controls was 21 years, with a range of 17–30 years for cases and 15–30 years for controls. The research subjects were better educated than the Kampala population as a whole. Sixty (92 percent) of the cases were literate, compared to 62 (95 percent) of the controls (and 55.4 percent of the Kampala female population, as reported in the Uganda Demographic and Health Survey [Kaijuka *et al.* 1989]).

In terms of income status, this group of women could be regarded as poor, with 37 (57 percent) of cases and 41 (63 percent) of controls reporting personal earnings of less than 3,000 Ugandan shillings a month (at the time of the study, equivalent to approximately U.S. $4.30). Of these, most (32 cases and 36 controls) reported that they engaged in no income-generating activity and that their personal income was zero. A subset of women with no income, however, did receive support from their husbands. Twenty-one (32 percent) cases and 30 (46 percent) controls were Catholic, 27 (42 percent) cases and 16 (25 percent) controls were Protestant, and 12 (18 percent) cases and 17 (26 percent) controls were of the Muslim faith.

The distribution of union types reported is given in table 6.2. Ninety-four (72 percent) women described themselves as currently in a union and living with a partner. Fifty (38 percent) reported that their husband had more than one wife (compared with data reported by Kaijuka *et al.* [1989] that indicated that 31 percent of urban Uganda women were currently in a polygynous union). In addition, 44 (68 percent) cases and 36 (55 percent) controls reported that their husbands had children with other women. Whether these children were born during the current union is not known, so it is not clear whether this indicates serial monogamy, extra-union partnerships, or both.

## AIDS Knowledge and Prevention

All the women in our study had heard of AIDS, with 63 (97 percent) cases and 100 percent of controls admitting knowledge that AIDS is transmitted through sexual activity. Sixty-three (97 percent) of the cases and 62 (95 percent) of the controls mentioned a way of protecting oneself from AIDS. For the majority, 47 (75 percent) of the cases and 42 (68 percent) of the controls, the primary method of protection mentioned was "sticking to one sexual partner." Abstinence was mentioned by 22 (35 percent) of the cases versus 14 (23 percent) of the controls. Condom use was mentioned as a means of AIDS prevention by 19 (30 percent) of the cases and 25 (40 percent) of the controls, but only 3 (5 percent) of the cases and 2 (3 percent) of the controls reported ever having used a condom either for protection against sexually transmitted diseases, including AIDS, or for contraceptive purposes. None of the 130 subjects reported that they currently used condoms.

Table 6.2
Marriage Status

|  | Cases (N=65) | | Controls (N=65) | |
|---|---|---|---|---|

Marital status[a] : (p-value = 0.808)

|  | N | % | N | % |
|---|---|---|---|---|
| Legal marriage | 21 | 32.3 | 24 | 36.9 |
| Consensual union | 26 | 40.0 | 25 | 38.5 |
| Visiting union | 14 | 21.5 | 10 | 15.4 |
| Formerly married | 2 | 3.1 | 4 | 6.2 |
| Single | 2 | 3.1 | 2 | 3.1 |

"Does your husband have more than one wife?" (p-value = 0.656)

|  | N | % | N | % |
|---|---|---|---|---|
| Yes | 25 | 38.5 | 25 | 38.5 |
| No | 33 | 50.8 | 40 | 61.5 |
| Unknown | 7 | 10.8 | 0 | 0.0 |

"Does your husband have children with other women?" (p-value = 0.149)

|  | N | % | N | % |
|---|---|---|---|---|
| Yes | 44 | 67.7 | 36 | 55.4 |
| No | 21 | 32.3 | 29 | 44.6 |

[a]Legal marriage is defined as one involving a religious or civil ceremony. Consensual unions exist when the couple lives together with no such ceremonies. Visiting unions exist when one partner comes and goes from the household. The remaining categories are self-explanatory.

## The Condom Attitude Scale (CAS)

To characterize the attitudes toward condom use held by the women in the study, a condom attitude scale (CAS) was developed using responses to the open-ended interviews. Since this scale was developed from open-ended questions rather than an array of Likert-scale variables, it does not represent a "scale" in the strict analytical sense. Rather, the CAS is proposed only as an ordered categorical classification scheme. Accordingly, all analysis on these data utilized chi-square contingency analysis. The CAS is specific to this study and has not been tested or examined in other study populations. Responses to questions about condom use were grouped according to willingness to use condoms in the future (since no women were currently using them). Interviews were reviewed by two independent persons to identify recurrent attitudes about condoms, and then twelve response categories were constructed. From these, the final ten-item CAS was constructed. The items in the scale were ordered from the most positive attitudes toward condom use to the most negative attitudes. The final CAS items were the following:

1. Unconditionally willing to use condoms
2. Willing to use condoms if the husband agrees
3. Willing to use condoms if an authority dictates it
4. Willing to use condoms for contraception
5. Unwilling to use condoms—no reason stated
6. Unwilling to use condoms because they are ineffective
7. Unwilling to use condoms because of a desire to conceive
8. Unwilling to use condoms because they are associated with "promiscuity"
9. Unwilling to use condoms because of fears for health and pain
10. Unwilling to use because of the husband's refusal

Attitudes were considered negative or positive based on the researchers' perceptions of how likely a woman would be to actually use condoms and how difficult it would be to change the stated attitude. For example, women who responded that they would never use condoms because their partners would not allow it were placed at the most negative end of the scale, indicating that they saw themselves as removed from the decision-making process. Education directed toward them will likely have minimal effect on this process. This attitude is distinct from others who expressed generally more favorable attitudes toward condom use, while still deferring to their partner. The term "promiscuity" was used by the respondents to express a negative category of behavior; therefore, this term is used to represent the subjects' values, not those of the authors. The final ordering of the categories of responses represents one interpretation of the available information, and it is recognized that others are possible. For example, it could be argued that the fear of being thought to be "promiscuous" would be more difficult to overcome than health fears or fears of pain. For the purposes of this discussion, however, the current order of CAS items is both appropriate and sufficient.

Each subject's response was assigned to a scale category. Women sometimes gave more than one response, but none gave contradictory responses. In the case of multiple responses, the response indicating the most negative attitude toward condom use was used. For example, if a woman responded that she was unwilling to use condoms because she felt both that they were ineffective and that she would be perceived as "promiscuous," her response would be placed in category 8: refusal to use condoms because of the association with "promiscuity."

This scaled variable was tested for significant associations with other variables, using chi-square contingency analysis. There were no significant associations between the scale variable and number of partners in the last five years ($p = .31$), religion ($p = .26$), house type ($p = .18$), income ($p = .19$), and education ($p = .50$). These results are not surprising, considering the sample size available and the dimensions of the contingency tables. Nonparametric tests of association are also not significant, although it is noteworthy that a Kendall's tau test of association between condom attitude and the number of partners over the last five years was marginally significant ($p = .063$). In addition, this relationship was negative, perhaps indicating that women with more partners over the past five years were more likely to express positive attitudes toward condom use.

The responses to the CAS were also dichotomized into "willing to use condoms" and "unwilling to use condoms." Thirty-four women (26 percent) expressed willingness to use condoms, while 96 (74 percent) were unwilling. Chi-square analysis found no significant difference between cases and controls for willingness to use condoms ($p = .55$). In addition, the dichotomous variable was compared to five variables: marital status, educational status, religion, housing type, and income. Three of these variables (religion, housing type, and income) have been shown to be significant predictors of HIV status in this population (Rwabukwali et al. 1991). There was no statistically significant association between willingness to use condoms and four of the variables: marital status ($p = .62$), religion ($p = .38$), housing type ($p = .35$), and educational status ($p = .20$). The association between women's income and willingness to use condoms was statistically significant ($p = .02$) when income was analyzed in six categories (as in table 6.2). Women reporting zero income or 5,001–7,000 shillings per month were more likely to be unwilling to use condoms. If income was collapsed to four categories, however (see Schumann et al., in preparation), statistical significance disappeared ($p = .71$). Therefore, we cannot state that income level and willingness to use condoms are significantly related.

Due to the lack of significant differences between cases and controls with respect to attitudes toward condom use, the rest of this discussion will consider the sample as a whole. Figure 6.1 presents the distribution of responses across the CAS. Ten (8 percent) of the women said that they would willingly and unconditionally use a condom in the future to prevent getting AIDS. A typical reply in this fashion was:

> I have never used condoms to prevent myself from catching AIDS, but I would use them very willingly if they were available. (Eighteen-year-old, Muslim, HIV-positive woman)

Figure 6.1
The Condom Attitude Scale

## Stated Attitudes

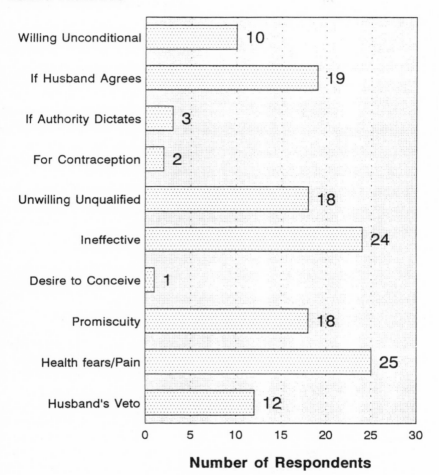

**Number of Respondents**

The critical role of the husband in the decision to use or not to use the condom is evident: 19 (15 percent) of the women interviewed stated that they would use a condom if their husbands gave them permission, and 12 (9 percent) said that they could not consider using condoms because their husbands would not allow it. As one women put it:

> I hear that people can use condoms to avoid catching the disease—AIDS—while having sex, but I have never discussed it with my husband. Though I have never used a condom, I would use it if my husband is the one who suggests it. (Twenty-one-year-old, Catholic, HIV-positive woman)

Three women (2.3 percent) said that they would consider using condoms if those in authority (e.g., doctors, churchmen, or leading politicians) suggested or even mandated it. Two (1.5 percent) said that if they used condoms, it would be for contraception, but not for disease prevention. This suggests that condoms are still perceived by a small percentage of women as contraception rather than disease-prevention devices. This finding is important, however, as willingness to use condoms as contraceptives suggests a way in which women may manage the fear of expressing distrust in a partner through requests for condom use (this will be discussed further in the concluding section).

As already indicated, the majority of the women did not wish to use condoms. Eighteen (14 percent) did not give any reason why they would not use condoms. However, 23 (18 percent) said that they would not use condoms because they perceived condoms as ineffective. In the words of one young woman:

> I have never used a condom and would not like to use one even if they were available because it is risky since sperm can pass through the condoms. (Twenty-two-year-old, Muslim, HIV-negative woman)

One woman said that she would not use condoms because she desired to conceive, but 18 (14 percent) stated that their objections to condom use were due to the association of condoms with "promiscuity" and risky sexual encounters. A typical response was:

> I have never used condoms to prevent catching AIDS. I can't use them even if they are available because for me, the implications of men who use condoms is that they are womanizers. (Eighteen-year-old, Protestant, HIV-negative woman)

The most common reason given for failure to use condoms was health fears and perception of pain associated with condom use (24 [18%]). (It should be emphasized that these perceptions were not based on personal experience, since only one of these women reported ever having used a condom.) Nevertheless, for these women the perceived risks were real. As one of them put it:

> I have never used condoms and I don't think I will ever use them because we are told that if you use condoms it sticks to your uterus and you will require an operation to remove it. This operation may result in your death. (Seventeen-year-old, Protestant, HIV-positive woman)

Many women had never seen a condom, let alone used one. It is, therefore, surprising that so many of them had such negative views about the condom. More research needs to be done to explore the origin of these negative feelings. It is also possible that the absence of condoms, especially in rural areas, has led to these myths about the condom. Recently, a nongovernmental organization, ARMSTRADE, supported by the U.S. Agency for International Development, began the social marketing of condoms. Perhaps the increased accessibility of condoms will serve to decrease the negative myths associated with condoms in this population.

## DISCUSSION AND CONCLUSIONS

Baganda women know about AIDS and the threat it poses to their lives. The response of this group of Baganda women to the AIDS epidemic has been to limit the number of sexual partners since they have been told that the most important route for HIV infection is through sexual intercourse (McGrath, Schumann, and Rwabukwali 1990; McGrath *et al.* 1992). However, many Baganda women still perceive themselves at risk of HIV infection because they are not sure whether or not their husbands are being faithful in their sexual relations with them (McGrath, Schumann, and Rwabukwali 1990; McGrath *et al.* 1992). Moreover, given the Baganda cultural norms that encourage men to have multiple sexual partners, women feel helpless to control their level of sexual risk. It is questionable, therefore, whether the female strategy of limiting the number of sexual partners will succeed in the long run. Increased use of condoms for protection from infection would, therefore, be a desired aspect of AIDS control programs.

The figures presented here indicate two major categories of objections to condom use. First, the largest category of objection relates to fears about condom safety and efficacy. Nineteen percent of the women feared the health consequences of using condoms, and 18 percent believed that they are not effective. Attitudes such as these suggest an emphasis on technical education about condoms, including how to use them safely and effectively. Because so few women in this population have ever used condoms, there is no body of "folk wisdom" about condoms. Only through increased education about what condoms are really like can these negative attitudes be overcome.

In addition, an important factor influencing decisions to use or not to use condoms is the belief that the partner would reject the use of condoms. Several of the women reported that if they suggested the use of condoms, their husbands would either beat them or ridicule them. This response occured for several reasons, prominent among which was the association of condom use with "promiscuity." Fourteen percent of the women refused condom use because they feared that if they requested condoms, their partner would either think that the woman must be "promiscuous" or that she did not trust him to be faithful. In either case there is a violation of trust in the relationship and the implication that inappropriate extra-union partnerships exist.

These data are of concern to those charged with the responsibility of designing programs to stem the spread of AIDS among Ugandans. It is helpful, however, to consider the conditions under which women stated their willingness to use condoms. First, 15 percent of the women stated that they would use condoms if their husbands agreed. This suggests that condom education for males may be successful in the long run. Eight percent of the women stated an unconditional willingness to use condoms. The fact that they were not using condoms is worrisome, but their stated willingness suggests that providing opportunities to obtain condoms and breaking the barriers to beginning use may increase condom use rates in this group.

As discussed earlier, the fact that a fraction of the women (2 percent) stated a willingness to use condoms for contraception suggests that women may be able to manage the stigma of association of condoms and "promiscuity" by referring to this alternative function. Since no couple desiring to conceive will use condoms anyway, allowing condoms to be perceived as contraceptives may permit women to request condom use without fearing the link to "promiscuity" and AIDS. This is not an optimal solution, of course, because it discourages couples using other forms of contraceptives from using condoms for protection from infection. For some women, however, the link to contraception may be important.

As stated earlier, in the absence of a vaccine or cure for AIDS, the only viable option is for the population to be given correct information and education for prevention and control. It is in this context that condom use should be promoted, since it is the most effective barrier method for stopping infection with HIV.

Under these circumstances, therefore, it is important that marketing skills and social science knowledge be brought to bear in the promotion of condom use among the Baganda. In particular, more intensive studies must be made of the range of variations in sexual practices as well as cultural meanings assigned to sexual behavior among Baganda men generally, but more specifically among young urban Baganda males (see McCombie *et al.* 1991). This is crucial because our data indicate that for women, the decision to adopt condom use is greatly influenced by the attitudes of the male partner.

Government policy, as well as policies of all development agencies in Uganda, should be geared toward empowering women with negotiating skills. This will enable women to assert their rights, including the right to refuse to have sex with a partner who they think might be putting them at risk of HIV infection. This is crucial if a breakthrough is to be made in increasing the number of couples using condoms. As Worth (1989:304) pointed out:

> Condom use has to be renegotiated with every sexual act. Women must address the issue of control over sexual-decision making every time they ask a male partner to use a condom.

It must be recognized, however, that skills training for women alone is seldom sufficient. The complexities of multiple relationships in this population (see McGrath *et al.* 1992) require recognition of the broad range of skills that women and men must acquire in order to reduce sexual risk.

Health education and sex education at all levels must be intensified, particularly to dispel negative rumors associated with condom use. The population must be reassured as to the safety and effectiveness of condoms. Ugandan physicians and other medical personnel should take the lead in the campaign to promote condom use since the general population is likely to find them credible. One suggestion for overcoming specific fears about condom effectiveness would be to manufacture condoms locally in Uganda. There have been reports of imported condoms spending days or even months stranded in customs warehouses and hence getting spoiled before being distributed to consumers. Some informants even reported rumors that Western countries (especially the United States) are sending defective or even viral-laden condoms to African countries. Although these rumors do not appear to have played a prominent role in the decisions of this group of women with respect to condom use, locally manufactured and distributed condoms may prevent concerns of this nature.

In the final analysis, it must be pointed out that in terms of prevention against infection with HIV, the ideal situation would be total abstinence from sexual encounters or mutual lifetime monogamy. It is unrealistic to expect either of these situations, and thus the condom is currently the only form of protection against HIV infection that is likely to find widespread acceptance. For this reason it is critical that negative views about the condom be replaced with more realistic appraisals of the appropriateness of the condom. In Uganda, where the AIDS epidemic will reach crisis proportions within the next decade, active promotion of condoms, short of broad cultural changes, is an essential strategy to reduce further spread of HIV infection. This effort will require assistance from all levels of Ugandan society, including the government and churches. For this reason it is essential that current debates concerning condom use be resolved immediately and that promotion of condom use become a major feature of AIDS prevention programs. Such programs will succeed, however, only if they are based on a concerted and united effort that recognizes the importance of condom use to AIDS risk reduction. Further delay in putting forth such an effort will further stall progress in reducing risk of HIV infection in this setting.

## NOTES

Support for the study upon which this chapter is based was provided by the International Collaboration on AIDS Research (ICAR) Program of the National Institutes of Health, grant number A02624-03, S. Okware, M.D., and F. Robbins, M.D., principal investigators; R. Mugerwa, M.D., and J. Ellner, M.D., co-principal investigators. The project "Family Structure and the Social Organization of Risk Behaviors" was awarded to Debra A. Schumann and Janet W. McGrath, co-project directors. The authors wish to thank Laura A. Guay, M.D., Patricia Ball, and the staff of the CWRU-Makerere pediatric follow-up clinic, who provided invaluable assistance in recruiting subjects.

1. Out of the 130 women interviewed, 116 (89 percent) were given second ELISA tests (for determination of serological status), and all were confirmed to their original status. Thirteen seronegative women (20 percent) and 47 seropositive women (72 percent) were given third ELISA tests, and all were confirmed. Ten seronegative women (15 percent) were given confirmatory Western blot tests. Of these, five (50 percent) were indeterminate (which is considered negative for clinical purposes), and five (50 percent) were confirmed negative. Fifty-five seropositive women (85 percent) were given Western blot tests, and all were confirmed positive (David Hom and Laura A. Guay, unpublished data).

2. The proportion of women requesting to know their serostatus has increased since the completion of data collection for this project as more women or their children show symptoms of HIV disease (Laura A. Guay, personal communication).

## REFERENCES

Ankrah, B. Maxine. 1989. AIDS: Methodological Problems in Studying Its Prevention and Spread. *Social Science and Medicine* 29:265–276.

Berkley, Seth F., et al. 1989. Risk Factors Associated with HIV Infection in Uganda. *Journal of Infectious Diseases* 160:22–30.

Berkley, Seth F., et al. 1990. AIDS and HIV infection in Uganda—Are More Women Infected Than Men? *AIDS* 4:1237–1242.

Brokensha, David. 1988. Overview: Social Factors in the Transmission and Control of AIDS. In *AIDS in Africa: The Social and Policy Impact,* ed. Norman Miller and Richard C. Rockwell, pp. 167–173. Studies in African Health and Medicine, vol. 1 Lewiston, NY: Edwin Mellen Press.

Caldwell, John C., Pat Caldwell, and Pat Quiggin. 1989. The Social Context of AIDS in Sub-Saharan Africa. *Population and Development Review* 15(2): 185–234.

Carswell, J. Wilson. 1987. HIV Infection in Healthy Persons in Uganda. *AIDS* 1: 223–227.

Carswell, J. Wilson, G. Lloyd, and J. Howells. 1989. Prevalence of HIV–in East African Lorry Drivers. *AIDS* 3:759–761.

Day, Sophie. 1990. Prostitute Women and the Ideology of Work in London. In

*Culture and AIDS,* ed. Douglas A. Feldman. pp. 93–109. New York: Praeger.

De Zalduondo, Barbara O., Gernard I. Maamanga, and Lincoln C. Chen. 1989. AIDS in Africa: Diversity in the Global Pandemic. *Daedalus,* v. 118, Summer, pp. 165–204.

Fallers, L. A., ed. 1964. *The King's Men: Leadership and Status in Buganda on the Eve of Independence.* London: Oxford University Press.

Fallers, Margaret C. 1960. *The Eastern Lacustrine Bantu.* London: International African Institute.

Feldblum, P. J., and J. A. Fortney. 1988. Condoms, Spermicides, and the Transmission of Human Immunodeficiency Virus: A Review of the Literature. *American Journal of Public Health* 78(1): 52–54.

Forster, Sarah J., and Kemlin E. Furley. 1988. Public Awareness Survey on AIDS and Condoms in Uganda. *AIDS* 3:147–154.

Frank, O. 1983. Infertility in Sub-Saharan Africa: Estimates and Implications. *Population and Development Review* 9:137–144.

Griffith, H. B. 1963. Gonorrhea and Fertility in Uganda. *Eugenics Review* 55(2): 103–108.

Hom, David, Laura Guay, F. Mmiro, Christophe Ndugwa, Johanna Goldfarb, and Karen Olness. 1991. HIV-1 Seroprevalence Rates in Women Attending a Prenatal Clinic in Kampala, Uganda. Paper presented at the VII International Conference on AIDS, Florence, Italy.

Kaijuka, Emmanuel M., Edward Z. A. Kaija, Anne R. Cross, and Edilberto Loaiza. 1989. *Uganda Demographic and Health Survey, 1988/89.* Entebbe, Uganda: Ministry of Health.

Kilbride, Philip L. 1979. Barmaiding as a Deviant Occupation among the Baganda of Uganda. *Ethos* 7(3): 232–255.

Kilbride, Philip L., and Janet C. Kilbride. 1990. *Changing Family Life in East Africa: Women and Children at Risk.* University Park: Pennsylvania State University Press.

Kisekka, Mere. 1972. Attitudes and Values Related to Love, Sex, and Marriage. In *Cultural Source Materials for Population Planning in East Africa,* ed. A. Molnos, vol. 1, *Review of Sociocultural Research, 1952–1972,* pp. 162–166. Institute of African Studies, University of Nairobi.

———. 1973. The Baganda of Central Uganda. In *Cultural Source Materials for Population Planning in East Africa,* ed. A. Molnos, vol. 3, *Beliefs and Practices,* pp. 148–162. Institute of African Studies, University of Nairobi.

Larson, Ann. 1989. Social Context of Human Immunodeficiency Virus Transmission in Africa: Historical and Cultural Bases of East and Central African Sexual Relations. *Reviews of Infectious Diseases* 11(5): 716–731.

Mair, Lucy P. 1965. *An African People in the Twentieth Century.* New York: Russell and Russell. (orig. 1934).

Mandeville, Elizabeth. 1975. The Formality of Marriage: A Kampala Case Study. *Journal of Anthropological Research* 31(3): 183–195.

Mann, Jonathan M., James Chin, Peter Piot, and Thomas Quinn. 1988. The International Epidemiology of AIDS. *Scientific American* 259(4): 82–89.

Mann, Jonathan M., Thomas C. Quinn, Peter Piot, Ngaly Bosenge, Nzila Nzilambi, Mpunga Kalata, Henry Francis, Robert L. Colebunders, Robert Byres, Pangu

Kasa Azila, Ngandu Kabeya, and James W. Curran. 1987. Condom Use and HIV Infection among Prostitutes in Zaire. *New England Journal of Medicine* 316(6): 345.

McCombie, Susan, Shem Bukombi, and Francis Rwakagiri. 1991. Changes in Condom Use among Women in Uganda. Paper presented at the VII International Conference on AIDS, Florence, Italy.

McCombie, Susan, Shem Bukombi, Francis Rwakagiri, and Paul Cohn. 1991. Sociodemographic Predictors of AIDS Related Knowledge and Practice in Uganda. Paper presented at the VII International Conference on AIDS, Florence, Italy.

McGrath, Janet W., Charles B. Rwabukwali, Debra A. Schumann, Jonnie Pearson-Marks, Sylvia Nakayiwa, Barbara Namande, Lucy Nakyobe, and Rebecca Mukasa. 1993. Anthropology and AIDS: The Cultural Context of Sexual Risk Behaviors Among Urban Baganda Women in Kampala, Uganda. *Social Science and Medicine* 36(4): 429–439.

McGrath, Janet W., Debra A. Schumann, and Charles B. Rwabukwali. 1990. Cultural Determinants of Sexual Risk Behavior among Ugandan Women. Paper presented at the Annual Meeting of the American Anthropological Association, New Orleans, Louisiana, December.

McGrath, Janet W., Debra A. Schumann, Charles B. Rwabukwali, Jonnie Pearson-Marks, Rebecca Mukasa, Barbara Namande, Sylvia Nakayiwa, and Lucy Nakyobe. 1992. Cultural Determinants of Sexual Risk Behavior for AIDS among Baganda Women. *Medical Anthropology Quarterly* 6(2): 153–161.

Ministry of Health. 1988. *Monthly AIDS Surveillance Report, September, 1988.* Entebbe, Uganda: Ministry of Health.

Ngugi, Elizabeth N., J. N. Simonsen, M. Bosire, A. R. Ronald, F. A. Plummer, D. W. Cameron, P. Waiyaki, and J. O. Ndinya-Achola. 1988. Prevention of Transmission of Human Immunodeficiency Virus in Africa: Effectiveness of Condom Promotion and Health Education among Prostitutes. *Lancet* 2(8616):887–890.

Obbo, Christine. 1980. *African Women: Their Struggle for Economic Independence.* London: Zed Press.

Okware, Samuel I., G. Giraldo, E. Beth-Giraldo, N. Clumeck, M. R. Gharbi, S. K. Kyalwazi, and G. De The. 1988. Epidemic of AIDS in Uganda. In *AIDS and Associated Cancers in Africa,* ed. G. Giraldo et al. London: Karger.

Parkin, David J. 1966. Types of Urban African Marriage in Kampala. *Africa* 36(3): 269–285.

Quinn, Thomas C., Jonathan M. Mann, James W. Curran, and Peter Piot. 1986. AIDS in Africa: An Epidemiologic Paradigm. *Science* 234:955–963.

Roscoe, John. 1966. *The Baganda: An Account of Their Native Customs and Beliefs.* New York: Barnes and Noble (orig. 1911).

Rwabukwali, Charles B., and Edward Kirumira. 1989. Decision Making, Sexual Behavior, and the Acceptability of Condoms to Ugandan Males. A Report to the Special Programme of Research, Development, and Research Training in Human Reproduction, World Health Organization, Geneva. Unpublished manuscript.

Rwabukwali, Charles B., Janet W. McGrath, Debra A. Schumann, Rebecca Mukasa, Sylvia Nakayiwa, Lucy Nakyobe, Barbara Namando, and Cindie Carroll-Pankhurst. 1991. Socioeconomic Determinants of Sexual Risk Behavior among Baganda Women in Kampala, Uganda. Poster presented at the VII International Conference on AIDS, June, Florence, Italy.

Rwabukwali, Charles B., Debra A. Schumann, and Janet W. McGrath. 1990. International Cooperation on AIDS Research: The Social Organization of Risk Behaviors in Kampala, Uganda. Paper presented at the Annual Meeting of the National Council for International Health, Washington, DC, June.

Schlesselman, J. J. 1982. *Case-Control Studies: Design, Conduct, Analysis.* New York: Oxford University Press.

Schumann, Debra A., Janet W. McGrath, Charles B. Rwabukwali, Jonnie Pearson-Marks, Barbara Namande, Lucy Nakyobe, Sylvia Nakayiwa, and Rebecca Mukasa. 1991. Culture and the Risk of AIDS: The Social Organization of Sexual Risk Behavior in Urban Uganda. Presented at American Anthropological Association meetings, November.

Schumann, Debra A., Janet W. McGrath, Charles B. Rwabukwali, Cindie Carroll-Pankhurst, Rebecca Mukasa, Barbara Namande, Lucy Nakyobe, and Sylvia Nakayiwa. In preparation. Social structure and the risk of HIV infection in Kampala, Uganda.

Schumann, Debra A., Charles B. Rwabukwali, and Janet W. McGrath. 1990. Maternal HIV Infection in Uganda: The Social and Cultural Context of High Risk Behavior. Poster presentation at the Annual Meeting of the American Public Health Association, New York, NY., October.

Southall, Aidan W., and Peter C. W. Gutkind. 1957. *Townsmen in the Making: Kampala and Its Suburbs.* Kampala: East African Institute of Social Research.

Southwold, Martin. 1972. The Baganda of Central Uganda. In *Cultural Source Materials for Population Planning in East Africa,* ed. A. Molnos, vol. 2, *Innovation and Communication,* pp. 171–180. Institute of African Studies, University of Nairobi.

―――. 1973. The Baganda of Central Uganda. In *Cultural Source Materials for Population Planning in East Africa,* ed. A. Molnos, vol. 3, *Beliefs and Practices,* pp. 163–173. Institute of African Studies, University of Nairobi.

―――. 1978. The Ganda of Uganda. In *Peoples of Africa,* ed. J. L. Gibbs, pp. 41–78. New York: Holt, Rinehart and Winston.

Sullivan, Louis W., and Ronald W. Roskens. 1991. *A Report to the President: Child Survival and AIDS in Sub-Saharan Africa: Findings and Recommendations of the Presidential Mission to Africa.* Washington, DC: Department of Health and Human Services.

World Health Organization. 1991. *Weekly Epidemiological Record* 66(1): 73.

Worth, Dooley. 1989. Sexual Decision-Making and AIDS: Why Condom Promotion among Vulnerable Women Is Likely to Fail. *Studies in Family Planning* 20(6): 297–307.

# 7

# AIDS in Ghana: Priorities and Policies

*Robert W. Porter*

Since the first AIDS cases were reported in Ghana, HIV/AIDS has come to be widely viewed as a disease of women, and more specifically of female prostitutes. This chapter reviews epidemiologic and other evidence for this construction and assesses its implications for setting policies and priorities in HIV prevention.

Ghana is still at an early stage in the HIV/AIDS epidemic, at least relative to countries in Central and East Africa. Yet recent evidence from Ghana's West African neighbors, particularly Côte d'Ivoire (where HIV prevalence among Abidjan's adult population is now estimated at above 10 percent), suggests that the AIDS problem in the region may soon be as serious as it is in the countries to the east and south.

In the now fairly extensive reportage on AIDS in Africa, Ghana has received little attention. The situation there is worth looking at, however, not only because the spread of HIV in the region may be accelerating more rapidly than had been anticipated only a short time ago, but because the way in which AIDS has been defined as a public health issue and the way it is now perceived and represented in Ghana's popular culture pose a set of issues that have wider implications for AIDS prevention policies and strategies.

## HIV/AIDS IN GHANA

The first cases of AIDS in Ghana were officially diagnosed and reported in 1986. In that year a serosurvey of STD patients in Accra found HIV prevalence to be 4.6 percent. Another early serosurvey of local sex workers in Accra placed HIV prevalence at 2.1 percent. Follow-up surveys of prostitutes in 1987 and 1988 found prevalence rates of 4.2 percent and 11.4

percent, respectively. HIV prevalence among blood donors and women attending antenatal clinics (ANC) ranges around 1 percent (see table 7.1). It must be emphasized, however, that these seroprevalence estimates have all been derived from convenience samples; consequently, they are not projectable, with any known degree of accuracy, to any wider population.

Nevertheless, official reports of AIDS cases are running at much lower levels than even these very tentative findings might suggest. For example, by the end of 1990, a cumulative total of only 2,237 AIDS cases had been officially reported to Ghana's National AIDS Control Programme (Asamoah-Odei 1991a). It is clear to everyone, however, that the official reports seriously underrepresent the epidemic's size and scope, although no data are available to estimate the extent of underreporting. Until population-based serosurveys yield more precise measures, it is currently estimated that somewhere in the range of 1 to 4 percent of the country's population is now HIV infected.

The official statistics deserve a closer look, however, because from the beginning, the reported cases of females with AIDS have significantly outnumbered male AIDS cases. In 1986 the ratio of female to male cases was 7.7 to 1 (see table 7.2.) By 1990, however, the ratio of female to male cases was 2.5 to 1. This shift suggests that the gender distribution of HIV/AIDS in Ghana is moving toward that of other areas in Africa, where the sex ratio is roughly 1 to 1. But for now, the official case reports still seem (at first glance) to support the construction of AIDS in Ghana as a disease of women, and more specifically, a disease of female sex workers. This is because the first official cases of AIDS occurred among women who apparently were infected abroad (see table 7.3). A significant proportion of these early cases were, by most accounts, sex workers, many from the Krobo traditional area east of Accra.

As a Ghanaian physician practicing in the United Kingdom wrote in a 1987 letter to the *Lancet,* after returning from a visit to Africa:

> It is common knowledge that all but two of the AIDS patients in Ghana were prostitutes who had been working in the Ivory Coast and had been sent home to die. The two non-prostitutes were a Ghanaian man and his German wife who had previously lived in Germany for 15 years. (Konotey-Ahulu 1987: 206)

This assessment by a Ghanaian expatriate may not be epidemiologically accurate, but it certainly is indicative of the general public's, particularly the educated public's, perception of AIDS. The National AIDS Control Programme (NACP) does not report on AIDS patients' social or occupational backgrounds, but official AIDS reports do indicate whether a person with AIDS has a "history of travel outside of Ghana." In the case of women

Table 7.1
Seroprevalence Data, Ghana, 1986–1991

| Year | Group | N | #Pos HIV-1 | Rate HIV-1 | #Pos HIV-2 | Rate HIV-2 | #Pos HIV-1+2 | Rate HIV-1+2 |
|------|-------|---|------------|------------|------------|------------|--------------|--------------|
| 1987 | Prostitutes, Accra | 72 | 3 | 4.2% | | | | |
| 1988 | Prostitutes, Accra | 35 | 4 | 11.4% | NA | NA | | |
| | | | | | | | | |
| 1986 | STD Patients, Accra | 64 | 3 | 4.6% | | | | |
| ---- | | | | | | | | |
| 1988 | STD Patients, Accra | 433 | 9 | 2.1% | | | | |
| 1989 | STD Patients, Accra | 347 | 15 | 4.3% | | | | |
| 1990 | STD Patients, Accra | 293 | 16 | 5.5% | 0 | 0.0% | | |
| | | | | | | | | |
| 1990 | ANC women, Accra | 300 | 2 | 0.7% | 0 | 0.0% | | |
| | ANC women, Sunyani | | | | | | | |
| | ANC women, Wenchi | | | | | | | |
| 1991 | ANC women, Agomanya | | | | | | | |

| Year | Category | | | | | | |
|---|---|---|---|---|---|---|---|
| 1986 | Blood donors, Accra/Tema | 288 | 0 | 0.0% | ND | -- | |
| 1988 | Blood donors, Accra/Tema | 13465 | 174 | 1.3% | ND | -- | |
| | Blood donors, Kumasi | 2304 | 25 | 1.1% | ND | -- | |
| | Blood donors, Akwatia | 123 | 0 | 0.0% | ND | -- | |
| 1990 | Blood donors, Accra | 10565 | -- | -- | -- | -- | 241   2.3% |
| | Blood donors, Kumassi | 9170 | -- | -- | -- | -- | 66   0.7% |
| | Blood donors, Tema | 1692 | -- | -- | -- | -- | 27   1.6% |
| | Blood donors, Tamale | 2463 | -- | -- | -- | -- | 2   0.1% |
| 1986 | Med. Cert. (travel) | 168 | 0 | 0.0% | ND | -- | |
| | Med. Cert. (travel) | 2578 | 22 | 0.9% | ND | -- | |

1990–91 Military (GAF):      "SAME AS NATIONAL RATE"

*Sources*: E. Asamoah-Odei, *HIV Surveillance in Ghana, 1986–1990* (Accra: Ministry of Health, 1991); USAID/Accra, *Technical Assessment—HIV/AIDS Situation in Ghana* (1991).

Table 7.2
Reported AIDS Cases in Ghana

| Year | No. Cases | Cumulative Cases | F:M Ratio |
|------|-----------|------------------|-----------|
| 1986 | 26 | 26 | 7.7 |
| 1987 | 35 | 61 | 4.8 |
| 1988 | 266 | 327 | 6.0 |
| 1989 | 899 | 1226 | 3.3 |
| 1990 | 1011 | 2237 | 2.5 |

Source: E. Asamoah-Odei, AIDS Status Report, Ghana: 1986–1990 (Accra: Ministry of Health, 1991).

(particularly poorer women) with AIDS who have traveled abroad, a history of foreign travel is assumed to mean a career in prostitution.

The epidemiologic data, then, have been widely interpreted in Ghana as proof that female prostitutes introduced HIV disease to the country. But by 1988, according to the Ministry of Health, it had become evident that HIV was being acquired and was spreading within Ghana. Over a third of AIDS cases officially reported in 1990 were autochthonous, among people who had never traveled abroad. However AIDS may have arrived, it is no longer a foreign disease.

EARLY RESPONSES

Early responses to AIDS in Ghana included the formation in 1985 of a Technical Committee on AIDS to advise the government and to work with the Ministry of Health and World Health Organization (WHO) consultants on developing a Short Term Plan for AIDS Prevention and Control. Antibody-testing and blood-screening facilities were introduced in 1987. An AIDS control program manager assumed duty in 1988, and by the end of that year a Medium Term Plan had been developed in collaboration with the WHO's Global Programme on AIDS.

An early pilot intervention involving seventy-five sex workers in Accra began in early 1987 and continued until the middle of 1988. Small-scale interventions targeting sex workers have continued intermittently up to the present. Educational activities aimed at the general public included sporadic public service announcements on television, leaflets, and posters (some of which recommended avoidance of sex workers). In the meantime, a Contraceptive Social Marketing Programme, implemented with funding from the United States Agency for International Development (USAID), had made condoms widely available through urban commercial channels at

Table 7.3

Reported AIDS Cases in Ghana and History of Travel Abroad, 1986–1990

| YEAR | RESIDENT OF GHANA WITH NO HISTORY OF TRAVEL ABROAD | RESIDENT OF GHANA WITH HISTORY OF TRAVEL ABROAD | NON-RESIDENT TEMPORARILY IN GHANA |
|------|-----|-----|-----|
| 1986 | 3 (11.5%) | 23 (88.5%) | 0 (0.0%) |
| 1987 | 11 (31.4%) | 23 (68.6%) | 0 (0.0%) |
| 1988 | 68 (26.0%) | 193 (72.6%) | 4 (1.5%) |
| 1989 | 306 (34.0%) | 574 (63.8%) | 19 (2.1%) |
| 1990 | 399 (39.5%) | 562 (55.6%) | 50 (4.9%) |

*Source:* E. Asamoah-Odei, *AIDS Status Report, Ghana: 1986–1990* (Accra: Ministry of Health, 1991).

*Note: One case for the year 1988 is unaccounted.

subsidized prices. In the last several years condom sales have increased markedly, presumably spurred by growing concerns about AIDS. Nevertheless, overall condom use remains low. Currently, the NACP is developing more comprehensive educational interventions, targeting a wider range of audiences.

## THE SOCIAL CONSTRUCTION OF AIDS

It appears now, however, that a major obstacle to educational programs aimed at youth, young adults, and other population segments is that AIDS in Ghana is highly stigmatizing, in part because of beliefs concerning its origin with female prostitutes. When people speak candidly of the disease, they do so with strong feelings of aversion. It is widely believed that most people with AIDS have only themselves to blame, and many Ghanaians find it extremely difficult to think about what it would be like personally to have HIV disease.

I was not really aware of how negatively people with AIDS were viewed until I assisted the NACP and a group of local communications researchers in designing and implementing an exploratory focus-group study in the three regions of Ghana where HIV/AIDS is most prevalent (according to official reports).[1] The overall purpose of the study was to assess AIDS-related knowledge, attitudes, beliefs, and practices among three populations: adolescents (both in and out of school), teachers, and parents. In addition, we wanted to see whether literacy, gender, and personal contact with the epidemic (knowing somebody with AIDS or HIV) were relevant variables for communication planning and audience segmentation.[2]

In all, thirty-six focus groups involving about 350 participants were conducted. Group discussions were facilitated by trained moderators using local languages, either Ga, Krobo, or Twi, depending on the ethnic
composition of the groups, with some switching back and forth into English.

Nearly all of the group participants knew that AIDS could be transmitted
through sexual intercourse and through contact with infected blood. But
many of these same people also reported a number of misconceptions about
the ways AIDS is spread. More specifically, the knowledge that AIDS can
be transmitted through sexual intercourse and by contact with infected
blood does not rule out the possibility—for many of the people interviewed—that it can also be transmitted through much more casual encounters with infected persons.

In short, very few people in the focus groups were able to accurately
assess their own risk of infection, and some were even adopting such inappropriate preventive measures as avoiding funerals or wakes (because the
deceased may have died of AIDS). Also, questions about what caused AIDS
led, in a number of focus groups, to spontaneous discussions of how AIDS
first came to Ghana. For example, out-of-school youth in the Krobo traditional area claimed that AIDS was brought to the community by "our
sisters who have travelled to Cote d'Ivoire and Paris who have been in-
dulging in sex with animals, with dogs and other pets." Parents in the
Krobo area (in a separate focus group) also claimed that AIDS was caused
by "prostitutes having sex with animals."

These kinds of accounts are not limited to Krobo. Parents in a Kumasi
focus group also reported, "We hear that when some of the women go
abroad, the white man pays them to have sex with animals, for example,
dogs. It is these animals who give the AIDS to the women." In these accounts AIDS is clearly associated with "unnatural" behavior: it is a product
of illicit sexual relations between animals and women, orchestrated by
white men (or white society, e.g., "Paris"). In this construction AIDS is
about sex, money, power, race, domination, and, of course, death. It en-
compasses a set of meanings and relations that are both potent and, for
most people, deeply disturbing.

It is not known at this point how widespread or how widely accepted
these origin myths may be. Nevertheless, they do inform the contemporary
discourse on AIDS in Ghana, particularly among the less educated and the
nonliterate, and they are clearly variations on the dominant, official construction of AIDS (i.e., that it was introduced by Ghanaian sex workers
sent home from Côte d'Ivoire). These popular accounts also help to explain
how it is that many Ghanaians invest AIDS with such negative meanings,
and why people living with AIDS are so heavily stigmatized.

The attitudes of youth, particularly school dropouts, toward people with
AIDS tend to be especially harsh. When asked how they would feel toward

someone they knew had AIDS, they said things like "I will advise the relatives to use the money to prepare for his funeral rather than to waste it on hospital charges"; "They should be thrown away"; and "If your friend detects that he is dying of AIDS, he may find ways and means of making you contract the disease. It is possible that he would cut himself with a fresh blade, hide it and if you unknowingly use it, you could also join him to die."

People who personally knew or had seen persons with AIDS expressed only slightly less negative attitudes. The following comments are typical: "The disease affected and changed her form so she became very ugly"; "I did not feel like getting near her because I was afraid"; and "I pitied her. I also began thinking and imagining that she was a bad person."

Residents of Somanya (our research site in Krobo) and nearby communities have probably been more directly affected by the epidemic than residents of other areas in Ghana. They tend to know people with AIDS, although they may not know for sure that someone was actually sick with AIDS until after he or she has died, when the immediate families of the deceased may speak more candidly about the nature of the illness. In Somanya there is evidence that people's anxiety and fear about AIDS are very high indeed. When parents report that they advise their children not to attend a wake because the deceased may have had AIDS, or when people say that the bodies of AIDS patients should not be released to their families for customary burial, then we know that AIDS-related fears and suspicions have reached critical proportions. The focus groups in Somanya also indicate that personal experience with AIDS does not, in and of itself, reduce the stigma of the disease. In Somanya local attitudes toward people with AIDS may actually be hardening. What implications can we draw from all this?

## EXPLANATORY MODELS

First, consider the question of prostitution and AIDS, and more specifically the idea that prostitution is responsible for the current distribution of AIDS in Ghana. Prostitutes in Africa have been singled out for targeted interventions in a number of countries, including Ghana, because they are often viewed as "high-frequency" or "core-group transmitters" of HIV, to use the idiom of STD control. (Of course, they are themselves at high risk of infection, but this seldom seems to be sufficient in and of itself to warrant special attention.)

It is reasonable to assume that a relatively small number of HIV-infected women having unprotected sex with a large and shifting clientele would result in a very high rate of transmission. However, if this were the dominant pattern of transmission in Ghana, the sex ratio of HIV infection and

AIDS would be just the opposite of what it is. That is, many more men than women would be infected with HIV.

So, given the gender ratio of AIDS cases (according to the official epidemiologic reports), one could actually make a better argument for a pattern of transmission in which a small number of infected men are having unprotected sex with a relatively large number of different female partners. Why has this alternative interpretation never been seriously considered?

Part of the answer is that both the collection of epidemiologic data on HIV/AIDS and its interpretation have been conditioned by an explanatory model of HIV disease in Ghana that took root early on in the epidemic and has been fairly resistant to change, even though the epidemiology is changing and becoming more complex. This model rests on three interrelated presuppositions: (1) HIV/AIDS is a disease of female prostitutes who were (2) originally infected elsewhere, returned home, and then (3) began infecting men who had not traveled abroad. Did the available epidemiologic data ever really warrant this interpretation? I argue that they have not. Rather, this model—we will call it the "prostitute model"—has largely determined how the epidemiologic data have been collected and read.

The clearest account of this explanatory model comes from a 1988 paper on the HIV/AIDS epidemic in Ghana by Dr. A. R. Neequaye and colleagues. Dr. Neequaye was an original member of Ghana's National Technical Committee on AIDS. In early 1988, at the time their paper was written, there were 277 seropositive cases officially reported in Ghana (see table 7.4 for their distribution among subgroups). Of the people screened for HIV, only blood donors and "healthy people seeking certificates for travel" were not, according to Neequaye et al. (1988:15), "preselected for risk behavior." HIV prevalence among these two samples was less than 1 percent (0.11 percent and 0.67 percent, respectively), while among sick prostitutes returning from Côte d'Ivoire it was close to 60 percent (59.4 percent). The blood donors and the applicants for travel certificates did not constitute probability samples, so HIV prevalence among these groups cannot be projected to larger populations with any calculable degree of sampling error; and this, of course, is true also for the estimate of HIV prevalence among prostitutes returning from Côte d'Ivoire. Still, the difference in HIV prevalence between these samples is striking indeed.

We must understand, however, that apart from blood donors, those seeking travel certification, and, more recently, attendees at certain STD, antenatal, and military clinics (i.e., serosurveillance sites), people are tested for HIV in Ghana only on their own initiative, or if they are recognized to present symptoms of AIDS. This policy is largely one of necessity. HIV testing in Ghana has been limited because Ghana's testing capabilities are themselves so limited. Test kits and people trained to use them, particularly in front-line clinics and hospitals, are in such short supply that an estimated 50 percent of blood transfusions are still not screened for HIV, even though

Table 7.4
Population Groups Tested for HIV in Ghana, 1987

| | Groups of People | No. Screened | No. HIV+ | % HIV+ |
|---|---|---|---|---|
| 1. | Blood donors | 5480 | 6 | 0.11 |
| 2. | Local prostitutes | 236 | 5 | 2.12 |
| 3. | Female prostitutes returning from Cote d'Ivoire with disease | 335 | 199 | 59.40 |
| 4. | Patients with sexually transmitted diseases | 107 | 5 | 4.67 |
| 5. | Infants from HIV positive mothers | 7 | 7 | 100.00 |
| 6. | Healthy people seeking certificate for travel | 300 | 2 | 0.67 |
| 7. | Other Ghanaians with history of stay in neighboring countries including Senegal, Nigeria, Togo and Burkina Faso | 215 | 33 | 15.35 |
| 8. | Patients reporting at the hospitals | 214 | 20 | 9.35 |

*Source:* A. R. Neequaye, L. Osei, J. A. A. Mingle, G. Ankra-Badu, C. Bentsi, A. Asamoah-Adu, J. E. Neequaye. "Dynamics of Human Immune Deficiency Virus (HIV) Epidemic—The Ghanaian Experience," in *The Global Impact of AIDS,* pp. 9–15, eds. A. F. Fleming, M. Carballo, D. W. FitzSimmons, M. R. Bailey, J. Mann, 1988.

protecting blood supplies is a much higher priority than serosurveillance (and ought to be).[3]

Hospital patients or clinic attendees are generally tested only to confirm symptoms that lead clinicians to suspect AIDS or HIV-related conditions. Here, for example, is the way candidates for HIV testing are selected at St. Martin's, a Catholic clinic at Agomanya, a Krobo market town in southeastern Ghana:

Staff at the out-patient clinics refer patients with symptoms of AIDS for pretest counseling and a blood test. Most patients have already been to traditional healers or "quack doctors" [*sic*] before they seek professional medical treatment at St. Martin's.

Patients diagnosed as HIV-positive at St. Martin's have an average of five typical symptoms of AIDS, the most common of which are persistent cough, fever and diarrhea. Some patients may have as many as eight such symptoms.

> When referring female patients for an HIV test, staff also take into account
> whether they have worked abroad, or are wearing unusually expensive
> clothes or jewelry. These are both indications that a woman may have
> worked in the "sex industry" and is therefore likely to have contracted HIV.
> (Hampton 1990:10)

In short, patients without symptoms of AIDS who pass through clinics or
hospitals in Ghana are not likely to be tested for HIV unless they either
admit to or are suspected of being sex workers or have traveled abroad,
for in the popular as well as the official epidemiology of AIDS in Ghana,
a history of foreign travel is treated as an index of prostitution, at least for
poorer, less educated women. In any case, few people (until recently) were
candidates for testing at all unless they were already symptomatic, meaning
that they presented symptoms that fit the AIDS case definition.

So HIV testing, and thus the epidemiologic data on HIV/AIDS in Ghana,
have come to focus on suspected cases of AIDS or symptomatic HIV disease
among women who have traveled abroad. Men and women who had not
traveled or who were not (or did not seem to be) sex workers were less
likely to be tested for HIV. Once this risk profile, "women with a history
of foreign travel," was established, there was little practical interest in
broadening it. Such a very narrow definition of risk helps front-line clinicians to decide how to ration scarce HIV test kits. "Foreign travel" as a
criterion for testing is still much too broad, since a very large number of
adult Ghanaians (perhaps millions), men and women alike, have lived outside the country. Ghana's economic crisis of the late 1970s and early 1980s
led to a massive outmigration. It is difficult to estimate its size, but the
forced repatriation of approximately 1.2 million Ghanaians from Nigeria
in 1984 offers some indication of the number of people involved. Today,
many other Ghanaians continue to reside and work in other West African
countries, as well as in Europe and North America. But the prostitute
model focuses only on a single category of migrant.

> During this period of exodus to neighboring countries a lot of young Ghan-
> aian women found their way to Cote d'Ivoire. Some went by their own efforts
> but others were actively recruited by other Ghanaian women who had been
> resident for some time in Cote d'Ivoire. Many went without knowing what
> work they would do, and finding no other means of support resorted to
> prostitution. (Neequaye *et al.* 1988:14)

The economic crisis was particularly severe in the Krobo traditional area.
The Krobo had already lost much of their most fertile lands when Lake
Volta was created in the 1960s (the Akosombo Dam across the Volta River
is just to the east). With the local agricultural economy in decline, young
Krobo increasingly entered the rural-urban labor migration stream. From

the 1960s onward, the migration of Krobo to Accra and to other urban centers in neighboring Francophone countries in search of employment accelerated.

> The local women call it "going to French." In one small Eastern Region hospital alone, by December 1987, 50 HIV positives, mostly AIDS cases, had been identified. Forty-five of these had a history of travel to Cote d'Ivoire and the rest to other neighboring countries. . . . In the course of time some of these young girls became sick. They could no longer work to support themselves. They are returning home in search of treatment which is expensive in Cote d'Ivoire. It is these young women who are returning with the disease [AIDS]. This explains why most of the cases are females from the Eastern Regions. . . . The majority of patients returning from Cote d'Ivoire have AIDS or AIDS Related Complex. (*ibid.*)

These women, according to the prostitute model, introduced HIV to Ghana:

> In Ghana, the first wave of HIV seropositives has been in female prostitutes who had worked in neighboring West African countries, in particular Côte d'Ivoire. Initially, the female/male ratio was 11:1. However, a trend towards a lower ratio is being observed as the infection spreads from these women into the local population. As in the East African countries, prostitution is likely to be a major factor in the spread of the disease. (*ibid.*:15)

One of the more obvious problems with this explanation, however, is that women with AIDS or symptomatic HIV disease are generally not able to continue earning a living through the commercial sale of sex. In other words, women who became sick with AIDS in Abidjan and have come home to Ghana for treatment are unlikely to be "high-frequency transmitters" of HIV within Ghana proper.

What about the transmission of HIV from returning prostitutes who are infected, but who have not yet developed AIDS? Neequaye *et al.* (1988:14) noted that "some of the asymptomatic seropositives who have no personal history of travel have had sexual links with prostitutes in neighboring countries who returned home on festive occasions and a few with prostitutes working locally." It is not clear from their report just who or how many HIV-infected men were being referred to, but they would appear to be a subset of the eight infected, but asymptomatic, blood donors and applicants for travel certificates (see table 7.4). This is a very small number of cases indeed.

So the epidemiologic evidence for any significant link between prostitutes returning to Ghana (either asymptomatic or already sick with AIDS) and local transmission of HIV is extremely tenuous. In sum, the available data do not lend much support to the view that returning female prostitutes are driving Ghana's HIV epidemic.

I am proposing here an alternative model of HIV transmission, perhaps best called the "networking model."[4] In this model there are two basic and largely independent patterns of transmission. In the first pattern, the loci of HIV infection are, for the most part, beyond Ghana proper. But HIV enters the satellite communities of migrant Ghanaians in Abidjan and elsewhere (i.e., Europe and North America). Female migrants with multiple sexual partners are among the most vulnerable to early infection. This risk category includes, but is not limited to, Ghanaian women who work in the commercial sex industry centered on the urban centers of West Africa—Abidjan in particular. When these women return to Ghana for medical treatment, their HIV disease is already quite advanced. Too infirm to make an independent living, they can still, once in their home communities, draw on the support of more concentrated networks of family and friends. These women are more properly part of the regional, pan–West African epidemic of HIV. Their role in Ghana's more local epidemic is probably very limited. These women have been at risk for HIV through exposure to the virus in the epicenters of the wider pandemic, but once they return to Ghana proper, they do not constitute a core transmission group—they are simply too sick.

At the same time, however, HIV is moving through Ghana's population via the kind of wider and more diffuse sexual networking that has been so clearly documented for Ghana and West Africa more broadly (Abu 1983; Bleek 1976; Caldwell and Caldwell 1987; Oppong 1983; Pellow 1977; Verdon 1983). In this second and largely separate pattern of HIV transmission, there is not much evidence of localized pools of infection. HIV and the risk of HIV infection do not appear to be equally distributed across all geographic or demographic segments of the population; but we simply do not know much about how the autochthonous epidemic is moving, largely because asymptomatic individuals are not being tested. This second HIV epidemic is only starting to surface as HIV testing expands and physicians become more familiar with AIDS case definitions.

New AIDS cases are coming in relatively greater numbers from the Ashanti Region (in central Ghana), where the cumulative incidence of AIDS is now second only to that of the Eastern Region. For the country as a whole, nearly 40 percent of the 1990 AIDS cases were among individuals who had no history of travel abroad (Asamoah-Odei 1991a). The female/male ratio for new cases has also dropped, but women still outnumber men. Yet it is safest to say that the epidemiologic data are still too fragmented and incomplete to offer any clear picture of core-group transmission, regardless of how "core group" is defined.

We know enough about patterns of HIV transmission elsewhere, however, to suggest that HIV/AIDS in Ghana has now developed into at least two quite distinctive epidemics, contiguous but largely unrelated. The first is more an epidemic of AIDS specifically than of HIV more broadly, at least by the time it reaches Ghana (with the return of Krobo women who had "gone to French"). Yet I suspect that this initial wave of AIDS was the temporal forerunner of the core HIV epidemic only in the sense that it was so visible and so geographically concentrated. In any event, it was largely self-limiting. For most of the women caught up in it (they are now deceased), the end stages of the disease process were played out in Ghana proper, while the early stages of viral infection and potential retransmission were played out abroad. So this "first" epidemic was more an epidemic of the Ghanaian diaspora and less of Ghana proper.

The second epidemic, the broader HIV epidemic, is much more widely diffused throughout Ghana and is still largely invisible. It is only now beginning to surface as a discernible pattern of morbidity. This epidemic is driven by people in the early asymptomatic stages of HIV disease, who are unknowingly transmitting the virus to others in Ghana proper. The people caught up in this epidemic will be less socially and economically marginal than the poorer Ghanaian migrants who developed AIDS in Côte d'Ivoire, and they will be harder to locate and categorize in epidemiologic terms because sexual networking continues to be a widespread strategy for female economic survival throughout much of the country, but particularly in urban areas. Note that we are not talking about "prostitution" here, a category whose analytic value outside of the Euro-American cultural sphere is limited at best, but of a more complicated and deeply seated pattern of sexual relations associated with (1) forms of indigenous social organization in which neither marriage nor monogamy is central to social reproduction; (2) the continued and widespread practice of postpartum female abstinence, in which mothers are enjoined from sexual relations to protect the health of the newborn, at the same time that their husbands may freely enter into outside sexual relationships; and (3) a breaking down of traditional forms of sexual education and initiation, managed by elder kin within the context of the local community, leading to more widespread sexual experimentation among adolescents at an earlier age (Abu 1987; Akuffo 1987; Hampton 1990; Oppong 1987; Porter 1990).

## IMPLICATIONS FOR PREVENTION

Why is it, then, that HIV disease in Ghana is constructed as a disease of women in both the popular culture and the medical community?[5] Women may have literally brought AIDS to Ghana when they came home from Abidjan to die, but these women are not the core of Ghana's HIV epidemic. It is more accurate, I suggest, to see them as scouts or sentinels. They have alerted us to what may be in store down the road. But have we misunderstood their message? And have we blamed them for being the first to bring the bad news home?

I have argued that the epidemiologic evidence does not support the supposition that prostitutes comprise the core transmission group for HIV in Ghana. I have not tried to answer two other questions that this argument raises: Why has the epidemiologic evidence, such as it is, been read in such a distorted manner? And how did the prostitute model of HIV transmission ever take hold so strongly within Ghana's professional medical community?

There are alternative ways of looking at the epidemiology, and different readings suggest the need for different prevention strategies. In the prostitute model the epidemic moves in a very linear fashion: returned prostitutes infect unsuspecting clients (i.e., men) who then transmit HIV to their other partners. Interventions are directed at prostitutes because they are the key link in the chain of infection. In the network model HIV is moving through the population in a much more diffuse and multilinear fashion, and it has probably been doing so from the beginning.[6] In this model, focusing prevention efforts on vulnerable groups certainly makes sense. But the supposition that we can identify and target "high-frequency transmitters" and thus keep the epidemic from spreading beyond "core groups" is another matter altogether.

In any case, local communities and kin groups in Ghana and elsewhere in Africa are ill prepared to care for people living with HIV/AIDS. It is not too soon to begin laying the foundations in support of more appropriate communal responses. The first step is to help people understand that AIDS is not a disease of others. This means, among other things, that educational campaigns that seek to effect behavior change through fear appeals, or that crudely target core transmission groups, are quite likely to intensify scapegoating and denial while doing little to stop the spread of HIV itself. Educational messages that imply that specific subgroups are "high-frequency transmitters" are especially to be avoided.

By way of conclusion, let us place the epidemic in Ghana in a broader context, for there are some clear parallels here to the response to AIDS in North America, Europe, and elsewhere. Above all, there is the issue of origins. While Western scientists and media have been quick to locate the origin of AIDS in Africa, Ghanaians speculate about the origins of AIDS in the West. In both instances AIDS is located elsewhere; it comes from the outside. In both instances it is identified with the first people to fall prey to the virus. In North America it was gay men, then, more transiently, Haitian-Americans, and more recently injecting drug users. In Ghana AIDS has been seen as a disease of prostitutes. In both instances HIV/AIDS is identified with socially marginal or stigmatized groups, and this identification is followed by widespread concern about its spread to the "general population." The more concrete lesson from Ghana, as from North America, is that the initial association of AIDS with whole categories of persons, particularly in the absence of any clear data on the actual distribution of HIV (which is still the case in Ghana), has made the very difficult task of responding in a responsible manner to these epidemics that much more difficult.

## NOTES

The author's work in Ghana was made possible through AIDSCOM, a project of the U.S. Agency for International Development and the Academy for Educational Development. Many thanks to Dr. Phyllis Antwi, Coordinator of Ghana's National AIDS Control Programme. This paper is in memory of my AIDSCOM colleague, Ken Dunnigan, M.D.

1. The research group in Ghana was led by Dr. Isaac Obeng-Quaidoo and Kwadwo Basompra, both of the School of Communications Studies, University of Ghana, Legon, and also by Kweku Rockson of the Ghana Institute of Journalism. Dr. Ken Dunnigan also helped guide the research.

2. I focused on these variables for the following reasons: Literacy is a good index of traditionalism and modernity; people who cannot read and write may have concepts of illness and take measures for its prevention and cure that will differ significantly from the concepts and health practices of the more literate and educated. Ghanaian society is also characterized by strong gender separations. Although there is regional and ethnic variation, men's and women's parental responsibilities, economic activities, residential arrangements, patterns of association, and links to wider kin groups are everywhere quite distinct. It is almost as if men and women live in two different, albeit overlapping, societies. Consequently, men's and women's views on a variety of matters relevant to risk behavior were, it was assumed, quite likely to differ. Experience in the United States and elsewhere also suggests that knowing someone with AIDS can have a significant impact on AIDS-related knowledge and attitudes and may often lead to sustained changes in risk behavior.

3. Physicians in regional hospitals told me in 1991 that they guessed that about 5 percent of their blood supplies were HIV infected. They could do nothing about it, except to limit blood transfusions as best they could.

4. This way of looking at HIV transmission in sub-Saharan Africa was first proposed, to my knowledge, by Caldwell, Caldwell, and Quiggin in an important 1989 article. Yet it seems that this paper generated little interest among epidemiologists working in Africa, who continued to be preoccupied with the concept of the core transmission group. There seems now, however, to be a growing recognition by some in the epidemiologic community that the core-group model (essentially a mathematical construct) cannot be successfully operationalized in much of Africa (Peter Piot 1991, personal communication).

5. In 1990 I was told a joke that was making the rounds of female medical staff at Korle Bu, Ghana's largest teaching hospital. The joke went like this: "It's a good thing that women brought AIDS to Ghana. If it had been men we'd all be infected by now." This is meant to be read as a sardonic (if grim) commentary on Ghanaian gender relations. Yet it also testifies to the tenacity of the notion that AIDS in Ghana is a female disease.

6. Hampton (1990) reported that some Ghanaian physicians were then beginning to think that they had seen local AIDS cases as early as 1981.

## REFERENCES

Abu, Katharine. 1983. The Separateness of Spouses: Conjugal Resources in an Ashanti Town. In *Female and Male in West Africa*, ed. C. Oppong, 156–168. London: George Allen and Unwin.

———. 1987. Report on In-Depth Study of Attitudes to Contraceptives among the Nonliterate in Tamale. SOMARC/The Futures Group.

Akuffo, F. O. 1987. Teenage Pregnancies and School Drop-Outs: The Relevance of Family Life Education and Vocational Training to Girl's Employment Opportunities. In *Sex Roles, Population, and Development in West Africa: Policy-related Studies on Work and Demographic Issues*, ed. C. Oppong, 154–164. London: James Curry.

Asamoah-Odei, E. 1991a. *AIDS Status Report, Ghana: 1986–1990*. Accra: Ministry of Health.

———. 1991b. *HIV Surveillance in Ghana, 1986–1990*. Accra: Ministry of Health.

Bleek, Wolf. 1976. *Sexual Relationships and Birthcontrol in Ghana: A Case Study of a Rural Town*. Amsterdam: Universiteit van Amsterdam.

Caldwell, John C., and Pat Caldwell. 1987. The Cultural Context of High Fertility in Sub-Saharan Africa. *Population and Development Review* 13(3): 409–437.

Caldwell, John C., Pat Caldwell, and Pat Quiggin. 1989. The Social Context of AIDS in Sub-Saharan Africa. *Population and Development Review* 15(2): 185–234.

Hampton, Janie. 1990. *Meeting AIDS with Compassion: AIDS Care and Prevention in Agomanya, Ghana*. London: ActionAid.

Konotey-Ahulu, Felix I. D. 1987. AIDS in Africa: Misinformation and Disinformation. *Lancet*, July 25, pp. 206–207.

Neequaye, A. R., L. Osei, J. A. A. Mingle, G. Ankra-Badu, C. Bentsi, A. Asamoah-Adu, J.E. Neequaye. 1988. "Dynamics of Human Immune Deficiency Virus (HIV) Epidemic—The Ghanaian Experience," in *The Global Impact of AIDS: Proceedings of the First International Conference on the Global Impact of AIDS*, eds. A. F. Fleming, M. Carballo, D. W. FitzSimmons, M. R. Bailey, J. Mann, 9–15. New York: Alan R. Liss, Inc.

Oppong, C., ed. 1983. *Female and Male in West Africa*. London: George Allen and Unwin.

———, ed. 1987. *Sex Roles, Population and Development in West Africa: Policy-related Studies on Work and Demographic Issues*. London: James Curry.

Pellow, Deborah. 1977. *Women in Accra: Options for Autonomy*. Algonac, MI: Reference Publications.

Porter, Robert W. 1990. AIDS and Youth in Ghana: A Report on Findings from an Exploratory Focus Group Study. AIDSCOM/The Academy for Educational Development.

USAID/Accra. 1991. *Technical Assessment—HIV/AIDS Situation in Ghana*.

Verdon, Michel. 1983. *The Abutia Ewe of West Africa: A Chiefdom That Never Was*. Berlin and New York: Mouton Publishers.

# 8

# Apartheid and the Politics of AIDS

*Virginia van der Vliet*

> How will we celebrate our liberation if up to 20 percent of the popu-
> lation may be HIV positive?
>
> Ivan Toms[1] (1990:13)

It is a cruel irony of South African history that the ending of apartheid
should coincide with the beginning of the AIDS epidemic. The political
transition now under way will complicate the process of formulating and
implementing a national AIDS policy. AIDS will run the risk of being al-
ternately highly politicized or ignored while leaders concentrate their energies on the process of transition itself. The conflicts and fears of the
apartheid years will affect the debate, and the depressed socioeconomic
circumstances in which the majority of South Africans live will make the
epidemic harder to contain.

There is no longer any doubt that South Africa faces a major AIDS epidemic. Failing a medical breakthrough or a significant change in sexual
behavior, AIDS will become one of the most important factors shaping
South Africa within the next ten years. Official statistics recorded only
2,027 AIDS cases between 1982 and January 1994 (*Epidemiological Comments* Vol 21(1)–January 1994:20). However, ongoing monitoring of HIV
incidence in sentinel groups, such as blood donors and people attending
antenatal, family-planning, and sexually transmitted disease (STD) clinics,
reveals a far more alarming picture. By late 1991 more than 1 percent of
the total adult population were estimated to be HIV positive (Centre for
Health Policy 1991:3).[2] An annual blood survey of all women attending
antenatal clinics in South Africa (excluding the independent states) charts
a growing epidemic. The 1990 survey showed 0.78 percent infected; the

1991 percentage grew to 1.49 percent. In 1992 the figure increased to 2.67 percent (Epidemiological Comments, Vol. 20(11) November 1993:191.) The 1993 survey reports 4.89 infected with the KwaZula/Natal area worst hit at 9.02 percent. Almost 600,000 of South Africa's 40 million people were estimated to be HIV positive by the end of 1993; 700 were being infected each day, and the doubling time of the epidemic was just over a year (The Argus 1994; Die Burger 1994.) In a recent authoritative model developed for the South African epidemic, actuary Peter Doyle described the country as being at an early stage of the epidemic phase, "so that very rapid spread of HIV is likely in the next few years" (1991:21). Doyle's model plots two future AIDS scenarios, one assuming no change in sexual behavior patterns, the other assuming that "changes in behaviour occur between 1995 and 2000" (ibid.:20). In the absence of change, the epidemic is predicted to peak at a prevalence of approximately 27 percent of the adult population by the year 2010. If change does occur, the epidemic will peak at approximately 18 percent sometime between 2000 and 2005 (ibid.: 22). "Doomsday" depopulation scenarios are ruled out, but Doyle's projections suggest that current population growth of 2.6 percent per annum (Health Trends in South Africa 1990 1991:2) will slow to between 1.2 percent and 1.7 percent per annum (Doyle 1991:23). South Africa, then, is in the throes of a "silent epidemic"—widespread and rapidly escalating infection, with only a tiny minority manifesting actual signs of illness.

Since 1987 the focus of infection in South Africa has gradually shifted from a pattern I epidemic in the homosexual community to a pattern II epidemic affecting mainly the black (African) heterosexual community. Given the size of the population at risk and the miserable social conditions in the black areas that will exacerbate the epidemic, this shift has grave implications.

Broomberg et al. (1991:71) in a sophisticated modeling exercise to assess the economic effects of the epidemic on South Africa, concluded that

> the total costs of the epidemic will grow to enormous proportions, with a noticeable impact on potential consumption, but that the overall economic impact is likely to be sustainable to the end of this decade. Thereafter, our estimates suggest that if significant prevention efforts and health service policies are not in place, the epidemic may begin to pose a serious threat to ongoing economic growth.

Health services in South Africa are already inadequate to meet the needs of a rapidly growing population. The Broomberg et al. study concluded that the AIDS epidemic will have a profound effect and "may well be devastating" (ibid.) unless there are urgent policy decisions that aim "to cut down on hospitalisation costs through the development of hospital admissions policies, and possible alternative treatment settings" (ibid.:66).

Whatever the direct and indirect costs of the epidemic may be, it will bring great personal hardship and suffering as families face the financial and emotional burdens of the ill and dying and the loss of members at the height of their productive lives, often leaving orphans and the elderly without breadwinners. There is the danger that a major epidemic could precipitate a crisis of confidence undermining the transition process, exacerbating racial conflicts, affecting domestic and foreign investment, trade, and tourism, and leaving the country politically and economically marginalized.

One might expect a looming human tragedy of these proportions to unite South Africans in a strategy to combat the epidemic. Instead, as people of all ideological persuasions interpret and manipulate it to suit their own political agenda, AIDS has become yet another stick with which to beat opponents. Politicizing AIDS is not unique to South Africa, but as Refiloe Serote of the Township AIDS Program (TAP) said, "Political and racial divisions, created and inflamed by apartheid, make everything to do with AIDS political" (*WorldAIDS* 1990:5).

This chapter explores the unfolding political dimensions of the epidemic and the implications of the politicization for effective control of the disease. It outlines state responses to the epidemic and looks at some of the criticisms of specific aspects of state policy and programs. It then examines the way government opponents from both the right and the left have interpreted and reacted to the epidemic, particularly as it moves into the black community. The chapter concentrates on the responses of major political players who have addressed the AIDS issue. Many other groups and organizations, such as local authorities, the gay community, churches, individual trade unions, employers, family-planning programs, and community-based organizations are actively involved in AIDS programs, but their role is beyond the scope of this chapter.

## STATE RESPONSES

Since the first case of AIDS was reported in 1982, the state has taken a number of steps broadly in line with international AIDS strategies. It has intervened to safeguard the supply of blood and blood products and to provide funding for education campaigns, training, counseling, and research. It has also established epidemiologic surveillance programs, including a nationwide antenatal HIV survey first carried out in October and November 1990 to serve as a monitoring baseline for regular surveys (*RSA Policy Review* 1991:66–79). More controversial was the alien control legislation passed in October 1987 that prohibited entry for people testing HIV positive. Aimed mainly at migrant mine workers from neighboring states, it brought outraged responses particularly from the National Union of Mineworkers (NUM). The NUM blamed the spread of the disease on the migrant labor system itself, which provided "fertile ground for an AIDS epidemic and the state and industry should bear the responsibility" (*Race Relations Survey* 1989:438).

Controversy and criticism are probably unavoidable whenever the state meddles in issues as fundamental as sex and death, but the deeply divided nature of South African society has intensified the conflicts surrounding campaigns. Inadequate state spending has been widely criticized. From the R1 million spent in 1987 (approximately U.S. $357,000), which George Watermeyer, spokesman of the Department of National Health and Population Development (DNHPD), dismissed as a "drop in the ocean" (*Financial Mail* 1988), to the R5.4 million (about U.S. $1.9 million) officially budgeted for 1991–1992,[3] state spending suggests that the state has underestimated the significance of the threat. Dr. Wilson Carswell, medical adviser to the DNHPD's AIDS unit, expressed the hope that evaluation over the next eighteen months would ensure a "more appropriate" budget (*Cape Times* 1991c). In the 1992/1993 budget, AIDS was allocated R21 878 000, almost R14 million that would be spent on education, and R500 000 to NGOs. The 1993/1994 budget was reduced to R21 764 000 with the education allocation reduced to less than R7 million and NGOs subsidized by R2 million. The surveillance budget jumped almost six-fold, and research funds trebled. The AIDS consortium, an alliance of sixty organizations working in the field of AIDS, protested that the sum allocated for 1993/1994 was less than a tenth of the annual budget of one academic hospital, and less than one sixteenth of the amount Zimbabwe was spending relative to GDP. The WHO's recommendations for South Africa was R143 million a year. (Race Relations Survey 1993/1994: 139–140). Shrinking funds and a growing epidemic stirs the suspicion that the government is not taking the matter seriously because it is going to affect blacks more than whites.

Early state advertising campaigns proved controversial. The 1988 campaign, for instance, featured two posters. One, directed at white South Africans, emphasized the need to limit sexual contacts; the other, aimed at black South Africans, showed black mourners around an open grave under the heading "AIDS is now in South Africa." While the information on the poster was unexceptionable, the picture itself was seen as trying to "scare people" (Toms 1990:14) and was dismissed by anti-apartheid groups as "typical of government racist propaganda." Critics argued that "if the government had consulted political organisations, trade unions and organisations such as NAMDA [National Medical and Dental Association], . . . it might have produced a more appropriate AIDS awareness programme" (Kelly 1991:9). Attempting such consultation may well have proved fruitless since anti-apartheid organizations have found it politically difficult to be seen to cooperate with government structures. Even pursuing the same strategies might be perceived as "collaboration" (Perkel and Strebel 1989: 77). Noncollaboration and pressures to keep the state isolated internationally have been part of the political strategy of opposition movements—a strategy that has created its own dilemmas, such as South Africa's exclusion from the World Health Organization's Global Program on AIDS (*ibid.*:79).

Introducing AIDS education into state schools has also been a source of controversy. The highly fragmented nature of the South African education system and the debate even within the departments about "appropriate" AIDS education have been major stumbling blocks. It was not until January 1991 that a government committee on AIDS prevention publicly announced strong support for an AIDS education program (*Cape Times* 1991a.) A compulsory program was due to start in all black and white secondary schools in early 1992, and a government-sponsored AIDS educational kit was released and then withdrawn later in the year amid controversy. The head of the Department of National Health and Population Development's AIDS unit, Natalie Stockton, reported that, "it had been too expensive and glossy. It was geared toward more developed communities, so it did not meet the needs of individual grassroots communities" (Race Relations Survey 1994: 143) Meanwhile, in a private sector initiative, a major insurance company and a publishing house have put together a package for black children in the sixth and seventh grades, consisting of books, teaching guides and training workshops for teachers. Dr. Rueben Shan, former head of the AIDS center at the South African Institute for Medical Research commented, "We have been trying unsuccessfully for years to get into schools to educate our children about AIDS and sexual awareness, but were thwarted by the powers that be. The acceptance of these books is a milestone" (*Ibid.*). State primary-school programs are also under consideration, and all programs will be field tested to develop "the most appropriate programme for a particular community" (*ibid.*: 73). Even though this is an internationally recognized strategy, it may also open the government to accusations of racism.

AIDS education will clash with a puritanical legacy that has resisted sex education in schools, believing that it promotes adolescent sexual experimentation—a curious attitude in a country where 330 out of every 1,000 births are to girls under the age of nineteen (*Health Trends in South Africa 1990* 1991: 51). A pilot AIDS program in the Transvaal Education Department (TED) in 1991, for instance, stopped short of teaching white children how to use condoms because parents refused to allow it (*Weekly Mail* 1991b). The report said that guidelines for the program stressed that the long-term goal was to encourage people to live a "healthy, biblically-based" lifestyle. Health educators questioned whether the TED is the appropriate body to train AIDS educators; its worldview was "not necessarily shared by everyone" and was seen by some as "totally out of line with reality." As Toms (1990:14) remarked of the early education posters, "moralistic" messages might have "no relevance to the community most at

risk—young sexually active blacks." British AIDS experts visiting South
Africa in 1987 accused the government of putting thousands of lives at risk
by catering to the whims of its constituency by not promoting condoms.
"The government is obviously responding to its power-base in the sense
that its power comes from a more puritanical minority" (*Race Relations
Survey* 1988:806). Such "puritanism" is not restricted to whites and could
make programs in black schools equally controversial. The present voluntary, after-hours programs running in some black high schools concede
parental veto rights (*Debates of Parliament* 1991).

Ultimately, however, the problems facing a state campaign in contemporary South Africa go beyond such specific criticisms and arise from the
bedrock of apartheid's legacy. Toms has argued that there is "no possibility
that the present government could, even if it has the inclination, run an
effective campaign to limit the spread of HIV infection. It has no credibility
or legitimacy whatsoever among blacks" (1990:14). Apartheid has created
a society where prejudice, mistrust, and fear haunt black/white relations.
This legacy will affect not only black perceptions of state AIDS campaigns,
but also right-wing constructions of the epidemic and, in the final analysis,
any alternative campaign devised by the anti-apartheid organizations themselves.

## RIGHT-WING RESPONSES

Since the beginning, the AIDS pandemic has been associated with a rising
tide of bigotry. Initially directed at gay men, the epidemic's first sufferers,
prejudice and discrimination rapidly spread to others who were associated
with the disease. Speculation about the African origin of AIDS led to African students abroad being HIV tested and subjected to racist taunts; people from Africa found themselves in the same taboo blood-donor category
as injecting drug users, prostitutes, and gay men. AIDS became yet another
"African disaster" story (Larson 1990:5). Africans and African analysts
reacted with outrage, interpreting suggestions of the African origin of AIDS
as an attempt to ascribe blame and responsibility, to vilify the continent
(*New African* 1990:9), to link the epidemic with bizarre sexual myths
(*Newsweek* 1987), or simply to perpetuate the "racist ideology" of the
West (Chirimuuta and Chirimuuta 1987:1).

Political groupings whose style embraces and even feeds on prejudice and
discrimination have already included AIDS in their own arsenal of bigotry.
To stir up fear against a group and then to offer protection against it in
return for support is an old political trick, particularly in times of uncertainty. In contemporary Central and Eastern Europe, for instance, as
"wrenching social and economic changes exacerbate ancient hatreds—
[u]ltra-nationalist and neo-Fascist parties, like Pamyat in the USSR, exploit
the situation by using AIDS as a new weapon in the battle to stigmatise

population groups, including homosexuals, drug users and refugees" (*WorldAIDS* 1991:12). In South Africa right-wing responses to AIDS so far suggest two interlinked patterns: on the one hand, overtly political responses designed to gain support and to outflank the National Party (NP) and the African National Congress (ANC); on the other, responses rooted in a deeply conservative mindset, nurtured by the apartheid years and threatened by the turmoil and loss of control in the current transitional situation.

## Political Ploys

Right-wing exploitation of the AIDS issue has been evident in parliamentary speeches and in right-wing publications. Among the latter are anonymous pamphlets emanating from that shadowy world of propaganda and disinformation in which sources are hard to trace. Some organizations on the left have asserted that these pamphlets come from the government and have warned the government not to "use AIDS for political purposes" (Workplace Information Group n.d.:19); in fact, given that the pamphlets often undermine aspects of the government's own reform plans, such as repatriating exiles and desegregating services and amenities, it seems far more likely that they have their origin somewhere in the tangled thickets of far-right organizations.

In Parliament AIDS has been a useful weapon in political infighting. For instance, Dr. F. H. Pauw, member of Parliament (MP) for the right-wing Conservative Party (CP), alleged that he was receiving reports from "throughout the entire country" of NP members and canvassers

> reassuring people that Black majority rule poses no threat to the Whites, Coloureds [those of mixed race] and Indians in South Africa. They are alleging that AIDS will be responsible for the large-scale elimination of the Black population, to such an extent that the Blacks in reality will become a minority within South Africa within five years. When one bases one's guarantees and one's hopes of solving the problems of our country on AIDS, this is a reflection of the level to which one has sunk. The CP dissociates itself from such speculation. We do not place our hope in AIDS. (*Debates of Parliament* 1990b)

Later in the debate, another CP MP insisted that Pauw's accusation was not hearsay; he had not two hours previously received similar assurances from two NP MPs (*Debates of Parliament* 1990c). In her reply, Health Minister Rina Venter repudiated the accusations, saying that they were more representative of CP attitudes, quoting CP MP Clive Derby-Lewis as saying that whites were tired of footing the bill for black wage demands: "If AIDS stops Black population growth, it would be like Father Christmas." Venter rejected outright "this fooling around with such a serious matter" and appealed to Parliament not to make AIDS a political issue (*Debates of Parliament* 1990d).

This incident was clearly a ploy to embarrass the government with a racist label from which the CP professed to disassociate itself. The CP's newspapers and pamphlets suggest otherwise. In October 1990, for instance, the CP newspaper *Patriot* quoted an anonymous doctor as saying that everyday casual contact can transmit AIDS. *Patriot* used this as an argument against abolishing segregated amenities, since whites paid for these amenities and had "the right to survive in an AIDS sea." An anonymous pamphlet traced to the CP, entitled "AIDS—The Facts" and distributed to households in some areas of the Transvaal in April 1991, also accused the government of "shockingly" increasing the risk of infection in "low risk groups" (i.e., whites) by desegregating facilities such as hospitals, schools, swimming pools, and blood banks. It demanded compulsory testing for certain categories, including health care workers and returning ANC exiles, and legislation to make AIDS a notifiable disease. A similar pamphlet circulated in Walvis Bay, the disputed South African enclave in Namibia, warned of "the threat of infection from heavily infected alien groups. Squatters and marchers can bring infection into your air, your streets and homes. Mixing is crazy" (*Sowetan* 1991). The fear and confusion generated by the pamphlets' dubious "facts" were undoubtedly intended to reap a political harvest.

In February 1991 *Die Afrikaner,* a newspaper of the right-wing Herstigte Nasionale Party (HNP), berated the government for only belatedly admitting the extent of HIV infection, despite warnings in *Die Afrikaner;* it pointed to increasing "evidence" that casual contact could transmit AIDS, accused the government of keeping silent on the issue because it threatened its policy of desegregating public amenities, and argued that "the government has a vested interest in concealing the facts" (*Afrikaner* 1991b). In January 1991 *Die Afrikaner* examined financial implications of AIDS for "medical aid schemes" (health care insurance) and denounced the government's plans to extend such insurance to all groups. This would result in white members, rather than the state, having to bear the costs of the epidemic in the black population and make such "medical aid schemes" unaffordable for whites by the year 2000 (*Afrikaner* 1991a).

The anonymous pamphlets carry similar messages; they differ only in the unrestrained viciousness of some of the attacks. One, entitled "Welcome to the New South Africa," having described gruesome episodes of violence and having pointed to the state's inability to protect citizens, went on to talk about AIDS, saying that "up to 25 million people will be dead or dying by the end of the century. And up to 7 million will be raving mad before dying." After painting a lurid picture of AIDS being transmitted in desegregated schools, in nonracial sports, and by domestic workers, producing a total collapse of the economy, it concluded: "There will be a *New South Africa* after the *Apocalypse* at the other side of the Valley of the Shadow of Death. Will you be there with us or will you have joined your 'new brothers' to their doom?" (emphasis in the original). Purporting to come from the White Consciousness Movement, it urged the reader, "If you have any survival instinct left, support those who fight for you, even if you do not always agree with them."

Other pamphlets link AIDS to Africa, to neighboring states, and to returning ANC exiles, presumably hoping simultaneously to create divisions in the black community, fear among whites, and embarrassment for the government. A pamphlet alleging that it came from the ANC and distributed in parts of Natal and the Transvaal advised black men to have sex with Indian women, because an "AIDS expert had proved that Indian women had antibodies [*sic*] to the virus." The pamphlet also claimed that South Africa had paid Israeli scientists R1 billion for the virus. It urged blacks to destroy white racists. Nelson Mandela, then deputy president of the ANC, publicly denied any ANC connection with the pamphlet, and a police spokesman, supporting Mandela's disclaimer, said, "The pamphlets are no more than an amateurish effort to create uncertainty and panic, especially in the white community" (*Sunday Times Extra* 1990).

### The Conservative Mindset

Apart from manipulating the AIDS issue for overtly political purposes, right-wing responses must also be seen against the background of a society that is prototypically conservative at many levels. The negative attitude to sex education in both the black and white communities is one of many indicators. Issues such as legalizing abortion and prostitution, advertising condoms through the media, and distributing them in prisons and educational institutions in an attempt to control AIDS have all created controversy (see, e.g., *Epidemiological Comments* 1990:9–10). Homosexuality is still a criminal offense, and homophobia is common in both the black and white communities. Early responses to the epidemic among gay men reflected this. Ivan Toms (1990:14) wrote: "The gay community is one part of the enfranchised white society that is legally and socially oppressed. It is a marginalised community, viewed by white society at large, and the government in particular as immoral and perverted."[4] The CP, for instance, ignoring the valuable role such publications have played in providing AIDS education, called for the banning of the gay newspaper *Exit*, arguing that it encouraged "sodomy and perversion as a normal way of life," and that this could not be justified with the "scourge of AIDS flaring" (*Sunday Star* 1989). Linking a "horribly frightening disease" with stigmatized groups has characterized the social construction of the disease elsewhere (Singer *et al.* 1990:72). In South Africa, where the disease is associated with groups already stigmatized by both homophobia and racism, the universal fears of contact and infection associated with AIDS are intensified.

Conservatism is reinforced by the role of fundamentalist churches in the formation of South African attitudes. They have not only subscribed to the view found elsewhere in the world that AIDS is a plague visited by God on the world's sinners, but have also intervened directly in AIDS campaigns. In preindependence Namibia, for instance, attempts by health authorities to educate the public about AIDS "were paralyzed by the objections of the Afrikaans Dutch Reformed Church to the mention of contraceptives" (*New Scientist* 1988:8). Dr. W. J. Snyman, a CP MP, criticized the purchase of twenty-one million condoms from the 1989–90 health budget funds, which he saw as encouraging "promiscuity" rather than raising moral standards. In support of his objections, he quoted an editorial in *Die Kerkblad* (the official newspaper of the Dutch Reformed Church of South Africa) that asked: "Must we now condone sin to fight AIDS? Condoms for 'safe' whoring?" (*Debates of Parliament* 1990a). In turning to the Bible for "insight and strategy," Pauw of the CP suggested "leper colonies" and tattoos to identify HIV-infected people. The suggestions brought strong criticisms from theologians, NP MPs, and the minister concerned (*Cape Times* 1991d), but such fundamentalist views are still heard in quarters where AIDS is seen as divine retribution for immoral ways, and these attitudes commonly appear in the letters-to-the-editor sections of white and black newspapers. As the number of AIDS cases among blacks increases, more conservative elements in the black population, such as rural people and those belonging to independent churches, may also favor supernatural interpretations, including sorcery. If there are no major biomedical breakthroughs in the search for a cure, they could well reject Western explanations and treatments in favor of traditional healers and folk strategies (see, e.g., Farmer 1990; Ingstad 1990).

An element in the conservative response among white South Africans that is difficult to document but that palpably exists is the profound feeling of unease, even despair, as the country moves away from the apartheid era in which they were socialized to a "new South Africa" in a transition turbulent with political confrontation and violence and burdened with massive problems of poverty, unemployment, rapid urbanization, and crime. To some who, in the past, tried to deny or control such South African realities, the specter of AIDS might be seen as a "solution," no matter how much rational analysis shows it to be a catastrophe in which all South Africans will suffer. Susan Sontag's remarks on American apocalyptic thinking could equally apply to South Africa:

> The taste for worst-case scenarios reflects the need to master fear of what is felt to be uncontrollable. It also expresses an imaginative complicity with disaster. The sense of cultural distress or failure gives rise to the desire for a

clean sweep, a *tabula rasa*. No one wants a plague, of course. But yes, it would be a chance to begin again. (Sontag 1988:87)

## RESPONSES FROM THE LEFT

Many anti-apartheid groups, including political movements, trade unions, civil-rights groups, churches, student organizations, health workers, and academics, are currently involved in developing AIDS programs, usually for their own constituencies. This chapter does not attempt to cover the numerous initiatives, projects, and policy statements that have come out of these groups. Rather, it looks critically at some emerging trends and problems in their responses as they begin to confront a growing epidemic in the black population.

Since 1989 a number of these organizations have indicated their intention of embarking on major initiatives. In 1989, for instance, the Congress of South African Trade Unions (COSATU), the country's largest trade-union body, which is predominantly black and allied to the ANC, passed a resolution to provide education and protection for workers' rights and to fight the social conditions associated with AIDS (*History in the Making* 1991b: 13–14). Some individual unions have at least rudimentary programs, but it was not until June 1991 that COSATU held its first conference devoted to developing an AIDS policy and program of action. David Morake, the conference organizer, criticized government and employer efforts as "racist" and "counterproductive": "There is recognition that worker education is now the responsibility of the unions" (*Weekly Mail* 1991c). By November 1991 there was still little evidence of a coordinated campaign. In April 1990, 250 delegates representing the ANC and other anti-apartheid organizations such as NAMDA and the United Democratic Front addressed the AIDS issue at a health and welfare conference held in Maputo. The resulting draft resolution on HIV and AIDS in South Africa urged delegates to play a leading role in AIDS campaigns "situated within the broader struggle for political change" (*History in the Making* 1991a:9). It recommended that "senior progressive political leadership" become involved to "help overcome suspicion and mistrust created by the South African state" (*ibid.*: 9–10). The resolution concluded that South Africa was facing a "crisis" and that urgent action by progressive organizations must be initiated immediately (*ibid.*:12). Although decisions to establish a program channeled through the existing National Progressive Primary Health Care (NPPHC) network, which already had strong links with community organizations, followed the Maputo conference, critics have noted that very little has yet resulted except the resolution itself (*ibid.*:4, 8). AIDS educator Mary Crewe wrote, "One has yet to hear any of the [ANC] National Executive Committee raise the issue of AIDS at a political rally or public meeting" (Crewe 1992:73). Toms's (1990:15) discussion of the initiatives suggested one source of the delay. He noted that despite the "imminent peril of the AIDS epidemic, such a campaign would lack community support if it was organized in too much haste." The participatory style of community decision making that developed during the apartheid era could make getting initiatives off the ground a slow and cumbersome process.

In arguing for alternative campaigns, anti-apartheid organizations invariably point to the lack of credibility of the state programs and the need for campaigns with roots in progressive organizations. Such alternative campaigns are not without problems of their own. In the early stages of the epidemic they too may face credibility problems associated with the invisibility of the epidemic (Mhloyi 1991), the overlap of their message with mistrusted government messages, the need to use state radio, television, and schools for programs, and their reliance on data from state or state-linked sources. The variable and contradictory nature of the statistics bandied about in the media and by government critics themselves adds to the confusion, with the state variously accused of underestimating and overestimating the danger.[5]

A major source of suspicion in any AIDS campaign will be the overlap with state family-planning messages and the associated genocidal conspiracy allegations of the past. In November 1988 *Sechaba,* an official publication of the ANC, contained an article questioning the African origin of the AIDS virus; it advanced the counterproposition that such a virus could have been developed "in the secrecy of the laboratories of many imperialist countries" (*Sechaba* 1988:28). Although more cautious in tone than the Soviet reports that unequivocally linked AIDS with a biological warfare research laboratory at Fort Detrick in Maryland (U.S. Department of State 1987), such speculation feeds suspicions already close to the surface in the black community. Rumors that the AIDS virus was spread in tear gas (McLean 1990:9), or that infected ex-ANC guerrillas now working for the police have been instructed to spread AIDS among black shebeen prostitutes (*New Nation* 1991),[6] will fit snugly into such conspiracy theorists' beliefs.

A countertheory—that the AIDS epidemic is a government fabrication devised to discourage blacks from having sex—has also surfaced and will no doubt persist until the disease becomes more conspicuous in the black townships. In Khayelitsha (near Cape Town), women who found it difficult to believe that AIDS existed at all commented, "It is mainly the government telling us. . . . No one is dying that we know of" (McLean 1990:9). The COSATU resolution noted that "the education and information programmes of the government and bosses are racist and have created suspicion amongst our members, and have even led to a doubt that AIDS exist[s]" (*History in the Making* 1991b:13). As has happened elsewhere, the AIDS acronym has been reinterpreted, here standing for "Afrikaner Invention to Deprive us of Sex" (*AIDS Analysis Africa* 1990:1), publicly attesting to their belief that AIDS had been concocted to discourage pre-marital sex and sex with multiple partners. The emphasis on condom usage has also raised suspicions of a link with the state family-planning program, a program itself bedeviled by politicization (Van der Vliet 1984). WorldAIDS (1989a:5) reported, "Some black South Africans are suspicious of condoms, believing that government is promoting them in a disguised attempt to curb the population." Surveys of black and "Coloured," (mixed-race) school and university student attitudes in the Western Cape reveal similar concerns (Argus 1991; Cape Times 1991b), and some union mem-bers of the Transport and General Workers Union (TGWU) are reported to believe that AIDS is "a plot devised by the government supported by the employers and pumped through a restricted press to convince black people to have less sex, and therefore fewer babies" (Cape Times 1989). Not pro-moting condom use, on the other hand, may lead to accusations of genocide by omission. "Why is the government so negligent about AIDS? . . . I think they are saying: 'let them die—it will help us control the population!' " (Southern Africa Report 1990:18). Others question whether a threat of similar magnitude among white South Africans would have evoked such half-hearted responses. Clearly, the government will be "damned if it does and damned if it doesn't" on the condom issue; this dilemma could also face campaigns organized by those opposing the government.

Alternative campaigns will also face resource constraints. AIDS education, counseling, and care will need enormous personnel and financial resources. Health workers in progressive organisations are already overstretched. Eliz-abeth Floyd (1990:6) described them as "consumed" by their multiple roles in conventional health care, working with detainees, ex-prisoners, and re-turning exiles, and participating in desegregation campaigns. She stressed that other progressive organizations have similar limitations. She was espe-cially concerned that youth organizations, whose members are particularly at risk, "tend to say that they are involved in a political struggle that de-mands all their energy." AIDS was relegated to the same low position ac-corded other health issues (ibid.:10).

Access to state financial resources for cash-starved alternative projects has been problematic. Accepting money from or working with state struc-tures could be branded as collaborationist and therefore suspect (WorldAIDS 1989b:4), and progressive organizations fear co-optation by the state (South 1990a; Vallabhjee 1991:1). Hopefully, a changing political atmosphere will ease some of these tensions. There are some signs of this. In March 1990 the government and the ANC made a joint request for funding to the World Health Organization (AIDS Analysis Africa 1990:9), and the government, recognizing its credibility problems, is beginning to make money directly available to nongovernmental organizations (NGOs) for developing their own AIDS programs (RSA Policy Review 1991:77). Funding for NGOs from organizations such as the U.S. Agency for Inter-

national Development (USAID) has also become available as they recognize
the need for strong prevention programs to avert a disaster of the proportions seen elsewhere in Africa (*AIDS Analysis Africa* 1991:2).

As the epidemic grows, AIDS must become a major issue in progressive
politics, and some have already voiced fears that it could become an area
of conflict within the organizations themselves. AIDS could attract considerable outside funding, setting off competing demands and offering the
prospect of people "building careers out of AIDS in the progressive sector"
(Floyd 1990:14). Presumably it is not committed AIDS workers, but rather
what Zimbabwe's minister of health, Dr. Timothy Stamp, has called "the
usual parasites that gather on the back of a new disease for the pickings"
(*Africa South* 1991:45), that dismay observers. Many interest groups such
as political parties, women's organizations, funding agencies, international
organizations, and NGOs will play important roles in future AIDS campaigns. As Gloria Waite (1988:156) noted of AIDS programs elsewhere in
Africa, "Conflicts can . . . be expected as these organisations attempt to
push their own mandates, and to do so in tandem with the changing policies of central government." A further political dimension of the epidemic
will be the power vested in those who control resources—funding, personnel, services, knowledge—and act as gatekeepers to those in need. They,
like the government, will need to monitor and evaluate their programs very
carefully to ensure that AIDS control, rather than political agenda, motivates their strategies.

The issue of priorities that Floyd raised in relation to already overcom-
mitted health workers is one that affects all the NGOs. Since the ANC and
other organizations were legalized in February 1990, liberation movements
have begun the difficult transition to political parties. In this volatile political climate, AIDS is unlikely to be seen as a top priority, although concerns
about the HIV status of returning exiles and the number of political prisoners found to be HIV positive have given the problem a higher profile.
Despite the Maputo resolution discussed earlier and repeated commitments
to "get involved in an AIDS program" (*South* 1990b) and to take AIDS
education "to every home" (*Sunday Times Extra* 1991), the ANC journal,
*Mayibuye,* admitted that the democratic movements' "deep commitment
and sense of urgency . . . [had not] translated into practice" (*Mayibuye*
1991a:37). Whatever their commitments, the practicalities of political factors, in which issues like housing, education, poverty, and violence already
vie for immediate attention, will most likely dictate that an invisible epidemic will be perceived as peripheral.

AIDS, with its unwelcome message of condoms and safer sex, is a topic
politicians might prefer to ignore. In many societies condoms are unpop-
ular. In South Africa that aversion is compounded by their association with
the state family-planning program. Their unpopularity with black users
(see, e.g., Preston-Whyte, Karim, and Zondi 1991:45) is reinforced by the

problems of obtaining, using, and dis
squatter communities where privacy an
9). Safer sex, too, will be a difficult me
militant youth whose lives have been br
schooling, social and political upheaval, vio
onment and death. AIDS, if they believe it ex
other of life's dangers. In a survey of Kwa
seventeen to twenty-three conducted in July 19
(KwaZulu Secretary of Health) found that a third
lieved that AIDS was a "joke," and 90 percent said
use a condom. For people caught up in political viole
a laughing matter. It's a case of eat, drink and be merr)
die!" (Hamilton 1991:13). Such youths are unlikely to be
sages of caution and moderation issued by "the enemy"
or even from parents and elders whose political caution has
butt of contempt and ridicule in the past. Political leaders h
the confidence and support of the militant youth might well
push these messages too vociferously.

One tactic in overcoming resistance and in making an AIDS c
more palatable is to deliberately politicize it. The National Progress
mary Health Care campaign is designed "to take advantage of po
networks and to 'politicise' AIDS prevention. . . . If exhortations to ∂
sexual behaviour became part of a political message, a significant respon
is much more likely" (Toms 1990:16). The ANC, too, has talked of situ
ating its AIDS campaign "within the broader struggle for sociopolitical
change" (*History in the Making* 1991a:9).

The strategy of politicization will influence the way organizations construct their explanatory model of the disease. A full explanation requires
three components: the viral, the social/contextual, and the behavioral. Politicizing AIDS requires that the model focus on the social/contextual element. In South Africa this would mean emphasizing causal factors such as
migrant labor, poverty, violence, poor housing, social disintegration, and
ill health, particularly the widespread occurrence of other STDs, all undoubtedly factors that greatly facilitate the transmission of AIDS. Addressing these issues as part of an AIDS strategy could give the strategy
legitimacy in black communities and allow it to be piggy-backed on existing
campaigns.

Some analysts believe that shifting the focus from personal behavior to
sociopolitical change is justified. American AIDS commentator Randall
Packard, for instance, writing on AIDS in Africa, accused social scientists
who have focused on the issue of risk behavior of prematurely narrowing
research on the etiology of AIDS. By underestimating the infection risks
posed by contaminated injections and not addressing the wide range of
social, political, and economic factors that may affect health, they have

"responsibility for transmission on the actors themselves" (Pack-
5). Even urbanization, with its frequent destruction of traditional
d controls, its rootless migrant workers and soldiers, and its im-
d women forced into prostitution, is challenged as an explanation
it implies the need "to modify urban sexual behaviour" rather than
ess the fundamental issues (*ibid.*:6). For Packard, an important part
solution must lie rather in changing the social context itself. "If a
ry risk factor is being poor and unemployed then our proposed in-
tion must address the causes of this condition. We must not allow
S to become one more symptom for which the West finds a cure with-
addressing the underlying causes" (*ibid.*:19).[8] In South Africa state-
nts by the ANC, the trade unions, and the progressive primary health
e movement have also strongly emphasized the sociopolitical context of
e epidemic. The South African Health Workers' Congress, for instance,
quated AIDS with diseases such as tuberculosis, measles, malnutrition, and
gastroenteritis, which attack those who are poorest and least powerful. It
concluded: "Any attempts to curb the spread of the disease without seeking
to address these factors would prove to be futile" (*Mayibuye* 1991b:31).

Social regeneration, however, is a long-term strategy; even if South Africa
were to become a model nonracial democracy tomorrow, the realities of
life would not change in time to prevent an epidemic. Emphasizing the
culpability of the apartheid system and the social conditions it precipitated
is understandable in organizations that are "as committed to ending apartheid as they are to fighting AIDS" (*WorldAIDS* 1989b:4). But unless this
is balanced by a very strong message that, in the short term, individuals
can effectively protect themselves from AIDS only by behavioral change,
such programs risk further disempowering people. Cast as victims of their
social circumstances, they could retreat into fatalism.

## CONCLUSION

The AIDS pandemic has opened political debates worldwide as issues
such as health policies, discrimination, legislation, education programs, and
the social conditions surrounding AIDS are addressed. As this chapter has
tried to demonstrate, the apartheid legacy and the transition to a "new"
South Africa have, paradoxically, both intensified the debates and made
addressing the issues politically hazardous.

State responses have been criticized as too little, too late. Curiously
muted, state reactions suggest that at least until recently, the potential size
and cost of the epidemic had not been realized. Resistance to sex education
in schools, prudishness in the media, and a state credibility gap in the black
community have all compounded the usual problems of implementing a
national AIDS program. The right wing has seized on the threat of an
epidemic in the black community to focus its racial prejudices and fears

into a call for renewed segregation, accompanied by a belief in some quarters that the epidemic might solve the country's political and demographic problems. Government opponents on the left, such as the ANC and the trade unions, are caught between blaming AIDS on the apartheid system and attacking state programs, and trying to devise credible and effective alternatives. At a time when their human and financial resources are stretched thin by the accelerating pace of political change, such organizations may be reluctant to prioritize such a controversial issue. A silent epidemic will not easily compete with the abundant problems clamoring for resolution.

Apartheid made it inevitable that AIDS would be politicized. Those who are devising South Africa's AIDS strategies are themselves products of the apartheid system, and the lack of consultation, adversarial posturing, and attempts to discredit each other's programs reflect the old era. However explicable these attitudes may be, South Africa stands on the threshold of a potentially devastating epidemic; the country cannot afford to have its leaders play political games with the disease.

Perhaps the time has come for an "AIDS summit" and some straight talking. It is essential to drive home the message that AIDS will affect every South African and to agree on a demystified message stripped to its factual essentials. South Africa needs a vigorous, sustained program with a realistic budget, access to schools, workplaces, community organizations, and the mass media, and unified, high-level public support from South Africans of every political stripe. Information will not of itself change behavior, but it is a critical first step in empowering people to make responsible choices.

While international experience has shown that particular risk groups—for instance, women, youth, drug users, and minorities—need specially tailored programs, these should flow from the central campaign and not attempt to discredit, contradict, or sidestep it. Such destructive strategies create confusion and ultimately undermine the program as a whole. Blaming the victims and blaming the apartheid system are equally dangerous. It enables those who consider themselves "morally pure" or not in "risk groups" to believe that they are safe, and those who are fighting the system to believe that they are fighting AIDS; in both cases they avoid confronting their personal risks. While the moral and political overtones that have marked South African responses to date are understandable, they could ultimately sabotage prevention programs and help to precipitate the very tragedy of which Toms (1990) warned.

## NOTES

My thanks go to Dr. Malcolm Steinberg for advice and information and to Professor Michael Savage and Professor David Welsh for comments and suggestions on earlier drafts of this chapter.

The statistics in this chapter were updated in April 1994. Some positive developments, such as the HIV/AIDS chapter launched in December 1992 and the establishment of the National AIDS Convention of South Africa (NACOSA), have occured since it was written. However, even those changes have been problematic. The general pattern described in this chapter remains the same. If anything, the enormous energy that has been channelled into the political transition and programs like voter education have absorbed most of the human and financial resources of South Africans. AIDS is not seen as a priority; a recent survey commissioned by *Reader's Digest* and carried out by Markinor, a leading research organization affiliated to Gallup International, found that only 1 percent of young South Africans believed that fighting AIDS should be an aim for the new government over the next five years (*Reader's Digest,* February 1994:19.)

1. Dr. Ivan Toms is a medical doctor, joint national coordinator of the National Progressive Primary Health Care Network, and long-time critic of the health care system in South Africa.

2. The estimated population of South Africa in 1990, including all "independent" and nonindependent homelands, was 37.5 million, of whom 28.3 million were officially classified African, 1 million Asian, 3.2 million "Coloured" (those of mixed race), and 5 million white (*Race Relations Survey* 1990:35).

3. Additional sums were made available in the course of the year. In an overview of state AIDS strategy, *RSA Policy Review* (1991:70) reported that the government had made R8 million (about U.S. $2.8 million) available in the 1991–92 financial year for its "direct educational AIDS programme." The official budget originally earmarked R1.7 million (about U.S. $607,000). A major information campaign was launched in August 1991 and another scheduled for November 1991. The November campaign had a budget of R6 million (U.S. $2.1 million) (*Finance Week* 1991). By May 1992 the minister of health stated that R12.9 million (U.S. $4.6 million) had been budgeted for the 1991–92 AIDS program, but to date only R10.3 million (U.S. $3.7 million) had been spent (*Cape Times* 1992). Allegations have also been made that R4.5 million (U.S. $1.6 million) of the AIDS funds had been redirected to other uses (*Weekend Argus* 1992). Whether or not such allegations are true, they raise suspicions in the public mind about government commitment to the program. (Figures are calculated at the May 1992 exchange rate of R2.8 = $1.)

4. Homophobia is by no means confined to whites. See, for example, the *Weekly Mail* (1991a) report on the trial of Winnie Mandela in which she was found guilty of kidnapping four youths and being an accessory after the fact to subsequent assaults. In her defense it was claimed that the kidnapped youths had been staying at a Methodist manse in Soweto and were involved in homosexual relationships with the (white) minister. Her supporters outside the court held posters proclaiming "Homosex [sic] is not in Black culture." The Gay and Lesbian Association of the Witwatersrand wrote an open letter to the ANC protesting the way in which Winnie Mandela's defense had persistently linked homosexuality to sexual abuse. They expressed alarm at the ANC's failure to respond to "the level of homophobia that has arisen both within and outside this court," raising doubts about whether the ANC had any serious commitment to the recognition of lesbian and gay rights. AIDS educator Dawn Mokhobo has said that homosexuality is perceived as being "largely non-existent" and "abhorrent" in black society. The linkage of AIDS with

homosexuality thus makes instituting programs more difficult (Mokhobo 1989:18). Systematic research on black homophobia is presently sparse and limited (Tshabalala and Isaacs 1990:1).

5. See, for example, the accusation by anti-apartheid activist Dr. David Seftel that the government is deliberately underplaying the size of the epidemic and not counseling infected blacks with hemophilia, allowing them to spread the disease in their communities. "South Africa's government is actively and passively creating a public health disaster—genocide by omission" (Seftel 1988:22). Given that only three cases of AIDS in blacks with hemophilia have been recorded (*Epidemiological Comments* 1992), such accusations only fuel mistrust and complicate the search for a rational AIDS strategy.

6. Shebeens are informal drinking establishments, resembling speakeasies, usually in black townships. Originally offering illicit home-brewed liquor or liquor obtained without a license when blacks had no access to commercial liquor supplies, they have been legalized in recent years. Apart from supplying liquor, they often provide music, dancing, and commercial sex.

7. Like the militant resistance to state family planning, particularly during the political violence of 1976 and 1985–86, rejecting the AIDS program could have political overtones.

8. It should be noted that African research suggests that the middle- and upper-middle-income groups are at least as vulnerable (Miller and Rockwell 1988:xxiv–xxvi). For a critique of Packard's views on both the social/contextual element and the role of hypodermics in the epidemic, see the comments following the published version of Packard's paper (Packard and Epstein 1991).

## REFERENCES

*Africa South* (Johannesburg). Health Minister Harnesses Literary Flair, August, 1991. 45.

*Die Afrikaner* (Pretoria). 1991a. January 16 (translated by Virginia van der Vliet).
―――. 1991b. February 6 (translated by Virginia van der Vliet).

*AIDS Analysis Africa* (Southern Africa Edition) (Rivonia, South Africa). 1990. 1(2), (August/September).
―――. 1991. 1(4), (December 1990/January 1991).

AIDS Consortium. 1992. AIDS and HIV Charter, *Critical Health*, September (40): 79–82.

*Argus* (Cape Town). 1991. June 12.
―――. 1992. October 23.
―――. 1994. March 30.

Broomberg, Jonathan, Malcolm Steinberg, P. Masobe, and G. Behr. 1991. Economic Impact of AIDS in South Africa. In Centre for Health Policy, *AIDS in South Africa: The Demographic and Economic Implications*, pp. 29–74. Paper no. 23, September. Johannesburg: Department of Community Health, Medical School, University of the Witwatersrand.

*Die Burger* (Cape Town). 1994. March 31.

*Cape Times* (Cape Town). 1989. June 28.
―――. 1991a. January 24.

————. 1991b. February 20.

————. 1991c. February 26.

————. 1991d. May 14.

————. 1992. May 27.

Centre for Health Policy. 1991. *AIDS in South Africa: The Demographic and Economic Implications.* Paper no. 23, September. Johannesburg: Department of Community Health, Medical School, University of the Witwatersrand.

Chirimuuta, Richard C., and Rosalind J. Chirimuuta. 1987. *AIDS, Africa, and Racism.* Bretby House, Derbyshire: R. Chirimuuta.

Crewe, Mary. 1992. *AIDS in South Africa: The Myth and the Reality.* London: Penguin Forum Series.

*Debates of Parliament* (Hansard) (Cape Town). 1990a. May 16, cols. 9402–3 (Translated by Virginia van der Vliet).

————. 1990b. May 18, col. 9761.

————. 1990c. May 18, col. 9783.

————. 1990d. May 18, col. 9797.

————. 1991. April 12, Parliamentary Question number 170, cols. 1007–8 in Questions and Replies section.

Doyle, Peter R. 1991. The Impact of AIDS on the South African Population. In Centre for Health Policy, *AIDS in South Africa: The Demographic and Economic Implications,* pp. 9–28. Paper no. 23, September. Johannesburg: Department of Community Health, Medical School, University of the Witwatersrand.

*Epidemiological Comments* (Pretoria: Department of National Health and Population Development). 1990. The Truth about AIDS. 17(3): 3–14.

————. 1992. AIDS in South Africa since 1982—As on 31 March 1992. 19(3): 57.

————. 1993. AIDS in South Africa: Status on World AIDS Day. 20(11): 184–203.

————. 1994. AIDS in South Africa. 21(1): 20.

Farmer, Paul. 1990. Sending Sickness: Sorcery, Politics, and Changing Concepts of AIDS in Rural Haiti. *Medical Anthropology Quarterly* 4(1): 6–27.

*Finance Week* (Johannesburg). 1991. October 17–23.

*Financial Mail* (Johannesburg). 1988. February 26.

Fleming, Alan. 1992. South Africa and AIDS—Seven Years Wasted. *Current AIDS Literature* 5(11): 406–420.

Floyd, Elizabeth. 1990. HIV and AIDS in South Africa Today. Draft paper presented at Conference on Health in Southern Africa, Maputo, April.

Hamilton, Robin. 1991. Special Issue on AIDS. *Social and Economic Update,* no. 14 (May). Johannesburg: South African Institute of Race Relations.

*Health Trends in South Africa 1990.* 1991. Pretoria: Department of National Health and Population Development.

*History in the Making* (Johannesburg: South African History Archive). 1991a. HIV and AIDS in Southern Africa: Draft Maputo Statement, 15/4/1990. 1(5): 8–12.

————. 1991b. 1989 Cosatu Congress: Resolution on AIDS. 1(5): 13–14.

Ingstad, Benedicte. 1990. The Cultural Construction of AIDS and Its Consequences for Prevention in Botswana. *Medical Anthropology Quarterly* 4(1): 28–40.

Kelly, Joe. 1991. *Social and Economic Update,* no. 12 (January). Johannesburg: South African Institute of Race Relations.

Larson, Ann 1990. The Social Epidemiology of Africa's AIDS Epidemic. *African Affairs* 89(354): 5–26.

*Mayibuye* (Johannesburg). 1991a. Campaigning against AIDS. April, pp. 37–38.

———. 1991b. Why Is AIDS political? September, p. 31.

McLean, Diarmuid. 1990. Communication Report on the Concerns of Women in Khayelitsha. *AIDS Scan* (Cape Town: Planned Parenthood Association and Sanlam AIDS Media Resource Centre Publication) 2(4): 9–10.

Mhloyi, Marvellous M. 1991. AIDS Transition in Southern Africa: Lessons to Be Learned. *Progress*, Spring/Summer, pp. 44–49.

Miller, Norman, and Richard C. Rockwell, eds. 1988. *AIDS in Africa: The Social and Policy Impact.* Lewiston, NY: Edwin Mellen Press.

Mokhobo, Dawn. 1989. Sexual Attitudes of Blacks towards AIDS Education. In *SANLAM Group Benefits Review: 1988–1989.* Belville, Cape: SANLAM.

*New African* (London). 1990. Africa and the AIDS Myth. No. 271 (April).

*New Nation* (Johannesburg). 1991. June 28–July 4.

*New Scientist* (New York). 1988. December 17.

*Newsweek* (New York). 1987. March 23.

Packard, Randall M. 1989. *Epidemiologists, Social Scientists, and the Structure of Medical Research on AIDS in Africa.* Working Papers in African Studies, no. 137. Boston: African Studies Center.

Packard, Randall M., and P. Epstein. 1991. Epidemiologists, Social Scientists, and the Structure of Medical Research on AIDS in Africa. (With comments by D. Feldman, C. Kendall, S. Minkin, P. Reining and B. G. Schoepf, and re-joinder by Packard and Epstein.) *Social Science and Medicine* 33(7) : 771–794.

Padayachee, G. N., and R. Schall. 1990. Short-Term Predictions of the Prevalence of Human Immunodeficiency Virus Infection among the Black Population in South Africa. *South African Medical Journal* 77:329–333.

*Patriot* (Pretoria). 1990. October 12 (translation by Virginia van der Vliet).

Perkel, Adrian, and Anna Strebel. 1989. AIDS. In *Social Services in a Changing South Africa*, ed. Mary Hazelton and N. Schaay, pp. 70–84. Proceedings of the Fourth OASSA [Organisation for Appropriate Social Services in South Africa] National Conference, University of the Witwatersrand, Johannesburg, September.

Preston-Whyte, Eleanor, Q. A. Karim, and M. Zondi. 1991. Women and AIDS— The Triple Imperative. *Critical Health*, no. 34 (June): 42–47.

*Race Relations Survey* (Johannesburg: South African Institute of Race Relations). 1988. 1987/88.

———. 1989. 1988/89.

———. 1990. 1989/90.

———. 1994. 1993/94.

*Reader's Digest.* 1994. What Young South Africans Think? February: 15–21.

*RSA Policy Review* 1991. (Pretoria: Bureau for Information). Strategy for AIDS. 4(5): 66–79.

*Sechaba* (Lusaka: ANC). 1988. AIDS and the Imperialist Connection. 22(11): 23–28.

Seftel, David. 1988. AIDS and Apartheid: Double Trouble. *Africa Report,* November–December, pp. 17–22.

Singer, Merrill, F. Flores, L. Davison, B. Burke, Z. Castillo, K. Scanlon, and M. Rivera. 1990. SIDA: The Economic, Social, and Cultural Context of AIDS among Latinos. *Medical Anthropology Quarterly* 4(1): 72–114.

Sontag, Susan. 1988. *AIDS and Its Metaphors*. New York: Farrar, Straus and Giroux.

*South* (Cape Town). 1990a. July 12–18.

———. 1990b. September 20–27.

*Southern Africa Report* (Johannesburg). 1990. Double Jeopardy: AIDS and Apartheid. 6(3): 18–20.

*Sowetan* (Johannesburg). 1991. October 7.

*Sunday Star* (Johannesburg). 1989. January 8.

*Sunday Times Extra* (Johannesburg). 1990. April 22.

———. 1991. March 17.

Toms, Ivan. 1990. AIDS in South Africa: Potential Decimation on the Eve of Liberation. *Progress*, Fall/Winter, pp. 13–16.

Tshabalala, M., and Gordon Isaacs. 1990. An Assessment of African Attitudes towards Homosexuality. Paper prepared for the Human Sciences Research Council, Pretoria.

U.S. Department of State. 1987. *Soviet Influence Activities: A Report on Active Measures and Propaganda, 1986–87*. August, chap. 5.

Vallabhjee, Krish. 1991. The Political, Medical, and Economic Challenges in Providing Health for All in South Africa. *Progress*, Spring/Summer, pp. 1–4.

Van der Vliet, Virginia. 1984. South Africa's Population Crisis. *Optima* 32(4): 147–153.

Waite, Gloria. 1988. The Politics of Disease: The AIDS Virus and Africa. In *AIDS in Africa: The Social and Policy Impact*, ed. Norman Miller and Richard C. Rockwell, pp. 145–164. Lewiston, NY: Edwin Mellen Press.

*Weekend Argus* (Cape Town). 1992. June 7.

*Weekly Mail* (Johannesburg). 1991a. March 15–21.

———. 1991b. March 28–April 4.

———. 1991c. June 28–July 4.

Workplace Information Group. n. d. *AIDS—Everybody's Problem*. Johannesburg: Workplace Information Group.

*WorldAIDS* (London: Panos Institute). 1989a. No. 4 (July).

———. 1989b. No. 6 (November).

———. 1990. No. 12 (November).

———. 1991. No. 15 (May).

# 9

# The Politics of International Health: Breastfeeding and HIV

*Dana Raphael*

HIV-infected mothers may transmit the virus to their infants via breast milk, but this fact has been toned down or denied by the world's major health organizations for economic and political concerns. Much like the sad story of the delay in recognizing AIDS as a serious pandemic disease, world agencies, advocates for mothers to breastfeed long and exclusively, that is, without any additional foods, have minimized this potentially negative effect due to historical and circumstantial pressures.

The process of discovery helps us understand the milestones in assessing whether or not babies do become infected with their mother's milk and why the research has been delayed. At first it was reported that between 13 and 39 percent of the babies born to HIV-positive mothers also tested positive for the HIV antibodies (Peckham *et al.* 1991). However, after a few weeks to a few months the antibodies in some babies appeared to "disappear," leading some investigators to hope that the infants were safe. Several months later, however, some of the babies became ill with AIDS-related symptoms, though they still did not necessarily exhibit the HIV-positive assay. Due to this situation, the percentage of at-risk babies now reported to have AIDS rose to 60 percent.

Infants are born with a weak antibody response, and their infection status cannot always be detected by current testing methods. The HIV antibodies had been acquired transplacentally from their mother's blood. Only later do babies produce their own antibodies that are then able to be detected. A similar pattern is found in rhesus macaque infants whose mothers are infected with simian immunodeficiency virus (SIV). These animals are born with SIV antibodies from their infected mothers. The antibodies disappear by six months of age, but the infants later seroconvert, showing a virus-positive response at nine to fifteen months (McClure *et al.* 1991).

Thus some of the questions to be solved during this decade remain: Were these human infants infected from birth, infected or reinfected by breast milk, or born HIV negative only to seroconvert after months of breast-feeding?

Tainted by association with a dreaded disease, breast milk is no longer the benevolent, therapeutic nutrient to which the major players—the International Pediatric Association (1991), the United Nations Fund for Population Activities (1991), the United Nations Children's Fund (UNICEF) (1992), the United States Agency for International Development (USAID) (1987), WHO (1990), the World Bank, and many others—had committed their resources. The contradictions behind the strategy of each agency can be best understood by scrutinizing the realities of the continuing politics of breastfeeding (*Lactation Review* 1977; Raphael and Davis 1985), for there we find public health officials pitting the practice of breastfeeding babies against formula-producing multinational companies, and health agencies basing their fiscal strategies and research agenda on expediency.

Factors unrelated to breast milk and breastfeeding have created a tragic process of institutional deceit and self-interest. The message is not that men are evil or that women are eager to kill off their infants with inappropriate feeding methods, but that a pattern of leadership exists that inhibits well-meaning people from accepting and then acting upon realities. They have moved far too slowly away from a worldwide absorption in a controversy involving the breast versus the bottle that engrossed these agencies for over a decade. Blocked by this distraction, they have delayed the critical research that could define or put aside fears regarding the risk of HIV transmission from mother to child, or, in extraordinary cases when the child was transfused with contaminated blood, from the child's saliva to the mother through an opening in the nipple.

A short history will help uncover the interference that led to the commingling of major world institutions and breastfeeding. It will help explain some of the forces that led to these culpable acts and how such life-giving nutrients as breast and cows' milk could have sliced deep rifts among nurses, advocates, physicians, researchers, newspaper reporters, and even politicians. We will also learn more about why breastfeeding, which had been taken for granted or ignored by the health community, suddenly loomed as the primary factor in infant survival, only to fade.

The story began in the mid-1970s in a small office on the third floor of a dilapidated building in a not-so-elegant area of London, where a small group of advocates, part of the now-defunct British charity War on Want, commissioned a pamphlet with a cover displaying a picture of a wailing, emaciated black child curled up like a shrunken doll inside a milk-formula bottle. In the accompanying statement, taken from a booklet entitled *The Baby Killer* (Muller 1974), this group condemned the formula companies for killing babies by influencing mothers to abandon breastfeeding and to use their products instead.

Deeply shocked, Nestle, with the largest share of the Third World market, made a move in response that was to cost it considerable time and effort and millions of dollars (see, for example, Nestle Infant Formula Audit Commission 1983). It sued the German equivalent of the accusing War on Want group, a few dozen well-meaning people, most of whom were university students, for libel when they titled the book *Nestle Kills Babies* (Edson 1979). Not surprisingly, the company won its suit, for such a claim was indeed unprovable. But Nestle lost the war, and the so-called breast/bottle controversy evolved into a campaign against the formula-producing multinational corporations that caught the imagination of tens of thousands of people all over the world, particularly in the United States. In fact, except for Ralph Nader's strategy against the auto industry, this controversy became the most notorious antimultinational effort in the United States.

Senator Edward Kennedy, responding to what was described as the most successful letter campaign on Capitol Hill, ordered hearings in Washington, D.C., that ended with the recommendation to turn the problem over to the World Health Organization (U.S. Senate Committee on Human Resources 1978). When WHO accepted the responsibility, it joined with UNICEF in 1979 for a joint meeting on infant and child feeding where approximately one hundred men and a few women, representing seventeen countries and various professional associations, industry, and consumers, came together to decide how to limit the marketing efforts of the multinationals and promote breastfeeding.

In 1981 WHO recommended a code for the distribution and sale of infant formula throughout the world, and a few dozen countries pledged to follow it. Hundreds of promotion campaigns were launched in dozens of ministries of health, clinics, public health centers, and hospitals internationally. Anyone questioning the desire of working mothers for a choice of feeding methods or the need of babies for additional food other than their mother's milk was immediately suspected of mistreating babies and, worse, of being seduced by multinational favors. These distortions and the misuse of power—in government or medical agencies—for economic or political ends are becoming all too familiar today as the result of revelation after revelation. Only when such patterns of behavior are understood can persons in power avoid them.

WHO began its work on breastfeeding early (Carballo 1979). UNICEF was more political in its approach and began a major campaign promoting breastfeeding that the agency claimed was being inhibited by the presence and use of milk formula (Grant 1982–83; UNICEF 1982, 1984, 1985), a charge it continues to attempt to substantiate. Millions of dollars were collected and distributed to hold seminars on breastfeeding and to back elaborate print advertising campaigns to promote it. Even UNESCO (1985) was swept up in this global project. One of its publications listed thirty-nine of its pamphlets encouraging mothers to breastfeed.

The U.S. Agency for International Development (USAID) sponsored the first international cross-cultural study of breastfeeding in 1975 (Raphael and King 1977; see also Raphael and Davis 1985), and several others followed from various sections of that agency. The explosion of interest in human lactation produced hundreds of research findings, some from advocates both in and out of the profession with very diverse levels of scholarship (USAID 1987).

During the 1980s many of these studies were beginning to confirm the Human Lactation Center's original findings that mothers gave their infants liquid and solids other than breast milk very early, sometimes from just a few weeks after birth (Raphael and Davis 1985; Raphael and King 1977). Nevertheless, health authorities continued to approve or relying exclusively on breastfeeding despite their own research that exposed the normal weaning patterns; "it was shown that although 99% of infants were breastfed in the first three months of life, 83% of them received water or tea in addition to breast milk" (WHO 1991b). Despite the published reports on how difficult breastfeeding is for poor women who must also work or are often physically unable to produce sufficient milk (UNICEF 1985), outspoken and well-meaning professionals continued to act as if mothers could be persuaded otherwise. The underlying assumption in many of these studies was that mothers were just ignorant or more interested in their own work, personal attractiveness, or freedom than in the health of their children.

Pressing for exclusive breastfeeding (commonly edicted for at least four to six months) can be extremely dangerous. The programs that were developed to persuade mothers to take up a new pattern of breastfeeding are mainly possible for those women who are well fed and well off. It would have been wiser to look at how most of the world's mothers in developing nations have survived so far without edicts and well-intentioned interferences.

In 1977 there was no more than a single shelf of references on breastfeeding and human lactation, and most of them had to do with comparative data between human and cows' milk. Only thirteen years later, a plethora of books, journal articles, seminars and field project reports, films and videos supporting and promoting breastfeeding, and codes and advocacy campaigns against the infant-formula industry had appeared worldwide, fueled by the availability of multimillions of yen, lira, pounds, dollars, and rupees.

UNICEF hosted a meeting where representatives from varied organizations, including the Swedish International Development Agency, were invited for the sole purpose of defining the word "breastfeeding" (Labbok and Krasovec 1988). WHO (1991a) had by now reduced this complex function—human lactation—to a cluster of Indicators for Assessing Breast-feeding Practices among both the poor and the well off. In 1990, guided by an underlying presumption that breastfeeding was in danger of being renounced, members from these great agencies held a conference in Florence, Italy, and released an "Innocenti Declaration" intended to protect, promote, and support breastfeeding. At that congregation the problem of the presence of HIV in breast milk was not addressed.

Happily, breastfeeding has finally been recognized among health professionals as a major force in infant survival, but not so welcome is the underlying premise that breast milk is a substance equal, if not superior, to lifesaving medicine. Breast milk was expected to inhibit or prevent serious diseases, and breastfeeding was said to have "a protective effect against breast cancer for lactating women" (Berg and Brems 1990).

But beginning in 1985, some startling evidence about breast milk came in from the field. Infected mothers were found to have HIV antibodies in their milk (Oxtoby et al. 1987; Pyun et al. 1987; Thiry et al. 1985; Wasserberger et al. 1986) and in some cases to transmit them to their infants (Hamosh and Hamosh 1988; Lepage 1987). Even more surprising were reports in the medical literature of cases where newborns whose mothers became HIV positive after childbirth as a result of the transfusion of contaminated blood were diagnosed with symptoms of AIDS. Breast milk was implicated (Senturia et al. 1987; Ziegler 1988; Ziegler et al. 1985).

Imagine the dilemma this presented for these agencies. Beginning as early as the late 1970s (Carballo 1979), WHO had become heavily involved in breastfeeding programs throughout the world. From 1982 on UNICEF had included the promotion of breastfeeding as one of four main objectives sought by that agency—no small budgeting matter (UNICEF 1982, 1984, 1985). Now, under pressure from the media and the medical professionals who were medicating desperate mothers, these agencies could no longer postpone facing this crisis. WHO (1987; see also WHO 1989) called for "A Consultation on Breastfeeding, Breast Milk, and HIV Infection."

Subsequent reports recognized the dangers. Breast milk could effect "intercurrent infections which could accelerate progression of HIV-related disease in already infected infants" (International Child Health 1991). Nonetheless, and here is the tragedy, WHO (1987) recommended that "particularly in situations where the safe and effective use of alternatives is not possible (and this includes the vast majority), breast-feeding by the biological mother should continue to be the feeding method of choice, irrespective of her HIV infection status."

The European Collaborative Study undertaken in 1992 did concede that "mothers with established infection can transmit HIV infection through breast milk," but still held out the possibility that there was no danger by concluding the sentence with "although the relative importance of this route remains to be defined." Other researchers and health protection agencies concurred (Radlett 1989; Ziegler 1988). Manciaurx (1992) commented sadly that "it would seem [to be] the lesser of two evils to encourage breastfeeding" while questioning if that was "ethically acceptable." Dunn et al. (1992) reported that the relative importance has now been defined and that "the additional risk of transmission through breastfeeding, beyond transmission in utero or during delivery, is 14%." How such a figure was reached is puzzling.

Looking back, we can see that the information had been available for several years. In 1985 the U.S. Centers for Disease Control (CDC) had already published its recommendation that women who tested HIV positive should not breastfeed. But the appeal—especially for the press—of this "new subject" with photographs and sentiment about breasts full of milk, emaciated babies, and the obvious villain, the multinational companies, was irresistible. The agencies were reluctant to give up the worldwide support for their efforts on behalf of mother's milk, which had become such a lucrative source of funds.

Many physicians agreed with the recommendation to breastfeed, even condemning the original findings that incriminated breast milk. One spokesperson for the CDC suggested that colostrum (fluid that appears in the breast prior to the appearance of breast milk) or breast milk itself might protect against AIDS (Peckham et al. 1989; Peckham et al. 1991). They argued that even if it were true that breast milk did infect 30 percent of the babies (Nestle Foundation for the Study of the Problems of Nutrition in the World 1989), most children of infected mothers do not acquire the virus (Baumslag 1987). Advocates for breastfeeding, no matter what the condition of the mother, further suggested that the milk could be safe after all since only the HIV antibodies had been detected, but the antigen could not be found: "Despite the best equipment they cannot replicate the claimed finding of intact HIV antigens in breast milk although antibodies can be demonstrated and PCR tests indicate that viral fragments are present" (Minchin 1990).

From Florence, Italy, WHO and UNICEF produced a document (WHO/UNICEF 1990) restating the goal that "all women should be enabled to practice exclusive breastfeeding [and] all infants should be fed exclusively on breast milk from birth to [four to six] months of age," a very dangerous edict. Radlett (1989) maintained that the nutritional superiority of breastfeeding, the bonding of mother and child, the contraceptive benefits of breastfeeding, and the potentially protective immunologic effects of breast milk continue to outweigh the potential risks of HIV transmission through breast milk.

Ignoring the CDC, counselors assured mothers that their babies were safe if nursed (Baumslag 1988; Baumslag and O'Gara 1989). As so often happens when absolutes are challenged by new evidence, researchers were able to turn the findings of the potentially lethal effect of breast milk, confirmed by their own research, to accommodate the overall political needs and economic status of their agencies. For instance, "If such transmission occurs, the relative contribution of this route [breastfeeding] is probably small" (WHO 1987; see also WHO 1989). The most recent work by these agencies (WHO/UNICEF 1992) finally conceded that infants are more likely to acquire the disease if the mother becomes infected during the breastfeeding period. The recommendation, however, essentially reaffirmed that "breast is best."

A sober risk/benefit argument has now been established, but with the intrusion of the virulent HIV factor, the remarkable emphasis on breastfeeding is over. No longer are the annual goals focused primarily on breastfeeding. One exception is that breastfeeding is seen as a valuable contraceptive, as a method to control population growth (UNICEF 1990, 1992; United Nations Fund for Population Activities 1992; WHO 1990).

Consider the realities of women in poverty. Most mothers throughout the world have no choice but to breastfeed. Even if they knew about the residue of HIV in breast milk or that their infants were or were not infected, they must nurse or let them die. Most families in the world cannot afford any form of milk, much less the very expensive infant formula (*Lactation Review* 1977; Raphael 1982; Raphael and King 1977).

However, there are families who can afford this option (Raphael 1973), and until the effects of breast milk are known for sure, they should be given that choice (Human Lactation Center 1988; *New York Post* 1988). Testing on a massive scale is unlikely. Testing methods are expensive even in the United States and more so in the developing world, so it is unlikely that health ministries, already overburdened, could use the limited financial resources to test infants except on an experimental basis. So while there is doubt, families with members who are HIV positive should be encouraged to use alternative foods if they can afford it. If it turns out that breast milk does not transmit the virus, it would be wonderful indeed; women who care to breastfeed would be able to do so.

The purpose of this analysis is not to confirm or deny the effect of breast milk, but to highlight the pattern of behavior that seems to have stymied these otherwise humanitarian institutions. The appropriate response would have included a statement encouraging those families that could manage to use alternative food, as well as a call for help from the infant-formula industry.

The Reagan/Bush position against abortion produced another curious conundrum. The World Bank's annual report for 1991 budgeted 1.5 billion dollars for population programs. McNamara (1992) projected 8 billion dollars for population work in annual expenditures by the year 2000. But for now, the World Bank, which had only lately become seriously involved in the issue of breastfeeding, recognizes the contraceptive benefits of lactation. In a recent publication by a senior nutrition advisor at that agency, breastfeeding was touted as a natural contraceptive (Berg and Brems 1990). It is likely that this was in deference to the politically delicate abortion issue that is related to the withholding of funds by the United States for the United Nations in general, and for population programs in particular.

Breastfeeding is an effective deterrent to unwanted births if and when it inhibits ovulation. When clearly understood and carefully practiced, the ovulation method combined with breastfeeding can be a very useful technique for determining fertility periods. It is particularly effective in areas where other methods of contraception are either too expensive or unavailable (Raphael 1988).

Since 1975 I have been an advocate of this natural family-planning method, especially after learning that rural Indian women (and women in many other cultures) were already expert in practicing abstinence during their fertile period. Women relied on the physical changes in their bodies to clue them in to the "safe time." Many of those same signals are part of the training in the ovulation method.

I had an inkling of the political stress that agencies are facing when I presented this method at a conference in India in the 1980s. Much to my dismay, in the middle of a presentation and before hundreds of people, an executive of one of the most powerful world population agencies condemned me for what she perceived as a Catholic viewpoint about contraception. Nothing could have been further from my mind. It is now very clear how an enormous investment in birth-control technology and the extensive paraphernalia committed to teaching programs caused these agencies to see this option as a threat.

Though it seems cynical to lay these patterns out so blatantly, we need to understand the pressures under which these important agencies are making decisions in the face of the obvious AIDS threat to the worldwide campaign for breastfeeding. For example, UNICEF (1990, 1992) is currently moving strongly into the population field. Breastfeeding, recently the central focus of its outreach, has now been repackaged and appears as part of a program entitled "The Baby Friendly Hospital Initiative."

At a conference at Johns Hopkins University (*Population Report* 1987; see also Labbok 1989) on natural methods of contraception, breastfeeding was mentioned primarily as a potential ovulation inhibitor, rather than as a nutritional benefit. In a summary of all USAID projects, not one word on breastfeeding or child nutrition was listed (USAID 1992).

UNICEF, a long-time exponent of exclusive breastfeeding, began to concede that "too much must not be expected of breastfeeding. It is only one part of the package that should be achieved as a minimal standard" (Grant 1989). An interesting spin-off is reflected in a reduction of the numerous photos by United Nations photographers of breastfeeding mothers with their breasts fully exposed. Unfortunately, too many of these photos served only to hype up editorial content.

But natural family-planning techniques, along with the value of breast-feeding to increase their effectiveness, do not sit well with all the agencies. The United Nations Fund for Population Activities (1991, 1992), already damaged by Reagan/Bush politics and reduced funding, is justifiably concerned that such a focus of interest could infringe on its current programs, so it has gone on the offensive. According to the September 1990 population newsletter, "Pledging UNFPA's wholehearted support" of efforts to promote breastfeeding, Executive Director Nafis Sadik warned that "we put at risk the interests of both mother and child if we fall into the trap of assuming that breastfeeding is a means of family planning."

Ethically, the HIV link is too important to wait for clear biological evidence about how, if, and when transmission occurs. A proactive stance is called for. In 1988 researchers at the Human Lactation Center proposed that the formula companies get involved in this worldwide crisis (see also Raphael 1990). It is probable that their contribution against this great scourge could be a means of delivering their formula to HIV-positive mothers despite the WHO directives and at affordable prices.

Sadly, no one listened then because media attention was still focused on condemning multinational companies for selectively chosen ills. To accept any plan that might be construed as benefiting the infant-formula industry was still premature and too revolutionary. For industry, the new concept of low-profit distribution is also hard won. Further, it is becoming clear to everyone that no matter how much powdered milk is delivered, without the fuel to boil the water (which is to be mixed with the substitute foods) making it potable, babies will still be in danger. On the other hand, none of the companies have made the gesture to participate in the solution to this gigantic tragedy. I once asked Margaret Mead why companies should do so. Her answer was "Because it is the right thing to do."

The problem continues to balloon. Millions of women throughout the world, whether they know their HIV status or not, whether they are in high- or low-incidence areas, need sensitively delivered information so they can make informed decisions as to whether or not to breastfeed. Once they know the facts, they will make the decisions that are best for them. The least we can do, whatever their choice, is to provide them with the means to achieve that end and the support they require to feel of value and to maintain some autonomy over their lives.

## REFERENCES

Baumslag, Naomi. 1987. Breast-feeding and HIV Infection. *Lancet* 2 (August 15): 401.

————. 1988. AIDS and Breastfeeding: Panic or Logic. *Breastfeeding Abstracts* (La Leche League) 7(4).

Baumslag, Naomi, and C. O'Gara. 1989. *Breastfeeding: The Passport to Life*. New York: NGO Committee on UNICEF and National Council for International Health.

Berg, Alan, and Susan Brems. 1990. Promoting Breastfeeding: A Means to Limit Fertility. In "A Case for Promoting Breastfeeding in Projects to Limit Fertility." *AAWH Quarterly* 4(3): 4–7.

Carballo, Manuel. 1979. World Health Organization Programs in Breastfeeding. In *Breastfeeding and Food Policy in a Hungry World*, ed. Dana Raphael, pp. 245–251. New York: Academic Press.

Centers for Disease Control (CDC). 1985. Recommendations for Assisting in the Prevention of Perinatal Transmission of Human-T-Lymphotropic Virus Type III/LAV. *Morbidity and Mortality Weekly Report* 34: 721–32.

Dunn, D. T., M. L. Newell. 1992. Risk of Human Immunodeficiency Virus Type I Transmission through Breastfeeding. *Lancet* (September 5) 340(8819): 585–588.

Edson, Lee. 1979. Babies in Poverty: The Real Victims of the Breast/Bottle Controversy. *Lactation Review* 4:1.

European Collaborative Study. 1992. Risk Factors for Mother-to-Child Transmission of HIV-1. *Lancet* 339: 1007–1012.

Grant, James P. 1982. *The State of the World's Children, 1982–83*. New York: UNICEF.

————. 1989. Foreword. In *Breastfeeding: The Passport to Life*, ed. N. Baumslag. New York: UNICEF.

Hamosh, Margit, and Paul Hamosh. 1988. Mother to Infant Biochemical and Immunological Transfer through Breast Milk. In *Perinatology*, ed. Wiknjosastro, Prakoso and Maeda, pp. 155–160. Amsterdam: Elsevier.

Human Lactation Center. 1988. Director of Lactation Center Urges Mothers Infected with the AIDS Virus to Consider Alternatives to Breastfeeding. Press release.

International Child Health. 1991. Why Does WHO Continue to Recommend Breast-feeding for Most HIV-infected Mothers? AIDS Prevention: Guidelines for MCH/FP Programme Managers. Global Program on AIDS, Maternal and Child Health Including Family Planning, AIDS Prevention: Guidelines for MCH/FP Programme Managers. May. 2(3).

International Pediatric Association. 1991. Report: Women, Children, Families and AIDS. *International Child Health: A Digest of Current Information* (In collaboration with UNICEF and WHO) 2(3): 66–68.

Labbok, Miriam, and Katherine Krasovec. 1988. Report of a meeting on Breast-feeding Definitions. The Interagency Group for Action on Breastfeeding, Hosted by UNICEF, Georgetown University, Washington, DC, April.

Labbok, N. H. 1989. Breastfeeding and Family Planning Programs: A Vital Complementarity. In *Breastfeeding: The Passport to Life*, ed. N. Baumslag. New York: UNICEF.

*Lactation Review*. 1977. Mothers in Poverty: Breastfeeding and the Maternal Struggle for Infant Survival. *Lactation Review* 2:3.

Lepage, Philippe, P. Van de Perre, M. Carael, and J. P. Butzler. 1987. Postnatal Transmission of HIV from Mother to Child. *Lancet* 2(August 15): 400.

Manciaux, Professor. 1992. Comments in the Provincional Summary Record, 7th Meeting, Committee B, 45th World Health Assembly, Infant and Young Child Nutrition, Geneva, May.

McClure, Harold, Daniel Anderson, Patricia Fultz, Aftab Ansari, Tamar Jehuda-Cohen, Francois Villinger, Sherry Klumpp, William Switzer, Ellen Lockwood, Anne Brodie, and Harry Keyserling. 1991. Maternal Transmission of SIV/SMM in Rhesus Macaques. *Journal of Medical Primatology* 20:182–187.

McNamara, Robert. 1992. Introduction. In World Bank, *Annual Report*. Washington, DC: World Bank.

Minchin, Maureen. 1990. Positive Prejudice: HIV and Breastfeeding. *Women's International Public Health Network News* 8(October/November): 2–3.

Muller, M. 1974. *The Baby Killer*. London: War on Want.

Nestle Foundation for the Study of the Problems of Nutrition in the World. 1989. *Annual Report*. Lausanne, Switzerland.

Nestle Infant Formula Audit Commission. 1983. Complaint Reports. Edmund S. Muskie, Chairman. *Quarterly Report No. 5*. Washington, DC.

*New York Post*. 1988. Breast-fed Babies Risk AIDS from Moms. June 14, p. 19.

Oxtoby, Margaret J., M. Rogers, P. Thomas, S. Manoff, and K. Winter. 1987. National Trends in Perinatally Acquired AIDS, United States. Paper delivered at the International Conference on Acquired Immune Deficiency Syndrome (AIDS), Sponsored by U.S. Department of Health and Human Services and World Health Organization, Washington, DC, June 1–5.

Peckham, C. S., M. L. Newell, A. E. Ades, and the European Collaborative Study. 1989. Vertical Transmission of HIV Infection–European Collaborative Study Update. Paper delivered at the V International Conference on AIDS, Montreal, Canada.

Peckham, Catherine, R. S. Tedder, M. Briggs, A. E. Ades, M. Hjelm, A. H. Wilcox, N. Parra-mejia, and C. O'Connor. 1991. Children Born to Women with HIV-1 Infection: Natural History and Risk of Transmission. *Lancet* 337(8736): 253–260.

*Population Report* (Baltimore: Johns Hopkins University). 1987. Family Planning for the Breastfeeding Woman. Series J, 36(December):26.

Pyun, Kwang H., et al. 1987. Perinatal Infection with Human Immunodeficiency Virus: Specific Antibody Responses by the Neonate. *New England Journal of Medicine*, 317(10): 611–614.

Radlett, Marty. 1989. Children at Risk: The Sorrow of Paediatric AIDS. *AIDS Watch, People* (Supplement) (London: International Planned Parenthood Federation) 4(8): 2–3.

Raphael, Dana. 1973. The Role of Breastfeeding in a Bottle-oriented World. *Ecology of Food and Nutrition* 2:121–126.

———. 1982. Weaning Is Always: The Anthropology of Breastfeeding Behavior. *Lactation Review* 6:1.

———. 1988. The Ovulation Method and the Politics of Contraception. In *Children and Families: Studies in Prevention and Intervention*, ed. Euthymia D. Hibbs, pp. 33–40. Madison, CT: International Universities Press.

————. 1990. *HIV and Breast Milk: Current Directions in Anthropological Research on AIDS.* AIDS and Anthropology Research Group Special Publication 1(January), ed. Douglas A. Feldman. Miami, FL: University of Miami, School of Medicine.

Raphael, Dana, and Flora Davis. 1985. *Only Mothers Know: Patterns of Infant Feeding in Traditional Cultures.* Westport, CT: Greenwood Press.

Raphael, Dana, and Joyce King. 1977. Mothers in Poverty: Breastfeeding and the Maternal Struggle for Infant Survival: Report to the Agency for International Development (AID). *Lactation Review* 2:3.

Senturia, Y. D., A. E. Ades, and C. S. Peckham. 1987. Breast-feeding and HIV Infection. *Lancet* 2(August 15): 400–401.

Thiry, L., S. Sprecher-Goldberger, T. Jockheer, J. Levy, P. Van de Perre, P. Henrivaux, J. Cogniaux-LeClrec, and N. Clumeck. 1985. Isolation of AIDS Virus from Cell-Free Breast Milk of Three Healthy Virus Carriers. *Lancet* 2(October 19): 891–92.

UNESCO. 1985. *Show and Tell: A Worldwide Directory of Nutrition Teaching-Learning Resources.* Paris: UNESCO Nutrition Education Programme.

United Nations Children's Fund (UNICEF). 1982. *The State of the World's Children 1982–3.* Oxford University Press.

————. 1984. UNICEF Has Four-Step Health Plan. *Population* 10(12): 4.

————. 1985. *The State of the World's Children 1985–6.*

————. 1990. Guidelines for Breastfeeding in Family Planning and Child Survival Programs. Institute for International Studies in Natural Family Planning, Georgetown University, Washington, DC, January.

————. 1992. Family Planning Saves, Improves Lives. *The State of the World's Children 1992–3.*

United Nations Fund for Population Activities (UNFPA). 1990. Pledging Support, Sadik Warns of Breastfeeding "Trap." *Population* 16(9): 1.

————. 1991. *The State of World Population.* UNFPA.

————. 1992. *The State of World Population.* UNFPA.

United States Agency for International Development (USAID). 1987. Position Paper on Breastfeeding. Prepared for the Office of Nutrition, Bureau of Science and Technology, October.

————. 1992. A.I.D. Research and Development Abstracts. USAID 17:2.

U.S. Senate Committee on Human Resources. 1978. *Marketing and Promotion of Infant Formula in the Developing Nations.* Hearing before the Subcommittee on Health and Scientific Research of the Committee on Human Resources, Second Session on Examination on the Advertising, Marketing, Promotion, and Use of Infant Formula in Developing Nations. May 23. Washington, DC: U.S. Government Printing Office.

Wasserberger, Jonathan, G. J. Ordog, and J. J. Stroh. 1986. AIDS and Breast Milk. *Journal of the American Medical Association* 255(4): 464.

World Bank. 1991. *Annual Report.* Washington, DC: World Bank.

World Health Organization (WHO).

————. 1987. Statement from the Consultation on Breast-feeding/Breast Milk and Human Immunodeficiency Virus (HIV). Special Program on AIDS, Geneva, June 23–25.

————. 1989. Ad-hoc Group of Experts Reaffirmed the Recommendations of June,

1987. Personal letter from Dr. Nicholas Dodd, Global Programme on AIDS, WHO, Geneva.

———. 1990–91. *Safe Motherhood* (Geneva: Division of Family Health), Issue 4 (November-February).

———. 1991a. Indicators for Assessing Breast-feeding Practices. Report of an Informal Meeting, Division of Diarrhoeal and Acute Respiratory Disease Control, Geneva, Switzerland, June 11.

———. 1991b. Breast-Feeding and the Use of Water and Teas. *Programme for Control of Diarrhoeal Diseases,* no. 9 (August).

World Health Organization/United Nations Childrens Fund (WHO/UNICEF). 1990. Innocenti Declaration: On the Protection and Support of Breastfeeding: Breastfeeding in the 1990s: A Global Initiative. Florence, Italy; Geneva: WHO, August 1.

———. 1992. Consensus Statement from the WHO/UNICEF Consultation on HIV Transmission and Breast-feeding, Geneva, April 30–May 1.

Ziegler, J. B. 1988. Breastfeeding and Transmission of HIV from Mother to Infant. Report to Fourth International Conference on AIDS, Stockholm, Sweden. Book 1, Abstract 5100, p. 339.

Ziegler, J. B., D. A. Cooper, R. O. Johnson, and J. Gold. 1985. Postnatal Transmission of AIDS-associated Retrovirus from Mother to Infant. *Lancet* 1(8434):896.

# 10

# AIDS Policy and the United States Political Economy

*Michael D. Quam*

As anthropologists have found themselves working in the contemporary societies of both the Western and the non-Western worlds, they have become more intrigued by the policy questions and the arenas of policy making that dominate public life. One response has been to incorporate the methodology of ethnographic research into policy research. Indeed several years ago the American Anthropological Association published a *Training Manual in Policy Ethnography* (Van Willigen and DeWalt 1985). A second approach has been to study policy makers in action, as evidenced in several of the chapters in Carole Hill's edited volume *Current Health Policy Issues and Alternatives* (Hill 1986). As the title indicates, the authors in this latter work were not content simply to describe or analyze the policy-making process; they were doing so "for the purpose of delineating alternative policies for health care organization and delivery" (Hill 1986:1).

In that same spirit, I would like to broaden the scope of inquiry and advocacy. The classic handbook in ethnographic methods, *Notes and Queries on Anthropology,* described the anthropological perspective this way:

> Modern social anthropology lays particular stress on the interdependence of the different aspects of social life in a given society. No sociological study of a particular problem can be complete without investigating its connection with the social structure, the economic system, religion, language, and technology. . . . The interdependence of the various aspects of culture is theoretically important, and must fundamentally affect the method of investigation. (Royal Anthropological Institute of Great Britain and Ireland 1951:38)

This holistic perspective is especially well suited to an examination of the basic issues and their ramifications in most questions of public health policy, and this breadth of vision is sorely needed during this second decade of the AIDS pandemic.

## THE U.S. POLITICAL ECONOMY

For many of those working in public health, the 1980s was the decade of AIDS, but seen more broadly, the 1980s was the decade of the so-called Reagan revolution. Within the United States, and also globally, this period was marked by a radical shift in the distribution of wealth. As Phillips (1990) so amply documented, the rich became enormously richer. In 1982 in the United States there were 38,335 decamillionaires (persons with a net worth over 10 million dollars), 400 centimillionaires (persons with a net worth over 100 million dollars), and 13 billionaires. By 1988 there were about 100,000 decamillionaires (more than a 150 percent increase), about 1,200 centimillionaires (a 200 percent increase), and 51 billionaires (a 292 percent increase).

This remarkable change in the fortunes of a relative few did not occur by chance, nor because of overall economic growth. Rather, it was the result of specific governmental policies designed to achieve precisely these ends. A key element was federal tax policy. Between 1977 and 1988 the effective tax rates for the lowest income decile (tenth) of the population increased 2.5 percent, while the highest decile's rates decreased 3.1 percent. The effective tax rates for the top 5 percent of the population were lowered by 4.2 percent, and the top 1 percent of the population received the greatest benefit, with a decrease of 7.8 percent in their tax rates. Furthermore, "by 1983 the percentage of federal tax receipts represented by corporate income tax revenues would drop to an all-time low of 6.2 percent, down from 32.1 percent in 1952 and 12.5 percent in 1980" (Phillips 1990:78).

Using data compiled by the Congressional Budget Office, Shapiro and Greenstein (1991: vii–viii) summarized the dramatic effects of this policy on income distribution.

From 1977 to 1988, the average *after*-tax income of the poorest fifth of households fell 10 percent, after adjusting for inflation.

The middle fifth of households experienced an average after-tax income gain of less than four percent over this period.

By contrast, the top fifth of households realized an average gain in after-tax income of 34 percent. At the same time, the average after-tax income of the richest one percent of Americans more than doubled from 1977 to 1988, rising 122 percent after adjusting for inflation. The average after-tax income of these households reached $451,000 in 1988, up from $203,000 in 1977.

In 1988, the total after-tax income of the richest one percent of all Americans was almost as great as the total after-tax income of the bottom 40 percent of Americans combined. In other words, *the richest 2.5 million Americans now have nearly as much income as the 100 million Americans with the lowest incomes.*

This is in sharp contrast to 1977, when the total after-tax income of the bottom 40 percent of Americans was more than double the total after-tax income of the richest one percent [emphases in original].

"Supply-side economics" had succeeded in generating an enormous supply of new income for the very wealthiest segment of the population.

A second basic element in the Reagan administration's economic strategy was the defunding of social programs that benefited principally lower- and middle-class citizens and a rapid escalation in defense spending, which primarily boosted corporate profits. In 1980 spending on "human resources" accounted for 28 percent of federal outlays, while defense outlays were 23 percent of the total. By 1987 these proportions had been reversed—28 percent for defense, 22 percent for human resources (Phillips 1990:87). The impact on the poor was especially severe.

> For households in the lower parts of the income scale, reductions in government benefit programs contributed to the decline in their before-tax incomes. The data [from the Congressional Budget Office] indicate that 43 percent of the increase in poverty between 1979 and 1989 was due to reductions in benefit programs at federal, state, and local levels.
>
> Especially sharp reductions occurred in the Aid to Families with Dependent Children program, the nation's basic cash assistance program for poor single-parent families. From 1970 to 1991, the maximum AFDC benefit for a family of three with no other income declined 42 percent in the typical state, after adjusting for inflation. In fact, AFDC benefits eroded so sharply that the average value of AFDC and food stamp benefits *combined* has now fallen to about the same level as the value of AFDC benefits *alone* in 1960, before the food stamp program was created [emphasis in original] (Shapiro and Greenstein 1991:ix).

The growth in the overall federal budget combined with the shrinking revenues (due in large part to the tax-rate cuts for the upper-income brackets mentioned earlier) created the burgeoning federal budget deficit. Federal expenditures on the interest on this debt rose from $96 billion in 1981 to $216 billion by 1988 (a 125 percent increase), and those who financed this debt benefited handsomely. "Not only were upper-quintile [those in the top income fifth] Americans collecting 80 percent of the federal interest payments made to persons, but the top tax rate applicable to these receipts was falling steadily (70 percent in 1980, 50 percent in 1982, 38.5 percent in 1987, 28 percent in 1988), so that less of the money spent on interest would come back to the U.S. Treasury as revenues" (Phillips 1990:90).

Had all or most of this newly created wealth been used as capital to invest in productive enterprises that employed working people for living wages and produced necessary goods and services, the great majority of Americans might have experienced the increased prosperity promised in President Kennedy's phrase "a rising tide lifts all boats" and in the supply-side chimeras of the Reagan administration's economic policy. Instead, much of the wealth supplied to the top 10 percent of the population was used not for productive business investment in the United States, but for conspicuous consumption, "high-roller" stock manipulations on Wall Street, and investment in production facilities abroad where wages are a small fraction of the American standard, and health and safety and environmental controls are nonexistent. In fact, during this period "most of the growth in income disparities has resulted from increased inequality in *be-fore*-tax incomes. . . . The average wage and salary income of the richest one percent of Americans more than doubled from 1977 to 1988, after adjusting for inflation, rising by $130,000 per household. By contrast, the average wage and salary income of the bottom 90 percent *fell* 3.5 percent or more than $800" (Shapiro and Greenstein 1991:viii–ix). Capital-gains income for the top 1 percent also doubled, from $72,000 in 1977 to $156,000 in 1988. The rest of the population experienced a decline in capital-gains income.

For the majority of Americans, the aspirations of middle-class life have become more and more problematic (Schmidt 1990; Wilkerson 1990). Falling income, periodic unemployment, and real-estate speculation by the wealthy have made home ownership less attainable, and declining tax revenues and fiscal crisis at the government level have caused higher-education costs to rise by 33 percent in public universities (Mattera 1990), pricing college, at least on a full-time basis, out of reach for many young adults (Grassmuck 1990).

But when times get hard, they always hit lower-income people the hardest. In the past decade, as the rich became the "super rich," the poor became the "underclass." Study after study has documented the deepening and more persistently grinding poverty that has descended upon lower-income people, and especially upon women, children, and minorities (Brown 1989; Harris and Wilkins 1988; Kotlowitz 1991; Sidel 1987; Wilson 1987). The deindustrialization of the U.S. economy—the result of lower rates of productive investment at home and the export of capital to foreign production facilities (Bluestone and Harrison 1982)—and the assault upon wages as many workers laid off from industrial employment are forced to take minimum-wage jobs in the service sector (Harrison and Bluestone 1988)—figure prominently in the generation of underemployment and unemployment and the development of persistent poverty, even among the "working poor" (Shapiro 1987; Wilson 1987). In fact, according to the

U.S. Census Bureau, the poverty rate increased sharply in 1990 as 2.1 million more people sank below the official poverty line (DeParle 1991).

These shifts in the distribution of wealth and income may not be a temporary aberration, for they are an integral part of a basic transformation in the national economy (Phillips 1990). In the first half of the 1980s high interest rates in the United States attracted foreign capital to finance the mounting national debt driven by the federal budget deficits. As a result, internationally the dollar rose in value, and U.S. exports became very expensive while foreign imports became cheaper, thus creating a large trade deficit and causing a further lowering of U.S.-based production. Hundreds of thousands of people lost their jobs and their hopes for the future. In 1985 the Reagan administration adopted a policy of devaluation of the dollar, and within two years the currency lost half its value. Now not only U.S. exports, but also U.S. factories and real estate were cheaper. But the "bargain-basement" acquisition of U.S. productive property by foreign investors added very little to the national economy.

> Foreign investment created relatively few *new* jobs—about 17,500 a year between 1984 and 1986. Most of the three million Americans who worked for foreign-owned companies in 1987 held jobs that foreigners had merely acquired, not created. Foreign investment also had some outright drawbacks. Several studies showed that roughly 80 percent of the profits of foreign-owned firms were sent home from the United States to the parent company. Companies in the United States owned by foreigners also used more imported goods than did American business, thus increasing the trade deficit. According to a Department of Commerce report, foreign-owned companies in the United States were responsible for almost half the U.S. merchandise trade deficit in 1986 and a net $73.8 billion drain on American trade [emphasis in original]. (Phillips 1990:123–124)

As a result, the foreign investment position of the United States changed drastically, from a plus $140.9 billion in 1981 to a minus $532.5 billion in 1988 (Phillips 1990:130). Ironically, whatever benefits the United States might gain from foreign investment appear to be in jeopardy, as recent reports indicate that Japan, fearing a long-term decline in the American economy, is cutting back on its U.S. investments in favor of Southeast Asia and Europe (Silk 1991).

The international wealth realignment has been dramatic. Using national assets (financial assets, including stocks, bonds, deposits, and insurance, and actual assets, including production facilities, housing, land, and inventories) as a comparative measure, in 1985 the United States stood at $30.6 trillion and Japan at $19.6 trillion. By 1987 the United States held $36.2 trillion, but Japan's national wealth had risen to $43.7 trillion. Much of Japan's new economic power is financial, as indicated by the fact that of the world's ten largest banks, seven are Japanese (only one of the top twenty-five is American). The international bank assets of England, France, Germany, Italy, and Switzerland have also grown considerably during this period (Phillips 1990:118, 134–135).

How has this dramatic change in the U.S. economy affected national health policy? The Bush administration had no comprehensive health policy, and although it promised to develop one, its Secretary of Health and Human Services, Dr. Louis Sullivan, stated that it would not be rushed into any such development. The closest the Bush administration came to any comprehensive statement on the nation's health was its issuance of the document *Healthy People 2000* (U.S. Public Health Service 1991), which contained in some detail nearly 300 health objectives for the nation for the 1990s, including an entire section on HIV disease. Compared to past attempts, this document was a great improvement and could have been useful for federal, state, and local health planning. But any serious commitment by the federal government to the achievement of these objectives appeared to be absent. At the September 1990 national conference for the unveiling of the document, federal officials gave no indication that these objectives would provide direction to federal health planning or funding. According to many of the conference participants, federal officials seemed to feel that their work was completed and that the task of meeting these national objectives was the responsibility of state and local authorities.

Although it appears to be quite comprehensive, many gaps can be found in *Healthy People 2000*. None is more glaring than the total absence of any recognition that poverty is a fundamental cause of many of the health problems outlined in the document. Instead, in his keynote address at the September 1990 conference, Secretary Sullivan chose to emphasize what he called the "culture of character." While he recognized that some people experienced problems of access to health care, he blamed most health problems on ignorance and bad personal choices and called for "a nationwide priority [to be] placed on personal responsibility and choices that maintain or improve health status" (Sullivan 1990). For many listeners, these phrases were reminiscent of the "culture of poverty" formulation, discredited more than twenty years earlier (Valentine 1968), and the persistent "blaming the victim" syndrome (Ryan 1976). This "culture of character" and "personal responsibility and choices" rhetoric also provides an implicit rationale for sharply limiting the federal government's responsibility for taking action to improve the health of the nation's people.

The Reagan administration used similar ideological devices as it sought to curtail federal spending on social programs and federal regulations that protected the health and safety of workers and consumers. Under the political rubric of "federalism," it devolved responsibility to the state level at the same time that it cut federal funding to the states. Realizing at the practical level their dependence on public programs and facilities, citizens have continued to demand services, and with the federal government in retreat from its responsibilities, the states and cities have had to pick up the pieces. In fact, because of the impoverishment caused by the policies of the past decade, local authorities are faced with increased demands for public support. The burgeoning costs of Medicaid are an excellent example of this dilemma. In a precarious financial juggling act, states have had to cut programs and raise taxes (Hinds 1991a, 1991b; Pear 1991). But taxpayers' anger, quite evident in the November 1990 elections (Pear 1990a), has sharply limited the state governments' capacity to increase funding even for the most desperately needy.

The outlook is made gloomier by the current precarious state of the nation's economic health as measured by establishment indicators: declining corporate profits and increasing debt burden, a fall in real-estate values and a rise in personal bankruptcies, the collapse of the savings and loan industry and the shakiness of many banks and some insurance companies, and, at the grassroots level, rising unemployment (Berg 1991; Hershey 1991; Holmes 1991; Hylton 1990; Peterson 1991; Rosenbaum 1991; Silk 1990; Wayne 1990).

## IMPLICATIONS FOR AIDS POLICY

In the context of the current political economy, we cannot realistically expect that the United States will make ever-increasing financial commitments to international AIDS programs. Indeed, as international economic power has shifted, Japan has surpassed the United States as the leading donor of aid to the developing nations (Phillips 1990:134). The unwillingness of the United States to make international health commitments was made starkly clear at the United Nations' World Summit for Children in September 1990. The deprivation and suffering experienced by millions of children around the world is widely recognized and deplored, and the need for large-scale international campaigns to improve the lives of these children is broadly acknowledged. Heads of state and ministers of health from virtually all United Nations member states participated in this historic summit. Yet even though the meeting was held in New York, extraordinary efforts had to be made to get President Bush to agree to attend. In his address to world leaders, the president of the United States expressed his personal compassion for the needs of children everywhere, but offered no financial support for any coordinated international efforts to meet those needs. The limits of President Bush's commitment to such efforts were evident in the news reports of his participation.

> Mr. Bush disappointed the summit's organizers by skipping Saturday night's dinner and making only a token appearance at today's opening session before racing back to Washington for the culmination of his budget meetings

with Congressional leaders. The President did not sign the final declaration and action plan on a new Convention on the Rights of the Child, approved by the United Nations General Assembly last year. The Convention lays down international norms for the protection of children that governments are bound to observe. Some American conservative groups have attacked the convention because it does not outlaw abortion while banning the execution of those under 18. (Lewis 1990:A12)

The Convention on the Rights of the Child has been signed by the great majority of the United Nations member states, and bipartisan resolutions in both houses of the U.S. Congress urged President Bush to sign the convention, but he continued to refuse to do so.

At the time of the summit, a number of observers were pessimistic about President Bush's actual commitment to improving the lives of children. As Representative George Miller, chair of the House Select Committee on Children, Youth, and Families, observed, "At the same time that President Bush was at the World Summit for Children, his agents were inside the budget summit trying to cut programs that assist children" (Pear 1990b). The symbolic import of the president's reluctant and half-hearted participation in this historic meeting is clear: the United States has in effect abdicated any leadership role in world health. During that same time period, Bush was expending great personal effort and national wealth to mobilize, in part through the United Nations, an international coalition for massive military actions against Iraq and in defense of the oil-rich kingdoms of Kuwait and Saudi Arabia. In policy, actions do speak louder than words.

In the United States, AIDS activists and policy makers must make basic changes in strategy. We cannot continue to press for special status, special funding, and special attention to the problems of HIV disease. We must understand that HIV/AIDS is one of many problems that threaten the lives of Americans. The AIDS epidemic has frequently been labelled a health emergency, but it is actually a part of a much larger and more complex life emergency that is engulfing substantial portions of American society.

This fact is nowhere more apparent than in impoverished minority communities. We are highly conscious of the inequitable burden of HIV disease that is being experienced by African-Americans and Latinos, but we must also be aware that other health problems are taking an even larger toll in these communities. The mortality data from Illinois (with the sixth highest number of reported cases of AIDS and the typical racial/ethnic disparities), for example, show that the largest epidemics, in terms of death rates and years of potential life lost, among nonwhites are infant mortality (most of it not AIDS–related), violence among teenagers and young adults, and heart disease, stroke, and cancer among middle-aged adults (Ferguson 1990). The national mortality statistics show the same profile of death at an early age for nonwhites (National Center for Health Statistics 1989). In the period from 1983 to 1988, "For blacks, death rates *not* due to AIDS have increased by 23.4 percent, 6.0 percent, and 7.6 percent for the three age groups [15–24, 25–34, 35–44], respectively—figures that are nothing short of shocking" [emphasis in original] (Mangano 1991:22).

When people in low-income minority communities are asked to assess their health problems, they do not place AIDS at the top of the list. After a lengthy community health needs assessment in a low-income black neighborhood in Chicago conducted largely by the community members, the residents' final choice of priorities was poverty, drugs, and violence (Knobloch 1990). In another example, Martha Ward (1989) reported on her work in an all-black low-income housing project in New Orleans. When she asked women about the problem of AIDS, they countered that the main problem was drugs.

In these communities, where it is indeed true that the AIDS epidemic is growing rapidly, the residents seem to have a better grasp of the big picture than do many researchers and public health officials. Seen from this broader and deeper perspective, AIDS is an outcome of a complex set of interrelated "vectors of disadvantage" (Haan and Kaplan 1985:84): unemployment and underemployment, hunger and malnutrition, a lack of social services, poor schools and low educational achievement, poor sanitation, environmental pollution, inadequate housing, a lack of personal safety in the home or on the streets, a high prevalence of substance abuse, the disruption of family life, desperation and despair, and high levels of stress caused by all of these adverse conditions. In a series of insightful articles, Rodrick and Deborah Wallace have shown the synergistic interaction of all these factors in the generation of social disintegration, the spread of "contagious urban decay," and the consequent breakdown in personal and community health and in health services (R. Wallace and D. Wallace 1990; R. Wallace 1990; D. Wallace 1990). AIDS is only one of the many deadly outcomes.

The special-issue approach to AIDS is failing strategically in impoverished minority communities. AIDS prevention requires behavior change, but AIDS education efforts will not succeed in adequately changing behavior unless the socioeconomic environment that conditions behavior is also changed to facilitate and reward different behavior. Why have so many white middle-class gay men changed their sexual behavior in response to AIDS? Because for the first time they are seeing their relatively young friends and acquaintances dying all around them. But that is already the normal experience in communities of the poor, where premature death from a variety of causes is not at all unusual. To be effective in these communities, AIDS prevention programs must be integrated into broader-scale community health programs (Williams 1986) that are grounded in community socioeconomic development programs (Freudenberg 1990).

The special-issue approach to AIDS is also losing ground politically. Political leaders must be sensitive to pressures from a variety of constituencies.

In a time of shrinking resources and expanding demands, the AIDS lobby becomes just another special interest, one that, because of the stigma of AIDS, may not be politically attractive. The erosion of political support became evident during the federal budget battles of 1990. President Bush then stated in a news conference that he was not convinced that spending more money on AIDS would have any additional effect in curbing the epidemic (Reuters 1990). Congress apparently did not think that more money was the answer, either. In the appropriations process it cut the funding for several major pieces of AIDS legislation ("Appropriations Panel" 1990; "Congress Agrees" 1990). One of the senators responding to criticism of these cuts said, "All of the sympathy doesn't go to AIDS patients." In the final 1991 federal budget resolution, requested increases for AIDS funding were sharply reduced ("Panel Adds" 1990).

Many of these funding cuts came in programs to support the unusually high costs of health care for persons with HIV disease. Attempts to estimate these costs and to predict their upward trend into the 1990s have been fraught with methodological difficulties and uncertainties about the contingencies of both medical interventions and the scope of the epidemic (Scitovsky 1988, 1989). Perhaps the best estimate of national medical care costs of AIDS in 1991, because it tried to take into account the impact of the drug AZT, was $6 billion (in 1988 dollars) (Hellinger 1988). The average lifetime medical care costs of a person with AIDS are currently estimated to be $50,000 to $60,000. This figure is based on patient populations of gay men, and other data indicate that the costs of infected drug users and of pediatric cases are probably much higher. Furthermore, most of these estimates are based primarily on hospitalization costs. The costs of therapeutic interventions at earlier stages of HIV infection may be more than $5 billion annually (Arno et al. 1989). The costs of testing have not been reliably estimated.

The impact of HIV disease on the health care system is skewed by the fact that the burden is being disproportionately borne by the public sector. Scitovsky estimated that "PWAs [persons with AIDS] in 1991 [will] require between 10 and 13 percent of all public hospital beds in New York City and about one-third of all beds in San Francisco General Hospital." She added, "Clearly there is a limit to the number of beds that public hospitals can provide for PWAs because they have the obligation to provide many other essential medical services to their cities' populations" (1988:38). Reports from other cities—for example, Cook County Hospital in Chicago (White 1990)—indicate the same pressures and dilemmas.

This reliance on public hospitals and clinics is driven largely by the financial status of most AIDS patients. "In addition to the strain on their physical resources, the public hospitals also face the most serious financial problems posed by the AIDS epidemic because of the high percentage of their AIDS patients either who are covered by Medicaid, which generally reimburses the hospitals for less than their costs, or who are self-pay [i.e., uninsured], which frequently turns into uncollectible bills" (Scitovsky 1988: 38). The results are near bankruptcy in the public hospital sector. "Members of the National Association of Public Hospitals (NAPH)—over 100 hospitals across the country—averaged 30 percent operating deficits in 1988" (McKenzie and Bilofsky 1991:10–11). Green and Arno (1990) found an increasing "Medicaidization" of AIDS among patients from all ethnic groups in New York City, San Francisco, and Los Angeles. They also documented the disparity between Medicaid and private insurance reimbursement rates, pointing out that the low Medicaid payments make access to office-based primary care very difficult for many persons with HIV disease. These financial and access problems will only intensify as private insurers find more ways to eliminate from coverage persons who are HIV infected (Eden 1988).

Obviously, more money is needed for AIDS. But just as obviously, more money is needed for a whole complex of health problems that are destroying lives, especially in low-income communities. The AIDS crisis has exposed the brutal failure of the current health establishment. After years of tinkering with various organizational and reimbursement gimmicks, all designed to keep the prevailing political and economic structure of the health care industry intact (Starr 1982), the only rational and humane alternative is the establishment of a national health program. A limited patchwork system of publicly funded health insurance, such as is suggested in the "play or pay" proposals for employer-based insurance, will not effectively solve the massive problems confronting institutions and people in need of services. At best, adopting such a policy would simply expand the number of people covered under an inadequate and stigmatized Medicaid-style reimbursement system. Even the more respectable insurance of Medicare has been eroded by its constantly expanding copayments and deductibles and now only covers about 60 percent of the health care costs of its beneficiaries (McKenzie and Bilofsky 1991:10). Instead, we must have a national health program that puts money into prevention and primary care and into rehabilitative services like drug and alcohol treatment programs, and that makes health services available upon demand when and where they are needed.

The key to such a program is the system for funding its implementation. One promising proposal is the Universal Health Care Act of 1991 (H.R. 1300), introduced by U.S. Representative Marty Russo and cosponsored by over 50 of his congressional colleagues. This act calls for the establishment of a system for universal access to comprehensive health care, including preventive services (e.g., annual checkups, screenings, immunizations, and dental care), prescription drugs, long-term care, and home care, with no deductibles or copayments. Drawing much of its inspiration from the Canadian system, the Russo plan mandates that all health care services be paid for out of a single National Health Trust Fund. The federal government would establish adequate and equitable reimbursement rates for all services, and no private insurance could be sold to cover services already covered under the national universal-access single-payer system, thus eliminating any incentive for providers to maintain a two-tiered system of care. As we have seen in Canada, centralized control of funding would make possible a national budgeting system for health care, which would not only provide a more rational control over health care costs but would also make possible some realignment of priorities in health programming. The National Health Trust Fund would be funded largely through the consolidation of existing health funding by the federal and state governments, payroll taxes on employers in place of the group insurance premiums they now pay, and some additional personal income taxes on the higher income brackets.

The advantages to low-income people, the uninsured and the underinsured, and most persons with HIV disease are obvious—equal access to high-quality health services would be guaranteed. The advantages to the nation in improved health services with effective cost controls are also apparent, especially when one considers the substantial savings in administrative costs under a single-payer system.

> In 1987 health care administration cost between $96.8 billion and $120.4 billion in the United States, amounting to 19.3 to 24.1 percent of total spending on health care, or $400 to $497 per capita. In Canada, between 8.4 and 11.1 percent of health care spending ($117 to $156 per capita) was devoted to administration. Administrative costs in the United States increased 37 percent in real dollars between 1983 and 1987, whereas in Canada they declined. The proportion of health care spending consumed by administration is now at least 117 percent higher in the United States than in Canada and accounts for about half the total difference in health care spending between the two nations. If health care administration in the United States had been as efficient as in Canada, $69.0 billion to $83.2 billion would have been saved in 1987. (Woolhandler and Himmelstein 1991:1253)

Under a universal-access single-payer system, financially beleaguered hospitals and clinics would become solvent. Indeed, with adequate reimbursement for all services to all clients and patients, health services might even flourish in currently underserved communities. The U.S. General Accounting Office, in a study comparing the U.S. and Canadian systems of health care, concluded that the adoption of a single-payer universal-access system in the United States would result in the newly insured increasing their use of health services, including prevention services (U.S. General Accounting Office 1991:75–77). With the elimination of out-of-pocket expenses for health services, most individuals would also experience substantial savings and, in effect, have more money for other essentials.

The Universal Health Care Act of 1991, like the Canadian system, would leave intact the current system of private medical providers. People would continue to have the choice of which physician, clinic, or hospital to use. In fact, for many people the range of choices would expand since financial barriers to access would be lifted. Hospitals would benefit from guaranteed adequate reimbursement, but physicians' fees would be controlled through the establishment of reimbursement rates. The organized medical profession has been less than enthusiastic about this prospect, even though a universal-access single-payer system would result in large savings for private practitioners through reduced administrative costs (e.g., eligibility determinations and multiple billings) and uncollectible bills. Of course, the health insurance industry would be decimated. Given its probusiness stance, it is not surprising that the Bush administration was openly hostile to proposals that would involve government intervention in the funding and control of the health care industry. Dr. Louis Sullivan stated that he believed that the studies showing potentially large savings through reducing currently high health care administrative costs are "flawed." Apparently speaking for the Bush administration in 1991, he remained opposed to the limited "play or pay" proposal to decrease the number of uninsured people and opposed to any system of national health insurance (Associated Press 1991). Despite this predictable opposition, it remains clear that a national universal-access single-payer health system is the only means of acquiring adequate financial support for the struggle against AIDS and transcending the zero-sum game that pits AIDS advocates against the legitimate health needs of other sufferers (Krieger 1988).

## CONCLUSION

Through the first decade of the AIDS epidemic thousands of individuals have given of their time, their money, and their compassion to help stem the tide of infection and to alleviate the suffering of those who are afflicted. Their efforts have been remarkably creative and, in many cases, sacrificial and courageous. They have made a tremendous impact, and their efforts will continue to be needed in the years ahead.

In this chapter I have argued that we must see the epidemic in the larger context of developments in the U.S. political economy over the last decade, national and international realignments in the distribution of wealth, and changes in control over production that have eroded the living standards of most American citizens and undermined the ability of the federal and state governments to meet the health needs of the American people, much less international health needs. AIDS policy dilemmas will only become more intractable unless we adapt our strategies to these new challenges. We must not accept the status quo of AIDS as a special interest in competition with other health interests for recognition and a share of an increasingly inadequate resource base. AIDS advocates will not find adequate support in local communities or at the state or national governmental level unless they also become advocates for broad-based community health programs and a national universal-access single-payer health system. They will not succeed as advocates for these programs unless they also become advocates for fundamental changes in the political economy—new policies in economic development that are designed to put people back to work at living wages producing goods and services needed for the health and well-being of everyone, and especially for those whose lives have until now been blighted by social and economic deprivation.

## POSTSCRIPT

Since the final draft of this chapter was submitted for publication, Bill Clinton has become President, a new administration has taken power over the executive branch of the Federal government, and several significant changes have occurred. The President has appointed Kristine Gebbie, a highly respected public health policy expert and a leader in the fight against AIDS, to be the AIDS "czar", and she will coordinate the various federal efforts dealing with the AIDS epidemic. Funding for AIDS programs has been significantly increased. The major health policymakers in the Clinton administration have consistently acknowledged AIDS as one of our most serious national health problems.

Furthermore, President Clinton has made health care reform the top domestic policy priority of his administration and has introduced a package of legislation to implement his complex plan. Clinton's proposed reform would provide universal coverage for a broad array of health care services, including primary care, through a system of HMO-like managed care conglomerates. Cost savings would be created—hypothetically—through market competition between these provider groups. As the political battle intensifies and the profitmakers in the health care establishment begin to wield their considerable power, many competing and opposing legislative proposals have been introduced. Some of these reduce the services covered, do not provide universal coverage, or gut reform of any governmental regulatory power over fees. Even the most generous proposals would phase in universal coverage, stretching its completion date out to the end of this century. A single-payer alternative is still alive in Congress and has the support of many public health organizations. It appears to be the only plan that provides to the individual patient full freedom of choice of health care provider, a basic concern of many middle-class voters. Furthermore, single-payer is the only universal coverage plan that would actually control health care costs, primarily by dramatically reducing administrative costs. This latter virtue strikes fear in the hearts of health care bureaucrats and insurance companies. (Under the managed care plans, the private sector managers would probably be the large health insurance companies who already have the corporate expertise and bureaucracy in place to handle these new corporate entities.) Thus, Clinton and the congressional leaders have dismissed the single-payer option as politically unfeasible.

While access to medical care may be expanded under whatever reform is eventually enacted, increased funding for prevention programs that are not based in the medical care system (e.g., community health education campaigns so crucial to HIV risk reduction,) are not guaranteed adequate funding. The pressure for ever-deeper budget cuts to deal with the federal deficit will undercut support for the comprehensive community health efforts necessary to deal with HIV in the context of the myriad risks encountered by the urban poor. With federal money drying up even further, cities will have to choose between health risk reduction programs and fire protection or funding for schools.

Finally, the United States economy is now showing consistent modest growth, but this recovery has not produced any growth in jobs that pay a living wage. Unemployment figures have not significantly decreased, and in a recent study the Census Bureau found that "the percentage of all Americans working full time but earning less that the poverty level for a family of four, about $13,000 a year, has risen by 50 percent in the past 13 years" (DeParle 1994). Some of the reasons cited for this lowering of living standards were the decline of manufacturing in the U.S., globalization of the economy, and the 23 percent decline in the purchasing power value of the minimum wage.

And the United States still has not signed the international Convention on the Rights of the Child.

## REFERENCES

Appropriations Panel Rejects AIDS Support for Cities, States. 1990. *Nation's Health,* October, p. 5.
Arno, Peter S., Douglas Shenson, Naomi F. Siegel, Pat Franks, and Phillip R. Lee. 1989. Economic and Policy Implications of Early Intervention in HIV Disease. *Journal of the American Medical Association* 262:1493–1498.
Associated Press. 1991. U.S. to Meet with Major Health Insurers. *New York Times,* September 24, p. A18.
Berg, Eric N. 1991. Problems Rising for Insurers, But No Wide Collapse Is Seen. *New York Times,* July 19, p. A1.
Bluestone, Barry, and Bennett Harrison. 1982. *The Deindustrialization of America.* New York: Basic Books.
Brown, J. Larry. 1989. When Violence Has a Benevolent Face: The Paradox of Hunger in the World's Wealthiest Democracy. *International Journal of Health Services* 19:257–277.
Congress Agrees on FY91 Funds. 1990. *Medicine and Health,* October 29, p. 3.

DeParle, Jason. 1991. Poverty Rate Ross Sharply Last Year As Incomes Slipped. *New York Times,* September 27, p. A1.

——. 1994. Sharp Increase Along the Borders of Poverty. *New York Times,* March 31, p. A10.

Eden, Jill. 1988. *AIDS and Health Insurance: An OTA Survey.* Washington, DC: Office of Technology Assessment, U.S. Congress.

Ferguson, Richard. 1990. Excess Mortality in Illinois. Springfield, IL: Illinois Department of Public Health.

Freudenberg, Nicholas. 1990. AIDS Prevention in the United States: Lessons from the First Decade. *International Journal of Health Services* 20:589–599.

Grassmuck, Karen. 1990. Fewer Students from Middle Class Enrolling in College. *Chronicle of Higher Education,* November 14, p. A1.

Green, Jesse, and Peter S. Arno. 1990. The "Medicalization" of AIDS: Trends in the Financing of HIV-related Medical Care. *Journal of the American Medical Association* 264:1261–1266.

Haan, Mary N., and George A. Kaplan. 1985. The Contribution of Socioeconomic Position to Minority Health. In *Report of the Secretary's Task Force on Black and Minority Health,* vol. 2, pp. 67–103. Washington, DC: U.S. Department of Health and Human Services.

Harris, Fred R., and Roger W. Wilkins, eds. 1988. *Quiet Riots: Race and Poverty in the United States.* New York: Pantheon Books.

Harrison, Bennett, and Barry Bluestone. 1988. *The Great U-Turn: Corporate Restructuring and the Polarizing of America.* New York: Basic Books.

Hellinger, F. J. 1988. National Forecasts of the Medical Care Costs of AIDS: 1988–1992. *Inquiry* 25:469–484.

Hershey, Robert D., Jr. 1991. Second Revision Puts G.N.P. Still Lower. *New York Times,* September 27, p. C1.

Hill, Carole, ed. 1986. *Current Health Policy Issues and Alternatives.* Athens: University of Georgia Press.

Hinds, Michael deCourcy. 1991a. Cash Crises Force Localities in U.S. to Slash Services. *New York Times,* June 3, p. A1.

——. 1991b. States and Cities Fight Recession with New Taxes. *New York Times,* July 27, p. A1.

Holmes, Steven A. 1991. Governments Out of Money, Public Employees Out of Jobs. *New York Times,* March 9, p. A1.

Hylton, Richard D. 1990. Real Estate Woes Seen Worsening. *New York Times,* November 19, p. C1.

Knobloch, Stephen. 1990. Interview, October 4, Illinois Department of Public Health, Springfield, Illinois.

Kotlowitz, Alex. 1991. *There Are No Children Here: The Story of Two Boys Growing Up in the Other America.* New York: Doubleday.

Krieger, Nancy. 1988. AIDS Funding: Competing Needs and the Politics of Priorities. *International Journal of Health Services* 18:521–541.

Lewis, Paul. 1990. World Leaders Endorse Plan to Improve Lives of Children. *New York Times,* October 1, pp. A1, A12.

Mangano, Joseph. 1991. Young Adults in the 1980's: Why Mortality Rates Are Rising. *Health/PAC Bulletin* 21(2): 19–24.

Mattera, Philip. 1990. *Prosperity Lost*. Reading, MA: Addison-Wesley Publishing Company.

McKenzie, Nancy, and Ellen Bilofsky. 1991. Shredding the Safety Net: The Dismantling of Public Programs. *Health/PAC Bulletin* 21(2): 5–12.

National Center for Health Statistics. 1989. Advance Report of Final Mortality Statistics, 1987. *Monthly Vital Statistics Report,* vol. 35, no. 5, Supplement. Washington, DC: National Center for Health Statistics, U.S. Department of Health and Human Services.

Panel Adds AIDS Money to HHS Bill. 1990. *Medicine and Health,* October 29, p. 5.

Pear, Robert. 1990a. Governors Facing a Fiscal Squeeze and Tough Choices. *New York Times,* November 11, p. A1.

———. 1990b. Will the Children Really Be Helped? *New York Times,* October 1, p. A13.

———. 1991. A Double Dose of Pain for the Poor: States Struggle, Needs Rise. *New York Times,* April 7, p. E1.

Peterson, Iver. 1991. Americans Confront the Debt the House Built. *New York Times,* August 11, p. E5.

Phillips, Kevin. 1990. *The Politics of Rich and Poor: Wealth and the American Electorate in the Reagan Aftermath*. New York: Random House.

Reuters. 1990. Bush Unconvinced More AIDS Money Will Curb Epidemic. *New York Times,* September 18, p. A13.

Rosenbaum, David E. 1991. Unemployment Is at Four-Year High with Jump to 6.5 Percent Last Month. *New York Times,* March 9, p. A1.

Royal Anthropological Institute of Great Britain and Ireland. 1951. Notes and Queries on Anthropology, London: Routledge and Kegan Paul.

Ryan, William. 1976. *Blaming the Victim*. New York: Vintage Books.

Schmidt, William E. 1990. Hard Work Can't Stop Hard Times. *New York Times,* November 5, p. A1.

Scitovsky, Anne A. 1988. The Economic Impact of AIDS in the United States. *Health Affairs* 7(4): 283–284.

———. 1989. Studying the Cost of HIV-related Illnesses: Reflections on the Moving Target. *Milbank Quarterly* 67:318–344.

Shapiro, Isaac. 1987. *No Escape: The Minimum Wage and Poverty*. Washington, DC: Center on Budget and Policy Priorities.

Shapiro, Isaac, and Robert Greenstein. 1991. *Selective Prosperity: Increasing Income Disparities since 1977*. Washington, DC: Center on Budget and Policy Priorities.

Sidel, Ruth. 1987. *Women and Children Last: The Plight of Poor Women in Affluent America*. New York: Penguin Books.

Silk, Leonard. 1990. Why It's Too Soon to Predict Another Great Depression. *New York Times,* November 11, p. E1.

———. 1991. A Japanese Shift Away from the U.S. *New York Times,* September 27, p. C2.

Starr, Paul. 1982. *The Social Transformation of American Medicine*. New York: Basic Books.

Sullivan, Louis W. 1990. Healthy People 2000: Promoting Health and Building a Culture of Character. *American Journal of Health Promotion* 5:5–6.

U.S. General Accounting Office. 1991. *Canadian Health Insurance: Lessons for the United States.* Washington, DC: U.S. General Accounting Office.

U.S. Public Health Service. 1991. *Healthy People 2000.* Washington, DC: U.S. Public Health Service, Department of Health and Human Services.

Valentine, Charles A. 1968. *Culture and Poverty: Critique and Counter-Proposals.* Chicago: University of Chicago Press.

Van Willigen, John, and Billie R. DeWalt. 1985. *Training Manual in Policy Ethnography.* Washington, DC: American Anthropological Association.

Wallace, Deborah. 1990. Roots of Increased Health Care Inequality in New York. *Social Science and Medicine* 31:1219–1227.

Wallace, Rodrick. 1990. Urban Desertification, Public Health, and Public Order: "Planned Shrinkage", Violent Death, Substance Abuse, and AIDS in the Bronx, *Social Science and Medicine* 31:801–813.

Wallace, Rodrick, and Deborah Wallace. 1990. Origins of Public Health Collapse in New York City: The Dynamics of Planned Shrinkage, Contagious Urban Decay, and Social Disintegration. *Bulletin of the New York Academy of Medicine* 66:391–434.

Ward, Martha. 1989. Toward an Ethnography of AIDS: Disease, Death, and Drugs in Desire. Paper presented at the Annual Meeting of the Society for Applied Anthropology, Santa Fe, New Mexico, April.

Wayne, Leslie. 1990. Investors Decline Government Deals for Failed S. and L.'s. *New York Times,* November 14, p. A1.

White, Nina. 1990. Chicago's War on AIDS: A Report from the Front on How the City Is Coping. *Inside Chicago,* July/August, pp. 18–22.

Wilkerson, Isabel. 1990. Middle-Class Blacks Trying to Grip a Ladder While Lending a Hand. *New York Times,* November 26, p. A1.

Williams, Linda Stewart. 1986. AIDS Risk Reduction: A Community Health Education Intervention for Minority High Risk Group Members. *Health Education Quarterly* 13:407–421.

Wilson, William Julius. 1987. *The Truly Disadvantaged: The Inner City, the Underclass, and Public Policy.* Chicago: University of Chicago Press.

Woolhandler, Steffie, and David U. Himmelstein. 1991. The Deteriorating Administrative Efficiency of the U.S. Health Care System. *New England Journal of Medicine* 324:1253–1258.

# 11

# Acting Up Academically: AIDS and the Politics of Disempowerment

*M. E. Melody*

With the stealth of a practiced cat burglar, HIV crept into America's urban, gay male enclaves sometime in the early 1970s.[1] Its long incubation period guaranteed that it would spread quickly before anyone could raise the hue and cry. It was not, however, America's first experience with a deadly epidemic. Yellow fever, cholera, smallpox, and influenza had preceded it.[2]

Yellow fever struck Philadelphia in 1793. The Pennsylvania state legislature dusted off its old, colonial quarantine law and fled from the city. It enacted the measure so hurriedly that it even neglected to change the term "province" to "state." During the epidemic, husbands often deserted wives and parents abandoned children. Orphaned children wandered the streets. City government broke down. The mayor declared that the citizens must govern themselves and form a committee. Composed of twenty-six men, the committee made policy and borrowed and spent money in the city's name. Other cities and states sent aid and established quarantines. In a pattern to be repeated nearly two centuries later, "Mayor Clarkson received his real help from artisans, radicals, revolutionaries, from those whom the gentry regarded as dangerous" (Powell 1965: 191). The committee asked the Elders of the city's African Society for aid. Since the malady had not yet struck the city's African-Americans, many thought them immune. The elders toured the city and noted the horrors.

They had seen many white people acting "in a manner that would make humanity shudder." They saw a white woman demand and get £6 for putting a corpse in a coffin. They saw four white men extort $40 for bringing it downstairs. They discovered a white nurse pilfering buckles and other valuables of Mr. and Mrs. Taylor, who died together in one night. They found the white nurse of an elderly lady who had died . . . lying drunk, with one of the patient's rings on her finger, another in her pocket. And they passed a white householder who threatened to shoot them if they carried a body by his house. Soon he himself was dead and in their coffin. (*ibid.*:106)

After articulating a litany of horrors, the African Society offered assistance which the committee accepted. This breakdown of the standard social barriers of the time highlighted the committee's desperation. Nearly half the city and almost all the gentry fled. Philadelphia served as the seat of the U.S. government at the time, and the pestilence quickly reduced its ability to govern. The fever struck six clerks at the Treasury Department, three at the Post Office, and seven at Customs. George Washington, then serving as president, hurried his own departure from the city.

Philadelphia's citizen committee established a hospital, an orphanage, and a supply system. It also provided for removal of the sick and for burials. Though many nurses and doctors fled with the gentry or turned away patients, the College of Physicians, especially Dr. Benjamin Rush, tried to provide leadership. Dr. Rush's cure, however, only added to the body count. He thought that salvation lay in bleeding. Rush mistakenly believed that the body contained more than twice the amount of blood it did. The newspapers announced instructions to draw "four-fifths, or 20 pounds, of blood from patients who [in reality] contained no more than twelve" (*ibid.*: 132). Rush's own recovery from yellow fever blinded him to reality. He had drawn only twenty ounces from himself and had taken only a few of the poisonous powders. His religious faith buttressed his confidence and courage, while popular acclaim led to scientific arrogance. Philadelphians blamed refugees from the West Indies for causing the epidemic (Powell 1965).

Cholera attacked New York City in 1832, 1849, and 1866. As had happened in Philadelphia, the gentry fled along with a great many doctors and ministers. Moral reformers in New York understood the disease as a lesson. Temperance advocates, for example, viewed alcohol as a predisposing cause. The pious, on the other hand, took cholera as an exercise of God's will. It provided punishment for the nation's sins. The view that cholera served as a natural governor upon passion and indiscretion sprang from this religious view. By 1866, however, cholera was understood primarily as a social problem, not a moral one, but the older moral approach still lurked within the concept of predisposing causes. All of these approaches attempted to "manage the unmanageable . . . [to] express and reinforce social values" (Rosenberg 1987: 239). The Board of Health proved ineffective, and quarantines, as usual, did little but disrupt commerce. Once officials understood that cholera was a water-borne disease, they launched vast projects to build water works (*ibid.*).

The great influenza epidemic of 1918 killed 550,000 Americans in a mere ten months, more than all the battle deaths since 1917. It attacked women and men in their prime, as well as the old, children, and the infirm. Institutional structures, such as boards of health, proved inadequate. As in the past, extragovernmental authorities took the lead in many cities. Philadelphia's Council for National Defense (a wartime body) organized and coordinated the city's efforts. San Francisco's reaction, on the other hand, presented a "macabre comedy" (Crosby 1989:91). The masking controversy, a struggle between the chief of the Board of Health, Dr. William Hassler, and the Board of Supervisors, preoccupied the city. Many believed that wearing a gauze pad over the mouth offered protection from infection. Eventually the supervisors voted to require masking, which, in turn, sparked the formation of an Anti-Mask League. The Red Cross busily made 30,000 masks a day, while the police arrested hundreds for mask violations. The masks did little to prevent the spread of influenza. San Francisco, unlike Philadelphia, did not have a coordinating body and, consequently, squandered its resources. As had happened with yellow fever in Philadelphia, burying the dead and providing for orphans presented problems (*ibid.*).

Once HIV-spectrum disease came to medical attention on June 5, 1981, many of these earlier patterns were repeated. Scapegoating began, and rhetorical patterns paralleled the discourse about cholera in 1832. Some saw HIV-spectrum disease as the wrath of God; others took the view that it resulted from indiscretion: a violation of mores. Public fascination with the number of sexual encounters reported by some of the first persons known to have AIDS reflected the latter view. As in the past, this understanding masked a religious presupposition. Like Pennsylvania in 1793, states revisited their quarantine laws, but neglected to study their effectiveness. Florida's efforts, for example, preoccupied activists and distracted people from more fundamental issues. Like influenza, AIDS assaulted people in their prime and as a consequence had a huge social cost. One medical doctor at the National Institutes of Health (NIH), Robert Gallo, occupied a role similar to that of Benjamin Rush. As HIV-spectrum disease spread among heterosexual injecting drug users (IDUs) and their sexual partners, newly orphaned children, often HIV infected, strained already burdened foster care systems.[3] No governments fled their cities, but, as in Philadelphia, extragovernmental organizations bore the burden. Washington provided little leadership and lacked a widely accepted, comprehensive policy (Anderson 1988; Parmet 1985; Perrow and Guillen 1990; Shilts 1987).

President Ronald Reagan, unlike George Washington, did not leave town in haste. Yet he did little. His typical response to briefings was to tell anecdotes. Many of his stories had nothing to do with the matter under discussion. He also had difficulty distinguishing fiction from fact. With Reagan, stories, like movie scripts, had their own reality. In many ways, he performed as president; the office provided a role just like Hollywood.

He mainly read his script for the day from index cards. Despite the scripted rhetoric, he had few agenda items of his own (Cannon 1991: 15–87).[4]

When Reagan took office in 1981, AIDS was not yet known to the medical community. By the time he left Washington, America had 82,764 reported cases, and 46,344 had died. Reagan first gave little thought to AIDS. The death of Rock Hudson, a well-known Hollywood actor, in October 1985 changed his mind, and the president consulted his White House physician. Awareness then broke through his languor. As Reagan said then, "I always thought the world would end in a flash, but this sounds like it's worse" (*ibid.*:814). Although he remarked to a reporter that AIDS was a "top priority," he did not mention it again until February 1986. In remarks he made to employees at the Department of Health and Human Services, he said, "One of our highest public-health priorities is going to continue to be finding a cure for AIDS" (*ibid.*). Yet on the very same day, the administration's budget proposal cut funds for AIDS research. The Office of Management and Budget (OMB), however, pretended that the budget figures represented an increase, since the numbers were higher than OMB's previous requests, but lower than the amounts actually appropriated by Congress. Reagan also announced that he was asking his surgeon general, Dr. C. Everett Koop, to prepare a report, though he never requested it formally. Koop, working through Jack Svahn at the White House, had earlier tried to get the president to tie AIDS in with Nancy Reagan's drug initiative. Later, a White House contact told him that Reagan was sold on linking the issues, but that the president's "advisors were simply not interested in the president's doing anything about AIDS" (Koop 1991:204, 211).

Once the surgeon general's report was drafted, Koop had to use a subterfuge to get approval from the Domestic Policy Council. As he put it: "I would have to skate fast on thin ice to get by political appointees who placed conservative ideology above saving lives" (*ibid.*:212). At this meeting Koop provided the council with only a superficial overview, and he sensed that they had not fully absorbed the report in any depth. He also presented them with copies printed on expensive paper, knowing that they would not want to make changes in order to save the cost of reprinting the first one thousand copies. After his press conference presenting the report on October 22, 1986, the White House informed Koop that further printing would be delayed until corrections were made. A few weeks later, Gary Bauer and another White House staffer visited him and suggested an "update" (*ibid.*:212–214).

The report divided Reagan's constituency. Some of the religious right, including the Reverend Jerry Falwell and others, supported Koop's sympathetic attitude toward people with AIDS. In their fundamentalist ideology, they could, as they often said, love the sinner while hating the sin. More secular groups within the new right, however, proved very hostile. They despised homosexuals and opposed sex education.[5] Phyllis Schlafly, leader of the conservative Eagle Forum, for example, denounced the report as "incredible, multimillion dollar free publicity" for condom manufacturers, who "want to go into the schools and teach children how to engage in safe sodomy and safe fornication by the use of these contraceptives" (Cannon 1991:815). Schlafly had previously made it clear to Koop "that she would rather see promiscuous young people contract and transmit AIDS than expose her own children to the existence of condoms" (Koop 1991:218). Her attack resonated with William Bennett, then secretary of education, with Gary Bauer, a former Bennett aide who became Reagan's domestic policy advisor, and with Patrick Buchanan, then White House director of communications.[6] Before he joined the White House staff, Buchanan had written in his newspaper column: "The poor homosexuals. They have declared war on nature and now nature is exacting an awful retribution" (Cannon 1991:816).

The triumvirate, Bennett, Bauer, and Buchanan, could accept sexual abstinence as policy, but they could not bring themselves to endorse the use of condoms. Such an endorsement would appear to legitimize sex outside of marriage as well as gay male sexuality. It would also ratify the earlier separation of sex from procreation, as indicated by the development of the birth-control pill in 1960. They responded, much as others did in cholera epidemics, by reinforcing their perception of social norms. They sought to support the traditional family, together with church and community.

Arguments about the surgeon general's report continued into "round two" at a Domestic Policy Council meeting called to discuss the government's role in sex education. According to Koop, the meeting went well until Gary Bauer spoke.

> He dug out his old white notebook containing examples of bad semi-pornographic sex education material. . . . I thought it must have made the rounds of every meeting in the White House. Bauer said that he did not want his . . . [three young daughters] to hear the lurid details of anal intercourse. No one had ever suggested that they should learn this, so I spoke up. (Koop 1991:221)

The meeting ended with the "usual admonitions" for the Departments of Health and Human Services and Education to work out their differences. The "sniping" at Koop continued at another meeting of the Domestic Policy Council. This time Koop defended the "integrity of his office" and attacked those who sought to "muzzle" him. Ed Meese, then the attorney general and chair of the council, denied any attempts to silence him. "Then those who had tried to muzzle me pretended they knew nothing about it" (*ibid.*:222). By the end of the meeting, the council agreed that the government should consult on sex education, but not provide it directly. Koop thought that "some crazies had gotten to some members of the cabinet" (*ibid.*:222). Later, Koop made a trip to the West Coast, where his AIDS message was warmly received. In a phone call, he reported to Bauer that the California press had intensified its attacks on the administration for its silence on AIDS.

> Bauer lashed out, saying that Reagan and he . . . had decided to move further away from me on issues like sex education and condoms. He said the president wanted to say only one thing about AIDS: The nation was facing the problem of AIDS simply because it had abandoned traditional morality, and it would not get out of the situation until we returned to that morality. (*ibid.*: 224)

Finally, on April 1, 1987, President Reagan declared AIDS "public health enemy Number One" in a speech to the Philadelphia College of Physicians (Cannon 1991:816). Koop, though, called this a brief and superficial reference (Koop 1991:224). As Reagan went up the ramp to Air Force One at the airport, reporters shouted questions about AIDS. His reply was "Just say no!" That night NBC news reported that Reagan had not read the surgeon general's report (*ibid.*:224).

By this time Reagan was thinking of taking more of a leadership role, but he was very reluctant to speak out. Bennett and Bauer reinforced his reticence. Nancy Reagan, on the other hand, prodded him to act. The president agreed to make a speech at a dinner for the American Foundation for AIDS Research (AmFAR). Since Nancy Reagan knew that the White House had a "reactionary" speech department, she called her own favorite speech writer. In the meantime, Edward Brandt, then an assistant secretary at the Department of Health and Human Services, kept Koop politically isolated. The surgeon general could not gain access to the president despite a dozen requests. Nancy Reagan, however, arranged for Koop to attend a cabinet meeting along with his superiors at Health and Human Services. At the meeting, Koop asked Reagan to denounce the fears sparked by HIV-spectrum disease.

Nancy Reagan's speechwriter, Landon Parvin, had to negotiate approval for his text. Though Koop had spoken with Parvin, he was not involved in drafting the text. Reagan's handlers struck a passage that said that AIDS was not spread by restaurant workers. The speech retained a softened passage that stressed the unlikelihood of casual transmission. Similarly, a reference to the heroic struggle of Ryan White, a teenager with hemophilia living with HIV at the time, was deleted and replaced with a vague reference to the Ray brothers, three Florida children, who had experienced extreme AIDS discrimination including being burned out of their home. At the dinner, the audience booed when Reagan said that AIDS would be added to the list of diseases that excluded immigrants and aliens seeking residence. They booed again when he proposed mandatory HIV testing for federal prisoners (Cannon 1991:817–818).

Koop's (1991) view differed from Cannon's (1991). Koop, however, was unaware of the negotiations over the draft speech. Koop called the AmFAR speech excellent and thought that it "laid to rest the danger of mandatory testing and kept the federal government off the wrong road on AIDS." The president, as Koop saw it, did not follow the advice of his staff. Looking back, he thought that the AIDS cabinet meeting and the AmFAR speech "kept the government from doing the wrong thing on AIDS. Whether they always did the right thing is a different question" (Koop 1991:230).

The triumvirate—Bennett, Bauer, and Buchanan—fashioned AIDS policy in the same manner as other White House policies. Reagan's passivity invited policy entrepreneurs to take charge. Given their mindset, Bennett, Bauer, and Buchanan might have figured that they should not thwart nature's "retribution." Besides, their new right constituency thrived on homophobia. As Koop simply put it: "A large portion of the president's constituency was anti-homosexual" (*ibid.*:204). President Reagan himself, a congenial man, did not appear to be especially homophobic. In 1978, for example, he had opposed an initiative in California that would have prohibited lesbians and gay men from teaching in public schools. He did not believe that HIV-spectrum disease embodied the wrath of God. Yet Reagan's approach consisted of "isolated displays of conflicting symbolism" (Cannon 1991:819). For example, when he appointed his presidential commission to study AIDS, its membership included opponents of AIDS education and excluded physicians who treated people with AIDS as well as scientists doing HIV research. Some of his appointees, like John Cardinal O'Connor of New York, were notoriously homophobic. Surprisingly, the commission wrote a report that gained wide acceptance. Among other things, the commission recommended that the government make available treatment on demand for IDUs. Injecting drug users typically had to wait several months for openings in existing programs. Yet little changed. Unlike the earlier yellow fever and cholera epidemics, HIV-spectrum disease did not spark costly projects for the general welfare (Perrow and Guillen 1990; Presidential Commission on the Human Immunodeficiency Virus Epidemic 1988).

Reagan's inaction presents us with a crime of omission. After leaving office, he said: "It wasn't easy. Here suddenly was a brand-new disease and you didn't have the facts or figures" (Cannon 1991:819). In reality, he never sought the "facts or figures." He mainly left the matter to his staff.

As with most things in the Reagan White House, staffers—in this case the triumvirate—took charge. As had frequently happened, once staffers took a position, they denied opponents any access to the president. After all, Reagan might say something to undermine their position. As Koop recalled, he was cut out of the loop for five and a half years (Koop 1991:

195). So the triumvirate, especially Buchanan and Bauer, let nature take its vengeance. The administration's failure to use the 1973 Rehabilitation Act (29 U.S.C. 794) provides an example. A generous, if not honest, reading of the act would take HIV-spectrum disease—from infection to end-stage disease—as a handicap within the meaning of the law. According to the act, even the perception of a handicap was a handicapping condition. Section 504 prohibited discrimination based on a handicap or the perception of one in federal programs or any program that received financial assistance.

Especially in the early years of the epidemic, people living with AIDS faced massive discrimination. Upon diagnosis, they often lost their jobs and, consequently, their medical insurance as well as their apartments. Many people perceived all gay men to be infected and discriminated accordingly. The Rehabilitation Act would have provided some protection. The Justice Department, however, took a different view. In a memorandum from Charles Cooper, assistant attorney general, Office of Legal Council, to Ronald E. Robertson, general counsel, Department of Health and Human Services, the department found that end-stage AIDS was a handicap, but that infection with HIV was not a handicapping condition. Even an irrational fear that an HIV-positive gay man could casually spread the disease to others was not a handicapping condition. The Rehabilitation Act, as previously remarked, defined the perception of a handicap as a handicapping condition. The memorandum's metaphor of a ship in port when typhoid fever breaks out seemed to invite states to consider quarantine (Cooper 1986:33). An earlier version of the memorandum, however, leaked to the press. This draft, written by the Civil Rights Division within the Department of Justice, held that the very perception of HIV infection served as a handicapping condition. This earlier version was written by Stewart Oneglia, chief of the Coordination and Review Section, Civil Rights Division, and sent to William Bradford Reynolds, assistant attorney general, Civil Rights Division (Oneglia 1986).

If the perception of HIV infection was defined as a handicapping condition and if gay men as a group were perceived as infected, then gay men were handicapped and should have received some protection from discrimination. The triumvirate, along with Ed Meese, then attorney general, had little desire to protect gay men. Koop noted that the conservative politics of the administration led to attempts "to stir up hostility towards . . . [AIDS] victims [sic]" (Koop 1991:198). Due to the Justice Department's recalcitrance, the federal courts had to decide the issue. All of this took time and resources. In 1987 the Supreme Court settled the matter in its Arline decision (School Board of Nassau County, Florida v. Arline, No. 85-1277). Though the case itself dealt with the application of the Rehabilitation Act to tuberculosis, the Court held that Congress intended to include diseases as handicapping conditions. Though the Court did not explicitly deal with whether or not the perception of contagion was a handicap, the Justice Department relented anyway (School Board of Nassau County, Florida v. Arline, No. 85-1277, n. 7).

Congress tried to fill the policy vacuum. Subcommittees held hearings and appropriated more funds than the administration requested. Administration officials, regardless of their private beliefs, testified that enough money had been requested for AIDS research. Congress then appropriated more anyway. Since the White House sent conflicting signals, government agencies such as the CDC and NIH sometimes used AIDS to further their own organizational agendas. On funding requests, sometimes the CDC and NIH worked at cross-purposes (Shilts 1987). Congress, with its 535 members, had difficulty setting policy or imposing discipline on the federal agencies. As is usual when congressional committees wish to prod an administration, they ordered their own watchdog groups to make reports (U.S. Office of Technology Assessment 1985). Despite pressure from Congress, the administration remained calm.

In the swirl of power and passion that defines Washington, policy entrepreneurs, as they say on Wall Street, put AIDS policy "in play" (Kingdon 1984: 92–95). The White House provided no agreed-upon or widely shared policy objectives. At this point, Reagan's crime of omission became one of commission. He allowed it to happen. In fact, his passivity allowed his most homophobic advisors to create paralysis. Paul Monette, writing from his perspective as a person living with AIDS (PLWA), termed this "genocide by indifference that has buried alive a generation of my brothers" (Monette 1992:172). Simon Watney, author of *Policing Desire* and director of the National AIDS Manual (NAM UK), suggested that "such aggressive indifference to the lives of gay men is profoundly structured in the roles and relations that make up 'heterosexuality' " (Watney 1992:359). In a kinder and gentler vein, Koop noted that "the Reagan revolution brought into positions of power and influence Americans whose politics and personal beliefs predisposed them to antipathy toward the homosexual community" (Koop 1991:198). The *Oxford English Dictionary* defines antipathy to include hostile feelings as well as settled aversion or dislike. Does political science, in the recent past a value-free discipline, have an appropriate discourse that can name this reality? Theodore Lowi's *American Political Science Review* article cited a lack of passion as one of the "sins of omission" of modern political science. As he argued, "We need not worry how to speak truth to power. It is enough to speak truth to ourselves" (Lowi 1992: 6; Kuhn 1970).

Funerals, not dates, now marked the calendars of gay men. Their friends died hideously from strange diseases that had unpronounceable Latin names. Besides immunocompromised gay men, sheep were similarly affected in an epidemic in Montana. When this sheep epidemic occurred, the remedy consisted of shooting the sheep. Reagan's indifference seemed murderous and helped fill many lives with pain and suffering. Gay men, aroused by their own wrath, soon struck back. As Paul Monette put it: "Warriors in pitched battle do not make their last will; they become it." Fighting back broke the back of despair, and gay men formed a "community of the stricken who would not lie down and die" (Monette 1988a:75, 103; Monette 1988b).

Milwaukee's experience with smallpox in 1894–95 demonstrates what occurs when medical issues become enmeshed in the political process, as they did in the Reagan administration. In Milwaukee the city's health commissioner, Dr. Kempster, first clashed with the Common Council on patronage issues. He controlled twenty-six jobs and disregarded political party affiliation when he filled them. Since it was a time of economic depression and many people were out of work, council members challenged Kempster's appointments and rejected a few. When smallpox began, it became another weapon to use against the commissioner. Some elected officials used recent immigrant groups, mainly Germans and Poles, to augment their political power. When the incidence of the disease increased in June 1894, the health commissioner took standard measures such as removing patients to an isolation hospital. At first, the public cooperated with the removal, but many cases still went unreported. The disease seemed to be localized in the city's south side, the site of the isolation hospital. Residents of this crowded, immigrant neighborhood came to view the hospital as the source of their troubles. On August 5, 1894, the Health Department attempted to take another sick child to the hospital. The family had recently lost a child at the facility, and they resisted having another one removed from their home. An angry crowd, armed with clubs, knives, and stones, gathered in defense of the family. Facing a mob of three thousand angry residents, the ambulance crew retreated.

Though the local alderman, a Mr. Rudolph, was not involved in the initial incident, by the next day he began to organize the enraged citizens. On August 6 he introduced a resolution in the Common Council removing the health commissioner's power to confine patients to the hospital. Rudolph also began attending rallies and made hostile, if not incendiary, speeches. Kempster stiffened his position and told the press, "But for politics and bad beer, the matter would never have been heard of" (Leavitt 1976:559). His insensitivity combined with hubris ignited the immigrant areas on the city's south side. Mobs roamed the streets and attacked health officials standing guard at quarantined houses. Kempster came to represent arbitrary authority understood as a threat to personal liberty. Crowds even called for his execution. As a local newspaper reported, the crowds claimed that the "people's rights were paramount and should be protected, if need be, at the point of a pistol" (ibid.). Attacks continued on ambulances as well as the police. "Mobs of women armed with baseball bats, potato mashers, clubs, bed slats, salt and pepper, and butcher knives, lay in wait all day for . . . the Isolation Hospital van" (*ibid.:560*). The south-side mobs prevented any patients from being taken to the hospital. Meanwhile, the epidemic intensified. Kempster was denounced at first for removing patients to the hospital and then denounced again when the disease spread. Cooler weather in the fall tempered mob activities, but the conflict merely shifted to the Common Council. Rudolph introduced another resolution to prohibit Kempster from removing patients, which passed. Rudolph, the only elected official in contact with the rioters, convinced his colleagues that the violence would continue unless his measure passed. He reminded the members who elected them in the first place: *vox populi supremus lex*—the voice of the people is the highest law.

In October 1894, Rudolph called for an investigation and presented a list of thirty-four charges against Kempster. Twenty-eight doctors agreed to the charges of misconduct, while leading physicians and the State Board of Health supported the embattled commissioner. Rudolph chaired the committee appointed to investigate, and he found support in the immigrant press. After taking testimony, the committee recommended impeachment on nine of the original charges. After a series of disorderly meetings, the Common Council voted to dismiss Kempster. Besides Kempster's hubris, the conflict reflected ethnic and class divisions fused with disputes over power and patronage. Milwaukee's experience demonstrates how leaders during an epidemic can use social cleavages and fear to increase their power at the expense of the afflicted, as well as the incendiary nature of arrogance like that of Benjamin Rush.

HIV-spectrum disease is comparable to Milwaukee's experience with smallpox. Some elected officials in Washington, like William Dannemeyer (R-CA), sought to gain power by mobilizing heterosexist voters against gay men as a medically stigmatized group. The congressman even advocated "homocide." In an evening call to Koop's home, Dannemeyer urged the mandatory HIV testing of the entire country. The surgeon general demurred, but asked the congressman what he would do if he had a list of all HIV positive Americans. Dannemeyer replied, "Wipe them off the face of the earth!" Koop noted in his memoirs, "This attitude, I realized as I conducted my interviews on the AIDS report, although not widely voiced, was widely held" (Koop 1991:208).

New Right organizations cooperated in the stigmatization of gay men. Some of them used AIDS to raise money for their crusade to protect the family. Ironically, capitalism, taken by the new right as a gift from God, had already "undermined the material basis of the nuclear family" (D'Emilio 1983: 108). The family no longer functioned as an integrated, intergenerational economic unit. But just as the Nazis used syphilis as a standard trope for anti-Semitic politics, AIDS became one for homophobic politics. Some gay male leaders, on the other hand, sought, like Rudolph, to gain power by playing upon the fears of their terrorized constituents.

Yet most leaders, elected or otherwise, did not embrace terror for their own advantages. Medical science had gained a great deal of authority since Milwaukee's smallpox epidemic of 1894–95. Though many contrary tendencies existed, medical opinion most often channeled and legitimized political action when it came to HIV-spectrum disease. This deference to medical authority, a case of science defining political options, most often blunted the most extreme abuses. It also gave vast power to National Institutes of Health researchers. Deference to medical authority, rooted in faith in science, also allowed arrogance like that of Rush's to blossom (Leavitt: 1976: 553–568; Sontag 1979: 59).[7]

Reflecting Washington's mixed signals and the consequent frustration, AIDS activists shifted their attention to state and local levels. Besides, many of the problems they encountered had to be dealt with in their own cities. Burials, for example, required them to find local funeral directors who would prepare deceased persons with AIDS for interment. Many would not, due to an irrational fear of contagion. Some dentists dropped patients perceived to be gay. Though some medical doctors acted heroically in the early phases of the epidemic, quite a few others did not. Dropping patients served as the equivalent of flight in earlier epidemics. In this context of terror, helplessness, and discrimination, bathhouses became a preoccupation first in San Francisco and later in New York City. Entrepreneurs, who had presided over lesbian/gay enclaves along with political activists, fought closure. The battle over bathhouses split many lesbian/gay political groups and preoccupied the established activists.

Shilts (1987) made the closure controversy a centerpiece of his important book *And the Band Played On*. He suggested that bathhouse owners manipulated the lesbian/gay rights movement for their own economic advantage and gave generously to emerging AIDS-related organizations to stifle criticism. The sexual bourgeoisie, in other words, cared little for their patrons, only their pockets. Shilts also indicted the lesbian/gay press for complicity in this calculated horror. The bathhouse owners most often controlled the lesbian/gay press by means of their advertising dollars. According to Shilts, the owners destroyed the very community that supported them. As one San Francisco entrepreneur told two medical doctors: "We're both in it for the same thing. Money. We make money at one end when they come to the baths. You make money from them on the other end when they come here [San Francisco General Hospital]." The owner of the St. Mark's Baths in New York City put the ethics of banality simply: "People can do what they want to do" (Shilts 1987:154f.). He said this as he rejected a plea that he encourage safer sex and close the orgy rooms. Eventually, San Francisco and then New York City closed nearly all of their bathhouses. The Sutro Baths in San Francisco had a three day "farewell orgy." At the climax of the event, employees burned AIDS brochures. Once the bathhouses closed, attention focused more directly on the issue of "uninhibited sexuality." Some had now come to view it as a new mental illness: sexual compulsion (Altman 1986:159f; Bayer 1989:1–71; Shilts 1987).

Though the bathhouse controversy distracted from more fundamental issues, it did signal the end of the sexual fast lane. William Hoffman's play *As Is* captured the end of the 1970's gay male ethos in a reminiscence:[8]

> *Rich:* God, how I love sleaze: the whining self-pity of a rainy Monday night in a leather bar in the early spring; five o'clock in the morning in the Mineshaft, . . .
>
> *Saul:* I miss my filthy old ripped-up patched button-fly jeans that I sun bleached on myself our first weekend on the Island. Remember? It was Labor Day—
>
> *Rich:* Memorial Day
>
> *Saul:* And we did blotter acid. Remember acid before they put speed in it? And we drank muscadet when we got thirsty.
>
> *Rich:* Which we did a lot.
>
> *Saul:* Remember?
>
> *Rich:* Remember Sunday afternoons blitzed on beer?
>
> *Saul:* And suddenly it's Sunday night and you're getting fucked in the second-floor window of the Hotel Christopher and you're being cheered on by a mob of hundreds of men. (Hoffman 1985:25–26)

The end of the sexual fast lane in urban, gay male enclaves created a major change in gay male sexual politics. It also loosened the hold of entrepreneurs on these enclaves. Into this leadership vacuum poured terrorized gay males. Leadership in the previously struggling lesbian/gay groups rapidly came to depend more upon organizational expertise than prior movement experience. These new leaders were also "more savvy in the ways of getting things done" (Altman 1986:105). Though lesbian/gay political groups had previously been marginalized within the larger disempowered group of "sexual minorities," they quickly gained critical importance. Existential terror had replaced the former delights of the urban enclaves. Gay men in massive numbers confronted death, probably for the first time. Without warning, many of them as well as their partners and friends had a life-threatening condition. Conversations came to focus on treatments and medications, much like the talk around condominium pools in South Florida's Century Villages. Many gay men began reading obituaries that now appeared with frightening regularity in the lesbian/gay press. In the heterosexist press they noted the deaths of young males without spouses that listed no cause of death. Hoffman's *As Is* captured the angst.

> *Saul:* [to his ex-partner Rich] Jimmy died, as you must have heard. I went out to San Francisco to be with him the last few weeks. You must have

heard that too. He was in a coma for a month. . . . Harry has K.S. [Kaposi's sarcoma, a common AIDS-related cancer], and Matt has the swollen glands. He went in for tests today. . . . I haven't slept well for weeks. Every morning I examine my body for swellings, marks. I'm terrified of every pimple, every rash. If I cough I think of Teddy. I wish he would die. He *is* dead. He might as well be. Why can't he die? I feel the disease closing in on me. All my activities are life and death. Keep up my Blue Cross. Up my reps. Eat my vegetables. Sometimes, I'm so scared I go back on my resolutions: I drink too much, and I smoke a joint, and I find myself at the bars and clubs, where I stand around and watch. They remind me of accounts of Europe during the Black Plague: coupling in the dark, dancing till you drop. The New Wave is the corpse look. I'm very frightened and I miss you. Say something, damn it.

*Rich:* I have it. (Hoffman 1985: 8)

The character Willie in *Longtime Companion* (Reme 1990) embodies the terror of AIDS. Willie begins to take AIDS seriously when his best friend dies in 1982. In June of the next year AIDS strikes Shawn, a member of his alternative family network. When Willie first visits Shawn in the hospital, he offers his cheek, not his lips, for a welcoming kiss. He then goes to the bathroom to scrub. By 1985 Willie has changed. After Shawn dies, Willie holds his hand and weeps as they wait for the undertakers. A year later Shawn's partner dies, and Willie speaks at the memorial service. The following year both Willie and his partner, Fuzzy, work as volunteers for Gay Men's Health Crisis (GMHC). Having dealt with his own terror, Willie now works as a "buddy." The movie ends with Willie and Fuzzy contemplating their own arrests during a political protest.

As *Longtime Companion* shows, after denial and terror came anger. Numerous funerals for formerly healthy and athletic men, as well as frequent visits to intensive care units, wonderfully focused consciousness. As in earlier deadly epidemics, extragovernmental organizations provided needed services and coordination. However, unlike these earlier epidemics, AIDS-related organizations represented the afflicted organizing to serve the afflicted. During Philadelphia's yellow fever epidemic, the Africa Society was asked for assistance because African-Americans were not ill at the time and were mistakenly thought to be immune. Local governments often were preoccupied with equivalents of San Francisco's masking controversy. Arguments about mandatory HIV testing for food handlers provide one example of such preoccupations.

Mainstream media, such as the *New York Times* and the television networks, largely ignored the suffering. The media only discussed AIDS when it seemed to threaten groups journalists perceived as their audience, or if they had a personal connection to its terrors. As opposed to this silence, journalists reacted with a cacophony of headlines to Legionnaire's disease in 1976 and the Tylenol scare of 1982. Legionnaire's disease took seven lives, while the Tylenol scare directly affected twenty-nine (Kinsella 1989: 1, 4, 29).

Some Americans smirked at the anguish of gay men and spoke of God's wrath. By breaking social conventions, they had, after all, sparked nature's balancing mechanism. Many other Americans proved indifferent early in the epidemic. A CBS News/*New York Times* poll asked a national sample of Americans, "How much sympathy do you have for people who have AIDS—a lot, some, or not much?" When the question was asked this way, 51 percent said a lot, 33 percent answered some, 9 percent said not much, and 2 percent replied none. Five percent did not respond. When the phrasing of the question was changed to include a reference to sexual transmission, the responses differed dramatically. When asked, "How much sympathy do you have for people who get AIDS from homosexual activity—a lot, some, or not much" only 19 percent said a lot, and 20 percent replied some. With the reference to homosexual activity included, 42 percent replied not much, and 18 percent said none. One percent did not respond. As an abstract, medical issue, 84 percent of the sample had some or a lot of sympathy for PLWAs, but only 39 percent had any sympathy for a gay PLWA (Sherrill 1991:14,15).

In 1982 Larry Kramer, Paul Popham, and others formed a committee in New York City to begin a counterattack. Over Labor Day weekend they tried to raise awareness as well as collect donations. They stood at the door of the Ice Palace, a large gay disco on Fire Island, a gay resort community on Long Island within commuting distance of New York City, from midnight till 8:00 A.M. They collected a mere $126 from the thousands of dancers. The committee also attempted to collect donations at other locations on Fire Island. Despite several appeals, the Pines Pavilion, another gay disco, would not allow them to solicit on the premises. All told, the committee's efforts brought in less than $800. The committee soon became Gay Men's Health Crisis (GMHC). The founders included Nathan Fain, Dr. Lawrence Mass, Paul Popham, Paul Rapoport, Edmund White, and Larry Kramer. As the body count grew, so did GMHC. Today, GMHC is the world's largest AIDS-related organization, owns its own building in Manhattan, and has a multimillion-dollar budget as well as a large staff. Million-dollar fundraisers are now common (Altman 1986:93; Kramer 1989:3–23).

GMHC attracted many new activists mobilized by this terror. It also had to confront both internal and external homophobia. Early disputes within GMHC included whether or not to print the full name of the organization on return envelopes or merely the initials. Though Larry Kramer and Paul Popham were good friends at the time, they found themselves on opposite ends of these disputes. Kramer almost always advocated a confrontational approach, especially with elected officials, while Popham wanted to work within the system. These constant disputes drove them apart, but they re-discovered their friendship before Popham died. Over time, GMHC came to focus primarily on a social service role, one Kramer called "pastoral," while political concerns mainly comprised secondary issues. Eventually, GMHC's board forced Kramer to leave the organization, and he then fo-cused more on what became a prophetic role. In his "Oh, My People" address to the Human Rights Campaign Fund dinner in 1987, Kramer eloquently called gay people to action (Altman 1986:86; Kramer 1985:57–59, 1989:186–192).

GMHC also helped struggling AIDS-related organizations in other cities by sharing its expertise. These AIDS-related organizations also attracted many women who already worked in social services or had organizational skills. The horrors faced by dying gay friends mobilized many more. Most of these women had previously had their consciousness raised. They knew, as radical feminists had said more than a decade earlier, that the personal was political, and that systems of oppression were rooted in consciousness as well as institutions.

Empowered by racial privilege, with many enjoying high incomes and social status, gay men had little trouble organizing corporations or raising large sums of money once most heard the alarm. But as the early disputes within GMHC demonstrated organizing around AIDS issues forced them to "come out." As empowered men, most of them privileged by race, they took action. In doing this, however, they confronted a heterosexist culture that forced them to deal with their disempowerment as a doubly stigma-tized minority. They were both gay and diseased. As a disempowered, dou-bly stigmatized group, gay men discovered, to an extent, that they were all devalued like women. Though disempowered, many gay men would not await death quietly or gently. Paul Popham, for example, a former Green Beret and bank executive, partially came to this truth in his near-death reconciliation with Larry Kramer.

Though he was forced by his fellow board members to leave GMHC, Kramer continued in his prophetic role, always stridently calling attention to the need for political action. A speech he delivered at New York City's Gay and Lesbian Community Center on March 10, 1987, led to the for-mation of the AIDS Coalition To Unleash Power (ACT UP). In this speech he quoted the then very ill Paul Popham: "Tell them we have to make gay people all over the country cooperate. Tell them we have to establish some way to cut through all the red tape. We have to find a way to make GMHC, the AIDS Action Council, and the other AIDS organizations stronger and more political" (Kramer 1989:133). Kramer went on to note that the con-servative surgeon general, Dr. C. Everett Koop, had become an ally.

Koop said, "We have to embarrass the administration into bringing the re-sources that are necessary to deal with this epidemic forcefully." He said a meeting has been arranged with the President several times, and several times this meeting has been canceled. His own Surgeon General is telling us that we have to embarrass the President to get some attention to AIDS. (*ibid.*: 136).

Two days after this speech, around three hundred activists held another meeting and launched ACT UP. The new organization originally intended to fight for release of experimental drugs. Within two weeks it had already staged its first demonstration attacking the Food and Drug Administration (FDA). Since 1987 ACT UP has launched more than fifty chapters in other cities. A strident, angry group, its members chant: "Act up/Fight back/Fight AIDS." During a protest march in Washington, they chanted: "Two, four, six, eight/Ronnie thinks his son is straight" as they passed the White House. As the organization grew, the agenda came to include all AIDS-related issues. As ACT UP members commonly say, they are "a diverse group of individuals united in anger and committed to direct action to end the AIDS crisis." They do not function, however, as a lesbian/gay rights group.

As an organization, ACT UP improves upon participatory democracy, an early New Left ideal in the 1960s. New York/ACT UP, for example, comprises a variety of caucuses and affinity groups. Individuals and sub-groups can undertake actions on their own. Approval is required only if a group wants to use ACT UP's name or requires money. Meetings are open. Facilitators, not elected officers, guide the discussions, and anyone can have the floor briefly. During one demonstration in New York City, a police captain asked a group of marchers, arms linked fifteen abreast, who was the leader. "We're all the leader. None of us is the leader. If you want to talk, you have to talk to all of us" (Minkowitz 1990:20). In addition to making infiltration difficult, ACT UP's organized chaos allows the full talents of its various affinity groups to shine without any bureaucratic mediation. ACT UP's structure also encourages participation, while it provides no structure to capture in a hostile takeover. Using facilitators, as opposed to elected leaders, also minimizes power struggles over microphones and other things. Hierarchical organizations, while probably more efficient, would tend to be oligarchic and nonempowering. ACT UP has also sparked the formation of CAN ACT, a group of cancer survivors. ACT UP now seeks to mobilize a "broad coalition of activist patients who face a range of life-threatening diseases" (d'Adesky 1991:158).

Gran Fury, one of ACT UP's subgroups, serves as its "unofficial propaganda ministry and guerrilla graphic designers" (Crimp and Rolston 1990: 16). Named after the car model New York City police use for undercover work, Gran Fury created ACT UP's now-familiar SILENCE=DEATH logo. On a stark, black background, the poster presents a pink triangle in the top center of the frame. In Nazi Germany's concentration camps inverted pink triangles identified gay men (Heger 1980). The image implicitly links

AIDS with Hitler's attempted extermination of gay men. Below the triangle in white letters, the image presents the seemingly simple equation SILENCE=DEATH. Silence in the AIDS epidemic, much like silence during the Holocaust, leads to death. Implicitly, the poster suggests that silence, on the part of those "at risk" as well as the "general public," is complicitous. Another poster designed by Gran Fury displays an erect penis in the center of the frame. At the top of the poster, above and to the right of the phallus, the text reads: "SEXISM REARS ITS/UNPROTECTED/HEAD." In smaller type, below the penis and to the left, the poster says: "MEN:/ Use Condoms/Or beat it" (Crimp and Rolston 1990:63). Queer Nation, which originally began as another ACT UP affinity group, specializes in antihomophobic actions and serves as a "strike force for gay and lesbian liberation" (Minkowitz 1990:22). Queer Nation has since separated from ACT UP and has rapidly grown into a new national organization with chapters in major cities.

Much like the African-American statement that black is beautiful in the 1960s, members of Queer Nation take a term of oppression ("queer") and turn it into an affirmation. Consisting mainly of younger lesbians and gay men, Queer Nation treats AIDS and homophobia as a single issue. In unifying these issues, Queer Nation has attracted a great many lesbians who have difficulty mobilizing around ACT UP's more narrow AIDS agenda. Queer Nation is "trying to combine contradictory impulses: to bring together people who have been made to feel perverse, queer, odd, outcast, different and deviant, and to affirm sameness by defining a common identity on the fringes" (Berube and Escoffer 1991:12, 14). In this new dialectic they are torn between affirming their "queer" identity and rejecting restrictive categories as well as assimilation, while seeking recognition by heterosexist society. In designing political actions, Queer Nation emphasizes individuals confronting individuals, not institutions like the FDA. Among other things, its members hold kiss-ins in heterosexist bars, and they chant, "We're here/We're queer/Get used to it" (Chee 1991:15–17, 19; Maggenti 1991:20–23; New York Times 1991b).

Looking back at these events in 1991, the National Commission on Acquired Immune Deficiency Syndrome framed America's choice starkly: either engage the issue or face an expanding tragedy. Front-line workers face constrained resources, and their logistics are crippled "by the sabotage of disbelief, prejudice, ignorance, and fear." "Worst of all, the country has responded with indifference. It is as if the HIV crisis were a televised portrayal of someone else's troubles." The commission reminded America to honor its fundamental social contract with all its citizens. It implicitly faulted the Reagan and Bush administrations. "Our nation's leaders have not done well. In the past decade, the White House has rarely broken its silence on the topic of AIDS." It went on to fault Congress for not fully funding programs. "Articulate leadership guiding America toward a proper response to AIDS has been notably absent." The commission found two destructive attitudes at large in the country. The first is the view that PLWAs somehow deserve what is happening to them, while the second comprises an indifference to their fate. The commission went on to call for the national leadership to overcome "governmental inertia" and insisted that the epidemic cannot be understood apart from the "context of racism, homophobia, poverty, and unemployment." HIV-spectrum disease represents a "synergy of plagues" (National Commission on Acquired Immune Deficiency Syndrome 1991:1–14).

Discrimination, as the commission noted, has not disappeared. It "reflects the racism and homophobia that pervade our society." Education efforts have been "stymied by an unwillingness to talk frankly about sexual and drug use behaviors." As the surgeon general tried to tell the Domestic Policy Council, "Constraints on discussions of sex whether imposed by law, political considerations, issues of morality, language, or culture, have been a substantial barrier to the creation and implementation of effective HIV prevention programs." Withholding potentially lifesaving information is what the commission termed a "serious ethical problem"—itself an interesting understatement (ibid.:14,21).

Ever since yellow fever arrived in Philadelphia in 1793, deadly epidemics have had a political dimension as well as a biological one. America, simply put, has never dealt well with epidemics. Extragovernmental organizations have typically borne the burden. City and state governments become preoccupied with equivalents of San Francisco's masking controversy. Despite the vast centralization of power in Washington following World War II, the national government has not performed remarkably better. The Tuskegee syphilis experiment (Jones 1981) as well as the swine flu panic of 1976 provide examples (Etheridge 1992:247–267). This inability to govern effectively according to rational public policy norms partially reflects the system's democratic nature. Elected representatives, often battered by terrorized constituents, enact measures to assuage inflamed public opinion. These measures may or may not prove scientifically sound. Thus San Francisco enacted a statute requiring masking, which, in turn, generated an antimasking league. The police made arrests. Yet AIDS adds a level of complexity to the typical pattern. HIV-spectrum disease, like smallpox in Milwaukee, presents us with a politicized epidemic. Unlike Milwaukee, this politicization reflects not only power issues, but also "moral" ones. This moral dimension precluded concerted political action by the Reagan and Bush administrations. AIDS also jolts America's collective memory of its Puritan and Christian heritage and, consequently, causes dissonant feelings, much like other sexually transmitted diseases.[9] HIV-spectrum disease represents a new pattern: power considerations conjoined with an implicit "politics of righteousness." This new pattern, along with idiosyncratic factors such as President Reagan's temperament, accounts for America's ambivalent response to AIDS.

Reflecting his early perception of the "politics of righteousness," Shilts (1987) argued that the epidemic was allowed to happen. His book became a listing of villains and an enumeration of their crimes. In many ways his claim is true. Once HIV-spectrum disease became politicized like abortion, norms other than those of rational policy making took hold. AIDS quickly became a partisan issue, though only a few officials would admit this.[10]

For the New Right and conservatives in general, AIDS became a marker for much of what was wrong with America. It symbolized the evils wrought by Columbia's turn from traditional values. To them, discouraging teenage sexual activity proved a higher value than protecting them from a deadly disease. They would not support a policy that distributed condoms to high-school students, regardless of the fact that most of these students were already sexually active. The 1992 Southern Baptist Convention provides an example. Delegates of the 15.2 million-member church resolved that "forced availability of birth control devices to minors . . . endangers the health and lives of children and is a violation of the rights of the family." Though Southern Baptists have always respected the autonomy of individual congregations, the delegates also ostracized two churches for "accepting homosexuality," while they praised the Boy Scouts for retaining the reference to God in the "Scout's Oath" and for barring gay adolescents from membership (*Miami Herald* 1992a). AIDS implicitly functions for conservatives as their God's wrath, as a penalty for immoral acts. As is widely known, the New Right consists mainly of Republican party identifiers. According to press accounts, Gary Bauer, in his new role as president of the Family Research Council, a Christian lobbying group, inspired Dan Quayle's speech to the Southern Baptist Convention. The vice president urged the delegates to fight to preserve traditional family values. The delegates gave Quayle a standing ovation (*Miami Herald* 1992b).

On a theoretical level, the religious right tends to conflate its religious community with the political one. For them, its supporters, the community of believers establishes the proper, God-given norms for the larger political community and serves as an exemplar of "the Way, the Truth, and the Life." They confound the city of (their) God with the city of Man—an enduring problem for groups defined by faith (Saint Augustine 1950)—and implicitly hold that the numerically smaller group of believers is the true representative of society. Their theocratic representation of truth is implicitly antidemocratic and antimajoritarian. At the extreme, the prolife group Operation Rescue demonstrates the clash between God's truth and a society grounded in individual rights. Truth, they believe, even by force, overrides an individual's choice. Believers not merely have an obligation to proselytize, but are also justified in using violence to prevent what they consider evil.

Liberals, mainly Democratic party identifiers, support AIDS research and social service programs, which allows them to shift the lesbian and gay rights agenda to medical issues, rather than political ones such as discrimination. This approach, with its focus on compassion, alienates fewer mainstream voters while it retains the support of lesbians and gay men. In reality, lesbians and gay men have few political options. Queer Nation's demonstration at the 1992 Academy Awards ceremony in Los Angeles provides an example. Queer Nation sought to use the occasion to protest Hollywood's sexism and homophobia. The academy responded by merely reversing a recent policy and allowed the stars to wear red ribbons to dramatize the plight of PLWAs. The original complaint about institutionalized sexism and homophobia got lost amidst a sea of red ribbons.

AIDS-related organizations will continue to bear an enormous social service burden. Even with a change in administration, the budget deficit, approaching 400 billion dollars in 1992 alone, will probably preclude massive funding for all that needs to be done. ACT UP will continue to use direct action to spark change. Unless new, effective therapies are approved soon, the anger of ACT UP's members, many of whom are HIV positive, will only grow more intense. Though some activists may drift into passivity, others may seek to escalate ACT UP's direct action approach as more and more of their partners and friends lapse into end-stage disease. ACT UP's decision-making system, however, will eventually limit direct action. The consensus-formation process can provide every assertive member with a veto over officially sponsored actions. Participatory democracy, an enduring organizing principle in radical groups, has never led to effective organizations in the long run (Epstein 1991). New reports, meanwhile, remind us that HIV-spectrum disease is a global catastrophe of immense proportions (*New York Times* 1992).

## NOTES

1. In this chapter I deal with HIV-spectrum disease not only as an epidemic—a medical or biological phenomenon—but also as a plague, the personal experience of a sudden, deadly epidemic. Though I originally intended to write a comprehensive study of the politics of AIDS, I have since abandoned this particular project. Besides issues of identity politics, the literature expands rapidly, and a comprehensive work requires the bridging of far too many academic fields. Even though the politics of AIDS explicated in this chapter impacts all the "risk groups," I am primarily focusing on the experience of gay white men. This chapter, though, is a part of a much larger work dealing with the politics of AIDS as it impacts on this group. An earlier version was delivered as a paper at the 1992 Annual Meeting of the American Political Science Association, Chicago, Illinois, September 3–6, 1992 (also see Melody 1993). This chapter is in memory of Craig Wanner.

2. For a contrary view on the use of these historical analogies, see Fee and Fox (1992:1–18). They argued that since HIV-spectrum disease is actually a chronic

condition, the appropriate analogies are to other long-term diseases such as cancer. As Fee and Fox acknowledged, their argument reflects one's personal perspective. Though studies of the politics of cancer and other chronic diseases are useful, HIV-spectrum disease, unlike cancer—according to present medical knowledge—is infectious. Deadly infectious diseases, especially sexually transmitted ones, produce a distinct style of politics (see Brandt 1985). Besides, in the early days of the epidemic that are dealt with in this chapter, gay-related immune deficiency (GRID), one of the earliest names for the syndrome now called AIDS, was not known to be chronic.

3. AIDS discourse often masks biases as well as distortions. For example, much more is implied in the term *injecting drug user* than the literal meaning of the words. Though this designation has become conventional and is certainly more acceptable than many others, it masks racist and classist biases. In a related manner, the term '*risk groups*,' strictly speaking, has no normative content.

4. It seems anomalous that such character traits could mark a person holding the presidency. Though President Reagan left office relatively recently and the record is not nearly complete, most of the reliable accounts support these observations. On the whole, I have followed Lou Cannon's (1991) detailed narrative of the Reagan administration. Cannon, a journalist for the *Washington Post,* has studied Reagan since his days as governor of California. Cannon incorporated interviews with Reagan, insider accounts of the administration, and the work of other journalists and informed commentators as well as his own observations.

Early intimations that something was different in the Reagan administration can be found in Stockman's (1986) insider account. In his role as director of the Office of Management and Budget (OMB), Stockman first drew notice to Reagan's lack of attention as well as his passivity. Though she wrote in a much friendlier tone, Peggy Noonan (1990), a White House speechwriter, corroborated some of Stockman's earlier observations. Even she, a true conservative, had to demur in some ways from the popular persona of Reagan. Garry Wills (1987), a journalist and writer for the *New York Review of Books,* first reflected upon some of the anomalies associated with Reagan's character, and also documents Reagan's confounding of fiction with fact. Cannon incorporated and expanded upon Wills's insights. Neither Reagan (1990) nor Meese (1992) listed AIDS, HIV-spectrum disease, or human immunodeficiency virus in their index or table of contents. For an insightful commentary based on Noonan's account, see Didion (1992:25–46).

5. The term *homosexual* flows from the medical model developed in the late nineteenth century. This view considers lesbians/gay men as mentally ill or, at best, deviant. Most lesbian and gay rights groups reject the term as embodying heterosexism's normative power. I am following Sedgwick (1990) in the use of the terms *heterosexist* and *heterosexism.*

6. Since leaving the White House, Buchanan has become a television commentator on Cable News Network (CNN) and then a presidential candidate, while Bauer serves as president of the Family Research Council, an influential, conservative lobbying group.

7. See *Miami Herald* 1991 for Rush-like politics and *New York Times* 1991a for scientific arrogance.

8. Gay male "promiscuity" (a term that badly needs an objective definition) must be viewed in the wider context of heterosexist "promiscuity" and serial monogamy as well as the generalized eroticization of our bourgeois culture. Sexualized

images of young girls, for example, are now commonly used to sell various products. In my larger study, I place this perspective within its proper context.

9. Whether or not America is (or ever was) a Christian nation has become an issue in presidential politics. For a view contrary to my own, see Wills (1990).

10. Besides writing a history of the early days of the epidemic, Shilts provided interwoven accounts of the lives of several PLWAs. In this sense, he wrote a novel as well as a history, and the novel is decidedly gothic and redemptive. His novel as well as his scapegoating of "Patient Zero" have been widely criticized. See, for example, Miller 1992:257–271.

## REFERENCES

Altman, Dennis. 1986. *AIDS in the Mind of America*. Garden City, NY: Anchor Press/Doubleday.

Anderson, Bonnie M. 1988. Locking Up AIDS Carriers Won't Solve the Problem. *Miami News,* February 5.

Augustine, Saint. 1950. *The City of God*. New York: Modern Library.

Bayer, Ronald. 1989. *Private Acts, Social Consequences*. New York: Free Press.

Berube, Allan, and Jeffrey Escoffer. 1991. Queer/Nation. *Outweek* 11(Winter): 12, 14.

Brandt, Allan. 1985. *No Magic Bullet*. New York: Oxford University Press.

Cannon, Lou. 1991. *President Reagan: The Role of a Lifetime*. New York: Simon and Schuster.

Chee, Alexander. 1991. A Queer Nationalism. *Outweek* 11(Winter): 15–17, 19.

Cooper, Charles. 1986. Application of Section 504 of the Rehabilitation Act to Persons with AIDS, AIDS-related Complex, or Infection with the AIDS Virus. Memorandum to Ronald E. Robertson, Department of Justice.

Crimp, Douglas, with Adam Rolston. 1990. *AIDS Demo Graphics*. Seattle: Bay Press.

Crosby, Alfred W. 1989. *America's Forgotten Pandemic: The Influenza of 1918*. Cambridge: Cambridge University Press.

d'Adesky, Ann-Christine. 1991. Empowerment or Co-optation? *Nation,* February 11, pp. 158–160.

D'Emilio, John. 1983. Capitalism and Gay Identity. In *Powers of Desire*, ed. Ann Snitow et al. New York: Monthly Review Press. pp. 100–113.

Didion, Joan. 1992. *After Henry*. New York: Simon and Schuster.

Epstein, Barbara. 1991. *Political Protest and Cultural Revolution*. Berkeley: University of California Press.

Etheridge, Elizabeth. 1992. *Sentinel for Health: A History of the Centers for Disease Control*. Berkeley: University of California Press.

Fee, Elizabeth, and Daniel Fox. 1992. *AIDS: The Making of a Chronic Disease*. Berkeley: University of California Press.

Heger, Heinz. 1980. *The Men with the Pink Triangle*. Boston: Alyson Publications.

Hoffman, William M. 1985. *As Is*. New York: Random House.

Jones, James. 1981. *Bad Blood*. New York: Free Press.

Kingdon, John. 1984. *Agendas, Alternatives, and Public Policies*. Boston: Little, Brown and Company.

Kinsella, James. 1989. *Covering the Plague: AIDS and the American Media.* New Brunswick: Rutgers University Press.

Koop, C. Everett. 1991. *Koop: The Memoirs of America's Family Doctor.* New York: Random House.

Kramer, Larry. 1985. *The Normal Heart.* New York: New American Library.

———. 1989. *Reports from the Holocaust: The Making of an AIDS Activist.* New York: St. Martin's Press.

Kuhn, Thomas. 1970. *The Structure of Scientific Revolutions.* 2nd ed. Chicago: University of Chicago Press.

Leavitt, Judith. 1976. Politics and Public Health: Smallpox in Milwaukee, 1894–1895. *Bulletin of the History of Medicine* 50: 553–568.

Lowi, Theodore. 1992. The State in Political Science: How We Became What We Study. *American Political Science Review* 86(March): 1–7.

Maggenti, Maria. 1991. Women as Queer Nationals. *Outweek* 11(Winter): 20–23.

Meese, Edwin. 1992. *With Reagan: The Inside Story.* Washington, DC: Regnery Gateway.

Melody, M. E. 1993. Breaking through to the Other Side: The Making of 'Erotic Politician,' unpublished paper presented at the annual meeting of the American Political Science Association, Washington, DC, September 1–5.

*Miami Herald.* 1991. AIDS Crusaders Spending Draws Fire As Agency Struggles to Pay Its Staff. June 30, p. 1A.

———. 1992a. Baptists Blast Distribution of Condoms at Public Schools. June 12, p. 4A.

———. 1992b. Churches Lead Campaign to Restore Traditional Values. June 14, p. 4A.

Miller, James. 1992. AIDS in the Novel: Getting It Straight. In *Fluid Exchanges: Artists and Critics in the AIDS Crisis,* ed. James Miller. Toronto: University of Toronto Press. pp. 257–271.

Minkowitz, Donna. 1990. ACT UP at a Crossroads. *Village Voice,* June 5.

Monette, Paul. 1988a. *Borrowed Time: An AIDS Memoir.* New York: Harcourt Brace Jovanovich.

———. 1988b. *Love Alone: 18 Elegies for Rog.* New York: St. Martin's Press.

———. 1992. *Becoming A Man: Half a Life Story.* New York: Harcourt Brace Jovanovich.

National Commission on Acquired Immune Deficiency Syndrome. 1991. *America Living with AIDS: Report of the National Commission.* Washington, DC: U.S. Government Printing Office.

*New York Times.* 1991a. American Drops Claim of Finding AIDS Virus. May 31, p. A8.

———. 1991b. Amid Hoopla, New York's Gay Parade Halts to Remember AIDS Dead. July 1, p. B12.

———. 1992. Researchers Report Much Grimmer AIDS Outlook. June 4, p. A1.

Noonan, Peggy. 1990. *What I Saw at the Revolution: A Political Life in the Reagan Era.* New York: Random House.

Oneglia, Stewart. 1986. Coverage of Acquired Immune Deficiency Syndrome (AIDS) under the Rehabilitation Act of 1973. Draft Memorandum to William Bradford Reynolds, Department of Justice.

Parmet, Wendy E. 1985. AIDS and Quarantine: The Revival of an Archaic Doctrine. *Hofstra Law Review* 14:53–90.

Perrow, Charles, and Mauro Guillen. 1990. *The AIDS Disaster*. New Haven: Yale University Press.

Powell, J. H. 1965. *Bring Out Your Dead: The Great Plague of Yellow Fever in Philadelphia in 1793*. New York: Time-Life Books.

Presidential Commission on the Human Immunodeficiency Virus Epidemic. 1988. *Report of the Presidential Commission on the Human Immunodeficiency Virus Epidemic*. Washington, DC: The Commission.

Reagan, Ronald. 1990. *An American Life*. New York: Pocket Books.

Reme, Norman. 1990. *Longtime Companion*. Companion Productions. Film.

Rosenberg, Charles E. 1987. *The Cholera Years: The United States in 1832, 1849, and 1866*. Chicago: University of Chicago Press.

Sedgwick, Eve. 1990. *The Epistemology of the Closet*. Berkeley: University of California Press.

Sherrill, Kenneth. 1991. Half Empty: Gay Power and Powerlessness in American Politics. Paper presented at the Annual Meeting of the American Political Science Association, Washington, DC.

Shilts, Randy. 1987. *And The Band Played On: Politics, People, and the AIDS Epidemic*. New York: St. Martin's Press.

Sontag, Susan. 1979. *Illness as Metaphor*. New York: Vintage Books.

Stockman, David A. 1986. *The Triumph of Politics: How the Reagan Revolution Failed*. New York: Harper and Row.

U.S. Office of Technology Assessment. 1985. *Review of the Public Health Service's Response to AIDS*. Washington, DC: U.S. Government Printing Office.

Watney, Simon. 1992. The Possibilities of Permutation: Pleasure, Proliferation, and the Politics of Gay Identity in the Age of AIDS. In *Fluid Exchanges: Artists and Critics in the AIDS Crisis*, ed. James Miller. Toronto: University of Toronto Press. pp. 329–367.

Wills, Garry. 1987. *Reagan's America: Innocents at Home*. Garden City, NY: Doubleday.

———. 1990. *Under God*. New York: Simon and Schuster.

# 12

# Ethnography, Epidemiology, and Public Policy: Needle-Use Practices and HIV-1 Risk Reduction among Injecting Drug Users in the Midwest

*Robert G. Carlson, Harvey A. Siegal, and Russel S. Falck*

In an article on HIV-1 in the United States, Curran and colleagues (1988: 613) perceptively stated that "the national course of HIV infection might best be viewed as a composite of many varied, partially overlapping 'subepidemics, each with its own rate of speed." The existence of numerous subepidemics, each with its own dynamic trajectory, is particularly evident among injecting drug users (IDUs), who make up the second largest risk group for HIV-1 in the United States as reflected in national AIDS statistics (Centers for Disease Control 1991:9; Des Jarlais and Friedman 1988). HIV-1 seroprevalence rates differ significantly among IDUs in localized geographic regions from a high of greater than 50 percent seropositive in some boroughs of New York City (e.g., Friedland 1989:159; Kleinman et al. 1990:346) to a low of 3 percent or less seropositive in places such as Seattle, Washington (Calsyn et al. 1991:187), and San Antonio, Texas (Hahn et al. 1989:2679; Zule, Vogtsberger, and Desmond 1990:38).

Regardless of the geographic variability in HIV-1 seroprevalence rates among IDUs, and in view of the absence of a vaccine or cure for AIDS, prevention of new infections has been a major public health initiative. Prevention among IDUs, their sex partners, and their unborn children has been based primarily on community outreach programs designed to educate those at risk about the very real threat of HIV-1 disease, to convince them to stop exchanging injection equipment (best achieved through a complete cessation of drug injection), to decontaminate their hypodermic needles by rinsing them with bleach, and to adopt safer sex techniques (see, e.g., Battjes and Pickens 1988; Brickner et al. 1989; Chaisson et al. 1987; Friedman, Des Jarlais, and Goldsmith 1989; Leukefeld, Battjes, and Amsel 1990; Miller, Turner, and Moses 1990; Newmeyer 1988). Additional interventions have included attempts to encourage the self-help organization of IDUs and experimental hypodermic-needle-exchange programs (see, e.g., Friedman, Des Jarlais, and Goldsmith 1989:104; Singer, Inizarry, and Schensul 1991).

Each of these intervention strategies raises policy issues in part because the risk behaviors themselves are either illegal and clandestine, or private and intimate, or both. AIDS has forced society to examine and attempt to alter behaviors that were largely ignored and left to thrive in the interstices and margins of what is generally thought of as "mainstream" American culture. AIDS evokes human emotions not only because it is a symbol of death but also because its transmission is associated with bodily fluids, substances that have long been recognized by cultural anthropologists as evoking emotions critical to the efficacy of symbolic meaning (see, e.g., Turner 1974:55–56). Although other diseases challenge the boundaries of biomedical efficacy, AIDS does so in a particularly invidious way since it is inextricably linked with basic aspects of being human—birth, the circulation and transfer of blood, and the intimate linkages between two individuals through sexual intercourse. As Singer, Irizarry, and Schensul (1991: 142–143) have emphasized, the emotions evoked by AIDS and HIV intervention strategies must be tempered with appropriate research so that reasonable policies can be formulated and acted upon. It is with this goal in mind that this chapter is written.

While currently low seroprevalence rates have been cast optimistically as providing "windows of opportunity" to mount prevention efforts through advocating safer needle use and safer sexual practices, much of the research on HIV-1 risk reduction among IDUs has focused on results in large metropolitan areas such as New York City (e.g., Des Jarlais *et al.* 1988; Kleinman *et al.* 1990; Neaigus *et al.* 1990), San Francisco (e.g., Feldman and Biernacki 1988; Newmeyer *et al.* 1989), Miami (e.g., Chitwood, McCoy, and Comerford 1990; McCoy and Khoury 1990), and Chicago (Wiebel 1988), where seroprevalence rates are already moderate to high. It is of great interest to examine how risk-reduction initiatives operate in low HIV-1 seroprevalence areas because AIDS is comparatively less salient in these locations. Such data will be increasingly relevant to the formation of public policy because low to moderate HIV-1 seroprevalence rates are probably more representative of the majority of IDUs around the country than are moderate to high seroprevalence rates in the hyperendemic Northeast and some other large metropolitan areas.

In this chapter we demonstrate the role and value of ethnography in understanding and addressing an epidemic such as AIDS, based on research conducted in west central Ohio, where the seroprevalence rate among IDUs is currently low. More specifically, we provide a case study of needle-use patterns and community outreach in the "drug-copping" (drug-purchasing) areas of Dayton and Columbus, Ohio. We argue, based on the case analysis, that the concept of needle sharing, as it has come to be known in

AIDS research, inaccurately proposes that IDUs value exchanging used hy- podermic needles for the purpose of expressing intimacy, friendship, and social bonding. We suggest that the term *needle sharing* should be replaced with terms such as *needle transfer* or *circulation*. Finally, we argue that the insights derived through ethnographic research on the epidemiology of HIV-1 seroprevalence rates and trajectories among IDUs in different geo- graphic locations have clear implications for policy formation in a Western, industrialized context.

The chapter is based on twenty-four months (September 1989–August 1991) of ethnographic research conducted by the principal author as part of the National AIDS Demonstration Research Program (NADR) initiated by the National Institute on Drug Abuse. Street observations, casual con- versations on the streets, and sixty-two tape-recorded, voluntary and con- fidential, informal interviews with injecting drug users form the ethnographic data base. Ethnographic interviews were conducted in the offices of a methadone treatment program, in the project site offices, and occasionally in a car, park, or residence.

Participants were recruited for ethnographic interviews initially through the assistance of indigenous outreach workers. The introduction of poten- tial interviewees by outreach workers from the local communities was a crucial stage in the development of the rapport required to elicit data on the private, if not illegal, aspects of people's lives. As the principal author became more familiar with local IDUs over time, he was also able to recruit individuals for interviews. Each person was given ten dollars after an in- terview in compensation for the time he or she devoted to research.[1]

Every effort was made to interview a "representative" sample of IDU lifestyles, and our understanding of the diversity of drug users' lives evolved over time. Forty-one people were interviewed in Dayton, and twenty-one people were interviewed in Columbus. Overall, 47 percent of the people interviewed were African-American males, 21 percent were African- American females, 14 percent were white males, and 18 percent were white females. Among African-Americans the mean age of males was 43.3, while the mean age of females was 37.9. Among whites the mean age of males was 40, and for females the mean age was 35.3. In the first part of the chapter we briefly review the current state of knowledge of various aspects of the transmission efficiency of HIV-1 among IDUs and the contributions that ethnographic research has made to our understanding of its epidemi- ology.

## THE TRANSMISSION EFFICIENCY OF HIV-1 AMONG INJECTING DRUG USERS

The transmission efficiency of HIV-1 through injection and/or sexual practices is based on the exceedingly complex interrelationship among biological, sociocultural, and behavioral parameters. Fundamentally, the risk of HIV-1 infection depends on the likelihood that a person with whom one engages in risk behaviors has been infected (McCoy and Khoury 1990:429).

A number of variables are thought to be relevant to the biological dimensions of the risk of HIV-1 infection, including at the very least (1) the immune functioning of infected and uninfected individuals (Levy 1989); (2) the biology of the virus itself (Cheng-Mayer *et al.* 1988); (3) the impact of the stage of infection on the amount of inoculum transmitted (e.g., Clark *et al.* 1991:958–959; Krieger *et al.* 1991; Von Reyn, Fordham, and Mann 1987:695); and (4) the presence or absence of various cofactors or risk modifiers for HIV-1 infection, including ulcerative sexually transmitted disease (e.g., Kaslow and Francis 1989:100–101; Levy 1989; Potterat 1987; Trapido, Lewis, and Comerford 1990:261). Perhaps other variables are still to be determined (e.g., Feldman 1990:46–49).

At the level of behavior, several broad domains have been addressed in assessing the transmission efficiency of HIV-1. Among these are (1) the type and frequency of various sexual behaviors and their relative impact upon females and males (e.g., Holmberg *et al.* 1989; Kaslow and Francis 1989: 98); (2) the patterns of used hypodermic needle circulation; (3) the sequential use of other injection paraphernalia, including cookers, cottons, and rinse water (Koester, Booth, and Wiebel 1990); and (4) the number of exposures and the amount of inoculum transmitted through various sexual and needle transfer routes (e.g., Friedland 1989:164; Von Reyn, Fordham, and Mann 1987:695).

Conflicting observations have been made on the relative impact of needle-use and sexual risk practices in the transmission of HIV-1 among IDUs. Some researchers (e.g., McCoy *et al.* 1990; Page *et al.* 1990:61) have suggested, based on the analysis of the correlates of risk practices and seropositivity among Miami IDUs, that needle risk practices are a more crucial means of virus transmission than are sexual behaviors. It seems intuitively plausible that direct intravenous exposure would be an extremely efficient means of transmission. Cases of single, accidental needlestick injuries resulting in HIV-1 infection among health care workers appear to support this view (see, e.g., Neisson-Vernant *et al.* 1986; Oksenhendler *et al.* 1986). Nevertheless, the risk of infection through accidental health-care–related needlesticks has been calculated to be low (Von Reyn, Fordham, and Mann 1987:695). Other researchers (e.g., Trapido, Lewis, and Comerford 1990: 259) have concluded that the sexual transmission of HIV-1 among IDUs may have been underestimated in the past. According to Friedland (1989: 165), needle and sexual risk practices among sexually active IDUs may have some currently unknown additive impact on viral transmission and infection.

## ETHNOGRAPHY AND THE EPIDEMIOLOGY OF HIV-1
## AMONG INJECTING DRUG USERS

Ethnographic research on regional variations in the social structural characteristics of needle-use practices, as well as laws and public health policies,
have become increasingly important in explaining the variability in HIV-1
seroprevalence rates among IDUs across geographic space and through time
(Friedland 1989:162; Page *et al.* 1990). Des Jarlais and colleagues (1989:
1010), for example, have posited that increases in the availability of heroin
and cocaine in the late 1970s that resulted in increased injection frequencies, along with the presence of numerous "shooting galleries" (places
where a fee is paid for the right to inject drugs and where used hypodermic
needles may be rented) that facilitated anonymous hypodermic needle circulation, were crucial to the rapid spread of HIV-1 among IDUs in New
York City from 1978 to 1981.

In a detailed comparison of the trajectories of HIV-1 seroprevalence rates
among IDUs in New York City and San Francisco, Watters (1989:18) attributed the moderate seroprevalence rate (15 percent) among San Francisco IDUs and the lack of an explosive increase in seroconversion to the
comparative absence of commercial shooting galleries. In San Francisco the
primary sites for injection are tenements and residential hotel rooms that
are conducive to restricted needle-transfer patterns among relatively isolated, small groups. Thus Watters (1989) proposed that the lack of overlap
of relatively closed social networks and the comparative absence of anonymous sharing through needle pooling may account to some extent for the
moderate seroprevalence rate among IDUs in San Francisco.

Other researchers (e.g., Hahn *et al.* 1989:2683; Siegal 1990:288) have
suggested that the insignificance of shooting galleries in various geographic
locations may be linked to low seroprevalence rates among IDUs. The importance of shooting galleries in local subepidemics was demonstrated by
Chitwood and colleagues (1990:151) through the seropositivity rate of hypodermic needles recovered from shooting galleries in Miami, Florida. Ten
percent of 148 used hypodermic needles were found to be positive for antibodies to HIV-1. It is interesting that high levels of shooting-gallery use
appear to be linked with high seroprevalence rates among IDUs in places
such as Miami and New York City where needles are unobtainable from
pharmacies without a prescription. San Francisco is an exception to this
observation because shooting galleries do not appear to be used extensively
even though hypodermic needles cannot be purchased from local pharmacies without a prescription.

Increasingly, local laws and public health policies are implicated in explanations of varying HIV-1 seroprevalence rates among IDUs. Calsyn and
colleagues (1991) have proposed that the ability to purchase hypodermic

190 Global AIDS Policy

needles without a prescription is associated with a lower frequency of anonymous sharing of injection equipment among IDUs in Seattle, which may partly account for the low HIV-1 seroprevalence rate (less than 3 percent) observed there (see also Siegal 1990). Similarly, Singer, Irizarry, and Schensul (1991:144) suggested that "the illegality of needle possession without a prescription in Connecticut, has contributed to the rapid diffusion of HIV infection among the state's IVDUs." The ability to purchase low-cost hypodermic needles from pharmacies without a prescription is not, however, always associated with low HIV seroprevalence rates. In Italy, where hypodermic needles can be purchased without a prescription, Nicolosi and colleagues (1991) reported very high HIV seroprevalence rates (30 to 50 percent) in 1989 among heroin users in the northern part of the country. The benefits for HIV-1 prevention that may accrue from the opportunity to purchase hypodermic needles without a prescription must be balanced against the presence and enforcement of drug paraphernalia possession laws.

Conviser and Rutledge (1989:117) have described how the variance in punitive attitudes of local police toward IDUs in Edinburgh and Glasgow, Scotland, may partially explain the disparity of seroprevalence rates of 50 percent and 5 percent (in the mid-1980s) in the two respective cities. Although hypodermic needles could be purchased legally at the discretion of pharmacists in both cities, police in Edinburgh strictly enforced needle possession laws that apparently drove addicts to use shooting galleries and presumably to engage in anonymous needle circulation. In contrast, addicts carrying hypodermic needles in Glasgow were not pursued aggressively by police, thereby enabling them to carry injection equipment with a diminished threat of incarceration and to inject drugs (and perhaps exchange injection equipment) primarily within small groups.

At this time it does not appear that the explosive increase in HIV-1 seroprevalence rates in New York City and other northeastern cities is representative of the trajectory of the virus among IDUs in most other parts of the United States. However, rapid increases in HIV seroprevalence have been observed among IDUs in other cities throughout the world. For example, until recently, HIV seroprevalence rates appeared to remain low over some time and then increased rapidly to about 50 percent seropositive among male IDUs in Bangkok, Thailand (see, e.g., Anderson 1990:415; Choopanya et al. 1991). The possibility that low seroprevalence rates will not increase exponentially in a short period of time cannot be discounted. Determining what accounts for rapid increases in HIV seroprevalence is an urgent research question. Determining what accounts for the apparent persistence of low seroprevalence rates is equally relevant, a subject to which we now turn in the case study of needle-transfer patterns and community outreach in drug-copping areas of Dayton and Columbus, Ohio.

## THE CULTURAL ECOLOGY OF INJECTING DRUG USE IN COPPING AREAS: A CASE STUDY IN WEST CENTRAL OHIO

The Dayton-Springfield and Columbus metropolitan statistical areas incorporate eleven counties in southwest and central Ohio, with a population of about 2 million people according to the 1990 census. Active project outreach has been focused primarily in the metropolitan areas of Dayton and Columbus, which have a total population of about 1.5 million people. The population of the city of Columbus (565,032) is more than twice that of Dayton (182,044), and the proportion of African-American and white ethnic groups in each city is different (Dayton: 58 percent white, 40 percent African-American; Columbus: 76 percent white, 22 percent African-American). Hispanic, native American, Asian, and other ethnic groups represent a very small proportion of the population. Current estimates from local law-enforcement and drug treatment agencies suggest that there are approximately 5,000–7,500 active injecting drug users in the Dayton and Columbus metropolitan regions.

The earliest known case of AIDS in the IDU population in Ohio was diagnosed in Columbus in July 1983. The twenty-six-year-old African-American woman died four months later. Contact with multiple sex partners was noted as an additional risk factor; unfortunately, no information is available regarding this person's mobility patterns (Joni Scolieri, Columbus Health Department, personal communication).

Studies of HIV-1 seroprevalence rates in Dayton and Columbus have revealed a relatively stable rate of less than 3 percent among IDUs since 1986. Based on the testing of 164 individuals enrolled in Dayton and Columbus methadone treatment programs in 1986, Hahn and colleagues (1989:2679) reported a seroprevalence rate of 1.7 percent; of 505 IDUs in methadone treatment in seven Ohio cities in 1986, the overall seroprevalence rate was 1 percent (see also Seligman et al. 1989). Of 855 active IDUs not in treatment who agreed to confidential testing of their blood for antibodies to HIV-1 from March 1989 through July 1990 in the Dayton and Columbus NADR project, 1.5 percent (13) were seropositive (Siegal et al. 1991).[2] The available epidemiologic evidence indicates that the seroprevalence rate among IDUs in west central Ohio is low and apparently has remained low for several years.

The characteristics of local shooting galleries, hypodermic needle availability, and attitudes toward sharing of injection equipment may explain, to some degree, the apparent persistence of a low HIV-1 seroprevalence rate among local IDUs (Siegal 1990). Drug injection has a long history with its own traditions in this part of the Midwest, as interviews with sixty- to seventy-year-old addicts have revealed. In their historical analysis of the diffusion of narcotic injection in the United States, O'Donnell and Jones

(1968:126) reported the case of a sixty-seven-year-old white woman from Columbus, Ohio, who injected heroin subcutaneously in 1925.

In both Dayton and Columbus a fundamental, and admittedly overgeneralized, contrast between the drug-using behaviors of African-Americans and whites has become apparent during the course of our research. The two major ethnic groups in the research location vary to some extent in their residential locations and in the extent to which drug dealing and use are "public" events. Both cities contain a rather small, five- to ten-square-block area in which African-Americans control the sale of heroin and some cocaine.

Copping areas thrive by the activities of a regular core group of African-Americans composed generally of low-echelon drug dealers, "runners" (people who make a sale for dealers in return for money and/or drugs), "holders" (people who hold drugs for sale), hypodermic needle vendors, and users who undertake various "hustling" activities to obtain the money needed to support their habit. The core group constantly changes its composition through what sometimes appears to be a rotational cycle of short- and long-term periods of incarceration.

The core group is complemented by transient users (primarily African-American) who come to the area to purchase their drugs. Members of this category of transient users may hang out in the area for varying lengths of time. This group tends to vary in size based on the season of the year. At any one time, ten to one hundred individuals may be congregated in the local copping areas. For the most part, African-Americans and those whites who drive through the copping areas to make their purchases generally leave with the drugs and inject in a private residence or in a car. Those whites who do drive through the area to cop heroin or cocaine are recognized as having a good sense of the street life. Some whites are able to take advantage of their ability to successfully negotiate a drug buy with African-Americans by reselling the drugs to whites who remain in other parts of the city. Occasionally, interstate truckers roll through the area to make a buy.

Although it is by no means always the case, African-Americans are generally known in the area for the use of heroin and "speedball" (a mixture of heroin and cocaine). Heroin is said by many African-Americans, and those whites who prefer it, to be extremely diluted through the "cutting" process it goes through before—and after—it reaches the drug injector in this region of mid-America. It is often considered a waste by older users especially, who recall "the good old days" when a "cap" of heroin costing three to four dollars was enough to keep a couple of people from experiencing withdrawal for an entire day. Although speedball has been used for many years, its purported increase in popularity appears to be related to the low quality of heroin; the mixture of heroin and cocaine is said to produce at least some alteration in perception. A bag of heroin costs between fifteen and twenty-five dollars, while a bag of cocaine costs seven to ten dollars. Variability in cost is a function of the quality of the drug, the quantity to be purchased, and the relationship between a runner and a buyer.

Whites who use opiates tend to prefer Dilaudid, a semisynthetic narcotic. According to most white opiate users, pharmaceuticals are preferred because, in contrast with heroin, they deliver a consistent effect. Dilaudid is generally sold out of private residences located throughout the metropolitan areas at a cost of thirty-five to sixty dollars per four-milligram tablet. Some Dilaudid dealers will travel to a buyer's house to deliver the merchandise. In this case, each Dilaudid tablet may cost as much as fifty to sixty dollars because of the extra effort expended by the dealer. In addition, prices sometimes increase on weekends. The Dilaudid trail therefore tends to lead white narcotic users outside of the copping areas. Similarly, whites who prefer cocaine most often purchase it from dealers outside of the copping areas. As a result, whites rarely use shooting galleries located in these areas.

Shooting galleries have too often been cast in the literature on AIDS and injecting drug use as though they were the same institution across the country. Regional variations in the style in which shooting galleries operate have important implications for prevention efforts and for understanding the variability in HIV-1 seroprevalence rates discussed earlier (see also Ouellet *et al.* 1991; Page, Smith, and Kane 1991). Generally, the term *shooting gallery* has been defined in reference to the characteristics of those found in New York City; that is, places where a user pays a fee for the right to inject his or her drugs, and where used hypodermic needles are pooled and can be rented from the manager.

To the best of our knowledge, in Dayton and Columbus hypodermic needles are very rarely rented in shooting galleries, largely, we surmise, because sterile needles and syringes are relatively easy to obtain. The extent of anonymous circulation of possibly HIV-1-contaminated needles through needle pooling is minimized as a result.

In Dayton, where more extensive ethnographic observations have been conducted, shooting galleries are few in number; the term is also used to describe abandoned buildings where users may congregate to inject drugs, most often without having to pay an entrance fee. From the fall of 1989 through the spring of 1991, six different shooting galleries (including two abandoned homes) were known to have been in operation; only two were in operation simultaneously for any length of time.

Although many more African-Americans than whites inject their drugs in shooting galleries, members of both ethnic groups look upon this institution with a great deal of derision and view its use as a last resort. Shooting galleries are viewed as dangerous and unclean; their use is viewed as a symbol of downward mobility in the drug-using world. They are dangerous because they are subject to constant police harassment (hence their relatively short life span), and because other users may attempt to rob a person, or worse. They are unclean because in many instances there is no running water, no toilet, no electricity (or light), and no heat in the winter. They are associated with social decline within the drug user's world because they signify that a person has "lost control" of his or her drug use; this is the primary reason why transient users would experience the unpleasant and dangerous aspects of the shooting-gallery scene. Those users who work the copping areas may use a gallery as a matter of convenience.

Ethnographic observations and data from interviews reveal that from fifteen to seventy-five different people use a gallery on any given day, with the average being twenty to twenty-five. The total volume of people can number one hundred or more since one individual may use a gallery repeatedly on the same day. In ten observations in shooting galleries, the number of people present ranged from two to forty-four (with a mean of twelve). Only three whites were observed using the galleries located in copping areas on these ten occasions.

A fee of one to two dollars, or a small amount of heroin or cocaine, is paid to a gallery manager (also called "the house") for the right to inject. Again, during the research study (1989–91), as far as could be determined, hypodermic needles ("outfits") were not being rented. Nevertheless, used outfits were sometimes available for purchase from the manager for one to two dollars, but this is considered a last resort by local users. In some instances managers sell outfits that are reportedly new. If a person buys a used hypodermic needle from the manager, he or she usually keeps it and does not return it to the owner. We emphasize that this practice tends to severely limit the extent to which used needles and syringes circulate anonymously.

Because hypodermic needle vendors usually present in the copping areas sell "new" outfits for one to two dollars, the need to purchase (or rent or borrow) a used hypodermic needle is greatly diminished. While it is true that a vendor can clean up a used outfit to make it look new, this practice is said not to be worth the trouble since sterile needles and syringes can be readily and inexpensively purchased at local pharmacies. In addition, experienced users claim that it is very difficult to be deceived. This is not to say that used needles are never sold as new, but this practice appears to be relatively rare.

State laws permit the purchase of hypodermic syringes without a prescription at the discretion of the pharmacist. A package of ten U-100 insulin hypodermic needles, the most popular "outfit" in this area, costs about two dollars at local pharmacies. Usually a person is required to sign for the purchase, but the effort made to verify a person's identity varies substantially.

Purchasing needles and syringes at a pharmacy is a hustling skill that must be learned; it is generally easier for someone who looks "straight" and knows the "diabetic story" to purchase them without a hassle than it is for someone who looks like he or she has just come off the streets. While IDUs lament that it is more difficult to purchase syringes at some pharmacies than others, they generally report little difficulty in obtaining a supply of sterile syringes (cf. Compton *et al.* 1992). With the profit that can be realized from needle vending, the trade has become a lucrative business that several individuals are said to use solely to support their habits in the copping areas of each city.

In some cases non-drug-using diabetics either provide needles and syringes for sale by themselves to make the extra profit or sell them in bulk to a vendor.[3] The majority of users interviewed claimed to have a diabetic friend or family member from whom they could obtain a new needle either for free or for a minimal charge.

We emphasize that in Dayton and Columbus users tend to have a variety of alternative strategies available through which to obtain sterile hypodermic needles. Perhaps this is related to the local attitudes of IDUs that place little value in the phenomenon that has become known as "needle sharing" in AIDS research.

Ever since the interrelationship between AIDS and injecting drug use was first recognized, needle sharing has been touted as a fundamental, morally driven feature of an injecting drug user's subculture across the country and abroad. Although many researchers (e.g., Friedman, Des Jarlais, and Sotheran 1986:385; Des Jarlais, Friedman, and Strug 1986:119) have mentioned the practical and economic aspects of needle transfer, the phenomenon is overwhelmingly cast as a valued means to express intimacy and friendship and even as a ritual of social bonding (Conviser and Rutledge 1989:116). Based on our research in Dayton and Columbus, what has been called "needle sharing" may be more accurately described as "a necessary evil" from the user's point of view. We propose that more accurate terms for needle-sharing behavior are *needle transfer* or *needle circulation.*

Once it is understood that the primary relationship in a user's life is between oneself, the drug(s), and the feelings it evokes, the phenomenon that has been called needle sharing becomes clearer. When IDUs in Dayton and Columbus describe drug injection with a hypodermic needle that has been used by someone else, they most often talk about borrowing an outfit or "shooting behind" someone, not sharing. Although shooting behind someone is not unavoidable, it certainly is not a practice that local IDUs desire to engage in to express "social bonding," friendship, or intimacy. No IDU who was interviewed said that he or she wanted to shoot behind someone else. Implicit in the term *sharing* is an attitude of altruism that is inconsistent with the self-centered nature of injecting drug use.

The primary reason why an IDU does not want to shoot behind someone else is because he or she has to wait for the other person to "fix" (inject the drug), which may take from two to sixty or more minutes depending on a user's ability to register a "hit" (puncture a vein) as signified by the aspiration of blood back up into the syringe. Shooting up behind someone is an expression of subordination that is most often found in the relationship between sexual partners, running partners, or between experienced and inexperienced drug users (see also Des Jarlais, Friedman, and Strug 1986:114–116). We have found that individuals who are involved in such relationships are more likely to exchange a used hypodermic needle with their partner, but the primary reason to do so is because another one is unavailable, not because the practice is a culturally prescribed means to express intimacy or solidarity. In addition, needles become dull or barbed with each use, making it more difficult to get a hit, which again increases substantially the waiting time before the euphoric feelings of the rush and high are perceived. All of this is not to propose that hypodermic needle transfer does not occur, but rather to clarify the observation that IDUs, at least in this region, do not view needle transfer as a valued means of expressing friendship or intimacy as is implied in the term *sharing*. Hypodermic needle transfer usually occurs only in situations of sterile needle scarcity, and even then, injecting with a used outfit is viewed as a necessary evil.

The principal reasons that used hypodermic needles circulate are either because money is short and one cannot afford to purchase a new needle, or because of the inability to purchase one in the setting of the injection event. IDUs are forced to borrow a used outfit when they do not have the extra one to two dollars to purchase a new hypodermic needle on the streets, when vendors are not present, or when it is late at night, pharmacies are closed, and it is too inconvenient to bother a diabetic whom they may know. Also, it is generally the case that when someone gives another user his or her outfit, it is not returned by the receiver. This kind of behavior, therefore, tends to minimize the cycle of needle circulation and may inhibit the possibility for transmission of HIV-1.

Anonymous circulation of hypodermic syringes tends to occur as a last resort when someone cannot borrow a used outfit from a friend or known acquaintance, or when someone cannot purchase an outfit and is forced to pick a used one up off the ground or out of the trash. In cases where an IDU finds an outfit hidden by its original owner, anonymous transfer can also occur.

IDUs typically hide their outfits in various places inside a gallery or outside in the copping area. Because they are in an area known to local police as a copping area, IDUs must be particularly careful not to be caught possessing a hypodermic needle. While police can prosecute someone for having a hypodermic needle without a legitimate medical reason under state drug paraphernalia laws, their willingness to do so appears to depend on the relationship between the user and the officer and on other aspects of the specific situation.[4] In many cases IDUs said that police merely destroy a confiscated hypodermic needle.

Two additional reasons that local IDUs disfavor shooting behind someone else are a general attitude of fear of disease that is partly associated with historical aspects of the impact of hepatitis B among IDUs, and attitudes concerning proper hygiene. As other researchers (see, e.g., McCombie 1989) have noted, hepatitis B has been a significant public health problem among IDUs for years. The Amsterdam needle-exchange program, initiated in 1984 through the efforts of local addicts, was originally designed to prevent the transmission of hepatitis B (van Haastrecht *et al.* 1991:60). In Dayton and Columbus many IDUs reported having friends who had hepatitis B and, most important, claimed a self-conscious effort to alter needle-exchange patterns years before the AIDS epidemic. A forty-two-year-old African-American male who used heroin for twenty years explained, "I caught hep' back in '68 by fixin' behind somebody else, and that taught me a lesson that I never use another needle behind somebody; I don't care who it is." A forty-year-old African-American male who used heroin and speedball for approximately eighteen years talked about needle sharing (when probed with this term) in these words:

> A lot of people got some misconception as far as sharin' syringes. People been leery of this syringe thing 'cause of hepatitis for years. Since they're leery of hepatitis and because of the AIDS thing too, there's not much sharing. I mean that's something real personal; you're exposin' yourself to someone else. So, like I ain't never had hepatitis, you know. I have shot behind a few people—not a lot—but a few, and I never had it.

Hepatitis B, of course, has had significant impact among IDUs across the country. The extent to which the historical impact of hepatitis on the needle-using behaviors of IDUs in Dayton and Columbus is related to the current low HIV seroprevalence rate is unknown. The ability of IDUs to react to the threat of hepatitis B exposure through needle transfer may have been related to local hypodermic needle availability. The desire of IDUs to alter needle-exchange behaviors may have some relationship with cultural attitudes toward illness, personal hygiene, and the perceived relationship between self and other. An excerpt from an interview with a white male who used opiates and cocaine for approximately twenty years provides some insight into these attitudes regarding health maintenance.

*Ethnographer:* How did you clean your outfits?

CZ: Well, we always had plenty of needles, we never worried about cleaning them. I would throw it away and use a new one.

*Ethnographer:* Really?

CZ: Yeah, we never, and these people saying we trade needles, we never done that much, *uh uh.*

*Ethnographer:* Really?

CZ: No, I use all my own needles; nobody uses my needles.

*Ethnographer:* Why?

CZ: Why? I don't know.

*Ethnographer:* Even since way back when?

CZ: Yeah.

*Ethnographer:* Why do you think?

CZ: Now I have used after somebody, don't get me wrong, I have, maybe it would be in a tight spot and couldn't get to some, but 99 percent of the time I have used my own. I didn't want you to use my needle.

*Ethnographer:* Why?

CZ: I just wouldn't, I mean . . . I don't want you drinking out of my cup neither!

*Ethnographer:* Really?

CZ: Yeah.

*Ethnographer:* Even if we were hustling together?

CZ: Yeah. I don't want you drinking out of it, you know, unsanitary, man.

*Ethnographer:* Really?

CZ: You know, I mean I take a bath too, and I don't want you in my bath water either!

Our preliminary findings indicate that similar attitudes regarding what is sanitary and what is unsanitary are common and are not limited to older users. Comparable ideas emerged during an interview with a white woman in her twenties as we discussed needle-use patterns.

*Ethnographer:* Who do you fix with most often?

CC: Well, my husband's not . . . he's been using, but he's not hooked. But when I was strung out real bad, I fixed with my husband.

*Ethnographer:* And so with that person, what would the situation be in terms of an outfit?

CC: We had our own.

*Ethnographer:* You each had your own?

CC: Yes.

*Ethnographer:* Really, why is that?

CC: It's just . . . well I didn't want him using mine because he would dull my needle! That's, I didn't know about AIDS then. So the purpose of that at that time was I didn't want him wearing mine out. Plus, nobody wants to wait. I wanted him to have his own, and he felt the same way.

*Ethnographer:* Where did you get your outfits?

*CC:* At the drugstore. You just go in and tell 'em that you've come to pick up some U-100's for your mother or that she's got diabetes and uses insulin and sign the book.

*Ethnographer:* Then, let's say before you came in to our project, how would you clean your outfits?

*CC:* Before I came in here, hot water.

*Ethnographer:* Hot water only. How often were you in a context where you fixed behind somebody else?

*CC:* None.

*Ethnographer:* Would you fix with a large group of people in any situation?

*CC:* None . . . just me and my husband, we would be together and fix. We would go cop with a bunch of people. But we go our separate ways; they would go home, and we would go home. We would get high, sit back and enjoy our highs.

*Ethnographer:* Before you got into the project, you just cleaned your outfits with hot water and then again you were never, if I understand correctly, you were never in a situation where you would share your outfit with anybody?

*CC:* Right.

*Ethnographer:* Why is that?

*CC:* See, before I knew about AIDS, there was hepatitis.

*Ethnographer:* Tell me about hepatitis.

*CC:* I've never had it. So I don't know what it's like. My brother-in-law had it and he was real yellow and he was in a lot of pain. It was from doing drugs, it was from dirty needles.

*Ethnographer:* You found out it was from a dirty needle?

*CC:* Yeah.

*Ethnographer:* Have you ever seen anybody shoot behind somebody else?

*CC:* Oh, yeah.

*Ethnographer:* In what kind of a context?

*CC:* I used to sell Dilaudids and people would come to my house and get off there and I would see 'em sharing needles. They asked me to use mine one time and I said nobody uses mine. They said—this has been two years ago—they said, "Well I don't have AIDS." I said, "So what, do you know if I do?"

*Ethnographer:* Even two years ago then, way before the project started?

*CC:* I just felt that that was mine. It was personal, you know, like personal things women have, just like you shouldn't wear another woman's underwear. Stuff like that, personal stuff. That was my personal [needle and syringe], personal to me and I felt like that nobody else had the right to use it, but me. It's just, you know, it's trifling to go and wear another woman's underwear, she could have, you don't know what she could have and you're gonna put somebody else's underwear on?

*Ethnographer:* Even if it was clean.

CC: Right, that's personal hygiene stuff. People aren't supposed to share stuff like that. Women, men, anybody, that's stuff that belongs to you.

We suggest, based on our research, that the term *needle sharing* is an inaccurate portrayal of the attitudes and values surrounding needle transfer and circulation among IDUs in this region. That IDUs do not value exchanging used hypodermic needles for the sake of creating a sense of intimacy, friendship, or social bonding is apparently not unique to the IDUs in Dayton and Columbus. Ethnographic research among IDUs conducted by Waldorf and colleagues (1990:324–325) in California, by Mason (Kane and Mason 1992:207, 210) in Baltimore, Maryland, by Clatts and colleagues (chapter 13 in this volume) in New York City, and by Koester (1992) in Denver, Colorado, makes it clear that from the perspective of IDUs, the transfer of used hypodermic needles occurs for pragmatic reasons in the overwhelming number of cases, not because the practice is a valued ritual in drug-using subcultures. Finally, ethnographers from various parts of the country (Houston, San Antonio, and Hawaii) who participated in a roundtable discussion of the concept of "needle sharing" at the Third Annual NADR Meetings sponsored by the National Institute on Drug Abuse (see Carlson, Siegal, and Falck 1991) expressed general agreement with the results reported here for Dayton and Columbus. More systematic research on this issue is needed.

These observations on the meaning of "needle sharing" have more than academic significance for understanding the culture of injecting drug users. They emphasize that keys to needle-use risk reduction are intimately related to local policies that govern needle availability, rather than to changing a value that is "thoroughly integrated into the IV [intravenous] drug subculture" (Des Jarlais, Friedman, and Strug 1986:119).

It is within this general context that community outreach interventions promoting the use of bleach for needle decontamination and condoms for safer sex must be understood. We emphasize that injection risk episodes are extremely diverse events (see Page 1990), and we have only briefly described those in copping areas, in particular, to the exclusion of other equally relevant contexts.

## COMMUNITY OUTREACH: THE DISTRIBUTION AND USE OF RISK-REDUCTION MATERIALS IN COPPING AREAS

From 1989 to 1991 seven outreach workers distributed risk-reduction kits among IDUs and their sex partners in Dayton and Columbus. The risk-reduction kits consisted of a brown, ziplock bag that contained (1) one two-ounce bottle of bleach and one two-ounce bottle of water, each of which had a label describing the contents and their proper use; (2) an assortment of twelve condoms along with a pamphlet on their proper use; (3) a coupon that could be anonymously redeemed for a package of twenty condoms in local pharmacies (see Falck *et al.* 1990); (4) two wallet-sized cards containing AIDS facts and a description of hypodermic needle sterilization procedures (including graphic representations); (5) a brochure on HIV and AIDS; and (6) a list of local treatment agencies and self-help programs.

Risk-reduction kits were given to individuals who participated in the structured intervention tracks of the project (see Falck and Siegal 1991). Kits were also distributed by the outreach workers to IDUs (and sexual partners) on the streets to reinforce, and hopefully to help maintain, prevention messages presented through the NADR Project. In addition, kit distribution was designed to reach those IDUs who either chose not to participate in the project, or who did not have an opportunity to do so because the quota of 1,200 people had been met. During an eighteen-month period outreach workers distributed 2,375 risk-reduction kits to IDUs and their sexual partners "on the streets" in Dayton and Columbus. Records indicate that 86 percent of these kits were given to African-Americans, primarily in the copping areas. Only 6 percent of the kits are known to have been given to whites, and 8 percent were given to people whose ethnicity was not recorded.

These data reflect the geographic dispersal of white IDU residence patterns, copping areas, and drug-use styles. Distributing kits to white IDUs was much more difficult primarily because whites do not tend to congregate in a comparatively public setting in large numbers, as do some African-Americans, either to cop or to inject their drugs. The exceptions are the extremely clandestine and difficult-to-locate residences where a number of whites may gather to inject their drugs. Most commonly, to our knowledge, this includes places where drugs are sold in varying amounts. This, of course, makes it even more difficult to gain access, to build trust and rapport, and to learn of their locations. Working IDUs of African-American and white ethnicity were the most difficult individuals to access.

By contrast, distributing kits to IDUs in copping areas was much more easily accomplished because people tend to gather in such locations for some length of time. Furthermore, kits and gallon bleach containers for refills could be left with cooperative managers of shooting galleries.

As other researchers have emphasized (e.g., Agar 1973; Page *et al.* 1990: 61; Preble and Casey 1969), hustling the resources necessary for drug injection is arduous work. Especially in copping areas, individuals usually have little time for long discussions because they are either hustling, copping, in the process of injecting, or enjoying their high. As a result, conversations surrounding the distribution of risk-reduction kits consisted of very short exchanges or were nonexistent. At times this was frustrating, but a key to the success of outreach activities has been respecting the major rules of the scene. Outreach activities must be as unobtrusive as possible. Most important, outreach activities must not interfere with "business."

People in copping areas literally flocked to the outreach workers to grab a kit, and it was not uncommon to hand out fifty or more kits at a time. Even in the best of circumstances, outreach workers were often unable to fulfill the demand for risk-reduction kits.

We have learned that IDUs generally prefer to keep the contents of one kit at home and to keep another one sequestered away within easy reach in the copping areas. We have also learned that the contents of the bleach and water bottles, which allow for thirty cleaning cycles, are often depleted in a short period of time. The two-ounce bottles of bleach and water should be enough for thirty decontamination cycles (two rinses in each cycle) if a one-milliliter syringe (U-100) is used. Sometimes the contents can be used completely in a matter of two to three days, especially if bleach and water bottles are used by two or more people. Interviews also indicated that most users in copping areas were hesitant to buy a large bottle of bleach to refill their bottle when it became empty. Price and inconvenience were usually offered as an explanation. We placed gallon bottles of bleach in the local galleries in an attempt to encourage refilling empty bottles.

It was extremely difficult to determine exactly what IDUs did with the contents of risk-reduction kits. This was especially true with condoms. Observations revealed that the condoms were sometimes sold to carryout stores to be resold to other customers. Although this was disconcerting, it also indicated a demand for condoms within the community. Interviews indicated a wide variety of attitudes toward condom use. Some people were willing to try them; others used them with anonymous sex partners, but not with their spouse or regular sex partner; and others simply would have nothing to do with them. Some people said that they gave the condoms that were distributed to sexually active friends and family members, including sons and daughters. There is some reason to believe that condoms were sold by IDUs to crack-cocaine sellers who commonly engage in high-risk sexual activities (see Carlson and Siegal 1991). Commercial female sex workers showed the most interest in obtaining condoms, and some stopped by the field sites regularly to obtain them.

Bleach bottles were a bit more easily followed. In the copping areas it was not uncommon to see individuals with a bottle of bleach in their shirt pockets. On several occasions people in local shooting galleries were observed using bleach and water bottles to decontaminate an outfit whether it was borrowed from someone else or not. Several gallery managers were even observed scrubbing the floors with the bleach we left in gallon containers in an effort to "keep the place clean." Many IDUs indicated in interviews that they made every effort to rinse their outfits with bleach if at all possible, even if the outfits had not been used by someone else.

Decontamination with bleach, then, sometimes takes on a symbolic meaning to keep things "clean" and remove symbolically the danger of HIV infection, even in situations in which the likelihood of HIV transmission is remote or nonexistent. Most IDUs claimed that they were much more likely to rinse their hypodermic needle with bleach when they were alone in the relaxed setting of their own homes, even if the outfit had not been used by someone else. IDUs said that they were correspondingly less likely to use bleach in high-risk settings such as when several people are injecting together and there are not enough hypodermic needles for everyone. In addition, the water bottles in the risk-reduction kits were valued as much as the bleach bottles. This was especially true when water was in short supply and was needed to mix with the drug(s). The following discussion of an injection episode illustrates some of these observations:

> *Ethnographer:* You've taken [risk-reduction] kits before that we hand out on the streets.
>
> *DD:* Yeah.
>
> *Ethnographer:* What do you do with the stuff that's in it?
>
> *DD:* I take mine home. I had one down there on the street hid. I had hid it, then a bunch of us went up there [to the gallery] to fix [inject drugs] and so nobody didn't have none. So I got mine out 'cause I had it hid near where we was. I got mine and I used it and I just left it there, and so I guess somebody else used it or picked it up. But I got my own personal one. I got two of 'em. I got one at home so I use that one at home. Generally as a rule I goes home to fix. And I try to keep a new outfit all the time 'cause it specifically states on 'em, "use once and dispose of." So if I don't have one when I'm at home I take my time. I run Clorox through it anyway 'cause I'm not in no big hurry or nobody's buggin' me about usin' it or anything.
>
> *Ethnographer:* Can you describe the events that happened when you said you were with a bunch of people and you went together to fix and you got a kit that was hidden? Then what'd you all do?
>
> *DD:* Well, we went to fix.
>
> *Ethnographer:* How many were there?
>
> *DD:* It was four of us altogether. And what really prompted me to get the kit, we didn't have no water, that's what prompted it. So I just got the whole kit, and we only had two outfits.
>
> *Ethnographer:* And there were four of you?
>
> *DD:* Yeah. I had mine [a hypodermic needle] and somebody else had one too, and somebody was gonna have to wait. Well I know they was gonna have to wait on me 'cause I had my own, I didn't have to wait. So that's what prompted it there. We didn't have water. So by me gettin' the

water, I just set the whole kit out.

And I really done it on purpose. After I fixed, I didn't clean the 'fit out. I left blood in it. I done that that day on purpose. So I don't know who it was that used my 'fit, but they had to run some water through it or the bleach. I don't know which one they done 'cause after I fixed, I left. I just left the 'fit, the kit, and the whole thing there. So I can't tell you if they used the bleach or not. But it was there at their disposal.

*Ethnographer:* I see. In a context like that is it assuming too much to say, for you to have said, "Hey there's this bleach here, if anybody uses my 'fit you better clean it with bleach?"

*DD:* Well, in my case the guys that I was with that day, they already knew that I was sick [craving the drug(s)], you know? Cause one of 'em had asked me, "Let me use the 'fit first man cause you gonna take all day." I told him, "Man, you know I'm sick and I'm not gonna let you use the 'fit first! And if I wasn't sick you ain't gonna use my 'fit 'for I do!" So here's all the stuff. I'm gone. After I fixed, I left.

*Ethnographer:* Why did you say you left blood in it purposefully?

*DD:* I don't know why I done that. I guess really for 'em to use the bleach. I guess that's really why I done it for whoever used the 'fit to use the bleach, you know, so that would be puttin' some kind a protection on 'em, or a blanket, or somethin'.

*Ethnographer:* Since you haven't come through the [NADR] Project yourself, how did you know how to use the bleach?

*DD:* Word of mouth. After the first kit was given out. Because out of all the years I been usin' drugs, bleach never was mentioned until this program here.

Public health initiatives designed to encourage IDUs to disinfect their injection equipment if they borrow a used hypodermic needle must always be tempered by an understanding and respect of the drug user's point of view. From a public health perspective, there is little apparent reason why an IDU should not want to clean a used hypodermic needle with bleach before he or she injects the drugs. This is especially the case because it is known that IDUs commonly rinse an outfit between needle uses or transfers with water. This procedure is practical since blood residue can clog a needle, and in part it is based on attitudes regarding cleanliness and the belief among IDUs that injecting even a small amount of another person's blood can cause a flulike illness IDUs call "the chills."

From an outsider's perspective, the suggestion that IDUs should rinse their syringes two times with bleach and two times with clean water to kill HIV-1 appears to be a small, reasonable addition to the ritual of injection. In many situations it appears to be a practice that people are willing to adopt. But one of the most important contexts in which IDUs should rinse with bleach (i.e., when two or more people want to shoot drugs and only one syringe is available) raises other problems. In the following excerpt from an interview with a thirty-year-old white male, an analogy was offered that clarifies why it is so difficult for an IDU to rinse his or her outfit with bleach in this context.

> *Ethnographer:* After all, you're going to rinse with water anyway, right? Why is using bleach such a problem?

> *ZZ:* Time, takes too much time. Let's say you are waiting in line to get your favorite food and you haven't eaten in days; you're starving. Not only do you have to wait in line, you have to wait while the other person eats *and* watch him eat your favorite food.

This simple analogy brings out some important aspects of the nature of the injection risk episode in question. The anticipation of the feelings that are about to be felt creates the illusion that relatively short periods of time are much longer than they actually are. In the context where people shoot immediately behind one another, the situation must be viewed from the perspective of the person who has to wait. Anything that adds time to an already anguishing waiting period is perceived as an added burden. Rinsing with water in such a context adds time. Adding two rinse cycles with bleach, if it is available, can appear to add an unbearable length of time in such contexts.

These observations emphasize that AIDS risk-reduction efforts among IDUs can diminish the spread of HIV-1, but they probably will not eliminate it unless drug injection ceases and safer sex techniques are always practiced. These two objectives, the former probably realistic and the latter somewhat idealistic, are both related to policy issues.

## CONCLUSION

A central point of this chapter is that injecting drug use and patterns of hypodermic needle risk taking are quite variable across the nation. As more detailed ethnographic research is undertaken in diverse regions, we will be in a better position to understand not only the regional dynamics of the subepidemics but also their interrelationships. Such analyses will also enable a more accurate understanding of local risk-taking patterns, thereby contributing to the design and implementation of culturally appropriate risk-reduction interventions.

Our ethnographic description and analysis of needle-use practices and attitudes toward needle transfer and circulation among IDUs in Dayton and Columbus appear to confirm the findings of Calsyn and colleagues (1991). Policies that allow the purchase of hypodermic needles without a prescription seem to be related to lower levels of needle exchange, lower levels of anonymous hypodermic needle circulation through needle pooling in shooting galleries, and lower HIV seroprevalence rates.

Our ethnographic case study emphasizes that relatively little is known about the variability of the daily lives of drug users in different regions of the country. As a result, stereotypical views of IDU subcultures that guided risk-reduction efforts in the early stages of the epidemic should be reconfigured. No longer can IDUs be cast realistically as drug-crazed individuals who have little concern for their health. No longer can shooting galleries and the patterns of needle circulation associated with them be cast as the same across the country. Furthermore, we have shown that in Dayton and Columbus, and probably much more widely, used-needle transfer and circulation occur for pragmatic and economic reasons in nearly all cases, not because IDUs value needle borrowing as a ritual necessary to express friendship, intimacy, or social bonding. These observations have clear implications for addressing policy issues and for designing intervention strategies.

Approaches to AIDS intervention strategies for IDUs generally take two forms. On the one hand, as preliminary findings have shown across the country (see, e.g., Des Jarlais *et al.* 1988; Neaigus *et al.* 1990; Newmeyer *et al.* 1989; Singer, Irizarry, and Schensul 1991:145), pragmatic initiatives such as community outreach that combine AIDS education with the distribution of risk-reduction materials can significantly reduce IDU risk behaviors, especially when the interventions are sensitive to issues of cultural diversity, sexual orientation, and gender (see, e.g., Singer 1991). Contrary to the initial fears that community outreach interventions would promote drug use, all the evidence to date suggests that they actually lead to a reported decrease in injection frequency or a cessation of drug injection in a number of cases (see, e.g., Friedman, Des Jarlais, and Goldsmith 1989: 106). The community outreach approach to intervention, by itself, can be viewed as "system-maintaining" because it does not address the macrolevel variables that structure the contexts within which a great deal of the high-risk drug and sexual practices take place across the country.

On the other hand, there are approaches to intervention that challenge and express frustration with the social conditions surrounding drug use, including why it occurs to the extent that it does in the first place, economic inequalities, poverty, homelessness, racism, gender inequality, and minority issues. A sense of frustration with the compelling evidence that these conditions are linked with HIV-1 transmission among IDUs, and with a corresponding limitation in risk-reduction options, is commonly added almost as a plea at the end of many AIDS prevention articles (see, e.g., Conviser and Rutledge 1989:124). For example, Weissman and the National AIDS Research Consortium (1991:61) stated:

It [risk reduction] is hardly a primary concern for a woman who is hungry, without a place to spend the night or to put her children to bed, or without clothing to keep her warm. Unless some of these basic and immediate needs can be addressed, it seems not only hopeless but also foolish to be talking about risk reduction and lifesaving measures.

Such pleas are often global in scope. Aral and Holmes (1991:69) concluded a recent article on the worldwide epidemic of sexually transmitted diseases and AIDS with this comment: "By themselves, the medical solutions to the prevention and control of STDs and AIDS are not enough: they must be coupled with the identification and correction of the societal factors responsible for the global pandemic."

Between the system-maintaining and "system-questioning" approaches to HIV risk-reduction interventions lie those strategies that combine pragmatic courses of action with recommending policy changes that do not entail what are currently unrealistic visions of the short-term future. We do not propose that the goal of addressing the fundamental social problems of our age is unimportant, but we emphasize that AIDS prevention entails an unprecedented degree of immediacy for action. The midrange intervention strategies to which we refer seek to combine community outreach activities with the modification of policies (where needed) through legislation to increase the availability of sterile syringes either by altering laws that restrict the purchase of needles from pharmacies without a prescription, or by instituting needle-exchange programs (see, e.g., Comerford et al. 1990; Singer, Irizarry, and Schensul 1991). Legislative policy modifications designed to decriminalize hypodermic needle acquisition and possession must be complemented with increased allocation of funding for community outreach and creative approaches to drug treatment.

It is becoming increasingly apparent that outreach efforts directed by ethnographers are needed for the long term so that risk-reduction techniques can be reinforced and consequently maintained over time (see, e.g., Becker and Joseph 1988; Miller, Turner, and Moses 1990:108–111). Given the current uncertainties in our knowledge of the transmission efficiency of HIV-1, we cannot overemphasize the necessity of maintaining outreach activities. This will be particularly important in areas of low HIV-1 seroprevalence where AIDS is comparatively less salient. Moreover, the success of the community outreach model holds significant promise for future efforts to work with people who have different lifestyles—if an effort is made to understand cultural diversity on its own terms—and perhaps tackle the issue of drug use and other health problems head on.

## NOTES

The research described in this chapter was supported by the National Institute on Drug Abuse Grant no. 1R18DA05757-01. In Dayton, NADR project outreach workers Riki Foster, Rocky Large, Oma Lombardo, and Brenda Wills were employed by Project CURE, Inc. (Abdur Zafr, director) and were supervised by Diana

Alexander (Combined Health District of Montgomery County). In Columbus, NADR project outreach workers Connie Goss, Carmen Marerro, and Walter Jamison worked for the Columbus Health Department (Ruth Frankenfield, site director). The ethnographic research could not have been completed without the support and encouragement of these individuals. We are also grateful to Carol Enigk and the staff at the Wright State University School of Medicine Word Processing Center for carefully transcribing and correcting the ethnographic interviews.

1. The data collected as part of the Dayton and Columbus NADR project are protected by a federal grant of confidentiality, which means that no local, state, or federal agency—or any other individual—may compel any project personnel to provide them with specific information regarding the participants. This was explained carefully to a person before beginning an interview. All participants were told that the interview was confidential, that their names or other identifying information would not be used in print or divulged to anyone, and that the interview would be tape recorded with their permission. Interviewees were encouraged not to use the names of others or to describe in specific detail events such as the locations of major drug deals. All of these efforts were necessary to protect the confidentiality of the participants. Fictitious initials are used in this chapter, and some details in quotations have been modified slightly to protect the confidentiality of participants, whose cooperation in the research was greatly appreciated.

2. Serum samples were initially screened using the Abbott ELISA. Confirmation tests consisted of Western blotting and were considered positive when antibodies to two of three bands were detected: p24; gp41; or gp120/160.

3. The needle-using behavior of diabetics and its interrelationship with injecting drug use has been largely overlooked. In one case, however, Nelson and colleagues (1990) reported a lower HIV-1 infection rate among diabetic IDUs compared to nondiabetic users in Baltimore, presumably because diabetics had easier access to sterile needles and exchanged needles less frequently (cited in Calsyn et al. 1991: 192). On the one hand, needle-use practices among diabetics may instill sterile-needle-using behavior among potential drug injectors, as some NADR project interviewees commented. At the same time, the phenomenon of diabetic injection conducted by non–drug users in the family context may socialize youths to the necessity of life-giving, daily, self-administered injections. This period of socialization to needle use may have some impact on the development of drug-using behaviors among youths raised in homes where diabetics live. Further research is needed on this topic.

4. See Pascal (1988) for a review of drug paraphernalia laws, their interpretation, and their implementation.

## REFERENCES

Agar, Michael H. 1973. *Ripping and Running: A Formal Ethnography of Urban Heroin Addicts*. New York: Seminar Press.

Anderson, Joe. 1990. AIDS in Thailand. *British Medical Journal* 300:415–416.

Aral, Sevgi O., and King K. Holmes. 1991. Sexually Transmitted Diseases in the AIDS Era. *Scientific American* 264(2): 62–69.

Battjes, Robert J., and Roy W. Pickens, eds. 1988. *Needle Sharing among Intra-*

*venous Drug Abusers: National and International Perspectives.* NIDA Research Monograph 80. Rockville, MD: National Institute on Drug Abuse.

Becker, M. H., and J. G. Joseph. 1988. AIDS and Behavioral Change to Reduce Risk: A Review. *American Journal of Public Health* 78:394–410.

Brickner, Philip W., Ramon A. Torres, Mark Barnes, Robert G. Newman, Don C. Des Jarlais, Dennis P. Whalen, and David E. Rogers. 1989. Recommendations for Control and Prevention of Human Immunodeficiency Virus (HIV) Infection in Intravenous Drug Users. *Annals of Internal Medicine* 110:833–837.

Calsyn, Donald A., Andrew J. Saxon, George Freeman, and Stephen Whittaker. 1991. Needle-Use Practices among Intravenous Drug Users in an Area Where Needle Purchase Is Legal. *AIDS* 5:187–193.

Carlson, Robert G., and Harvey A. Siegal. 1991. The Crack Life: An Ethnographic Overview of Crack Use and Sexual Behavior among African-Americans in a Midwest Metropolitan City. *Journal of Psychoactive Drugs* 23(1): 11–20.

Carlson, Robert G., Harvey A. Siegal, and Russel Falck. 1991. The Ethnography of "Needle Sharing" among Injection Drug Users in the Midwest. Paper presented at the Third Annual NADR Meeting, October 29–31 [*Summary Minutes: Third Annual NADR National Meeting*, pp. 49–50. 1992. Bethesda, MD: NOVA Research Company].

Centers for Disease Control. 1991. *HIV/AIDS Surveillance.* June, pp. 1–18.

Chaisson, Richard E., Dennis Osmond, Andrew R. Moss, Harvey W. Feldman, and Patrick Biernacki. 1987. HIV, Bleach, and Needle Sharing [Letter]. *Lancet* 1(8547): 1430.

Cheng-Mayer, C., D. Seto, M. Tateno, and J. A. Levy. 1988. Biologic Features of HIV-1 That Correlate with Virulence in the Host. *Science* 240:80–82.

Chitwood, Dale D., Clyde McCoy, and Mary Comerford. 1990. Risk Behavior of Intravenous Cocaine Users: Implications for Intervention. In *AIDS and Intravenous Drug Use: Future Directions for Community-based Prevention Research*, ed. C. G. Leukefeld, R. J. Battjes, and Z. Amsel, pp. 120–131. NIDA Research Monograph 93. Washington, DC: U.S. Government Printing Office.

Chitwood, Dale D., Clyde B. McCoy, James A. Inciardi, Duane C. McBride, Mary Comerford, Edward Trapido, H. Virginia McCoy, J. Bryan Page, James Griffin, Mary Ann Fletcher, and Margarita A. Ashman. 1990. HIV Seropositivity of Needles from Shooting Galleries in South Florida. *American Journal of Public Health* 80:150–152.

Choopanya, Kachit, Suphak Vanichseni, Don C. Des Jarlais, Kanokporn Plangsringarm, Wandee Sonchai, Manuel Carballo, Patricia Friedmann, and Samuel R. Friedman. 1991. Risk Factors and HIV Seropositivity among Injecting Drug Users in Bangkok. *AIDS* 5:1509–1513.

Clark, Stephen J., Michael S. Saag, W. Don Decker, Sherri Campbell-Hill, Joseph L. Robertson, Peter J. Veldkamp, John C. Kappes, Beatrice H. Hahn, and George M. Shaw. 1991. High Titers of Cytopathic Virus in Plasma of Patients with Symptomatic Primary HIV-1 Infection. *New England Journal of Medicine* 324:954–960.

Comerford, Mary, D. Chitwood, C. McKay, R. Anderson, and J. B. Page. 1990. Attitudes of IVDUs toward Needle Exchanges and Over-the-Counter Purchase of Syringes. Paper presented at the Sixth International Conference on AIDS, San Francisco, June.

Compton, Wilson M., III, Linda B. Cottler, Scott H. Decker, Douglas Mager, and Roosevelt Stringfellow. 1992. Legal Needle Buying in St. Louis. *American Journal of Public Health* 82:595–596.

Conviser, Richard, and John H. Rutledge. 1989. Can Public Policies Limit the Spread of HIV among IV Drug Users? *Journal of Drug Issues* 19:113–128.

Curran, James W., Harold W. Jaffe, Ann M. Hardy, W. Meade Morgan, Richard M. Selik, and Timothy J. Dondero. 1988. Epidemiology of HIV Infection and AIDS in the United States. *Science* 239:610–616.

Des Jarlais, Don C., and Samuel R. Friedman. 1988. Transmission of Human Immunodeficiency Virus among Intravenous Drug Users. In *AIDS: Etiology, Diagnosis, Treatment, and Prevention,* ed. Vincent J. DeVita, Samuel Hellman, and Steven A. Rosenberg, pp. 385–395. 2nd ed. Philadelphia: J. B. Lippincott Company.

Des Jarlais, Don C., Samuel R. Friedman, David M. Novick, Jo L. Sotheran, Pauline Thomas, Stanley R. Yancovitz, Donna Mildvan, John Weber, Mary Jeanne Kreek, Robert Maslansky, Sarah Bartelme, Thomas Spira, and Michael Marmor. 1989. HIV-1 Infection among Intravenous Drug Users in Manhattan, New York City, from 1977 through 1987. *Journal of the American Medical Association* 261(7): 1008–1012.

Des Jarlais, Don C., Samuel R. Friedman, Jo L. Sotheran, and Rand Stoneburner. 1988. The Sharing of Drug Injection Equipment and the AIDS Epidemic in New York City: The First Decade. In *Needle Sharing among Intravenous Drug Abusers: National and International Perspectives,* ed. Robert J. Battjes and Roy W. Pickens, pp. 160–175. NIDA Research Monograph 80. Rockville, MD: National Institute on Drug Abuse.

Des Jarlais, Don C., Samuel R. Friedman, and David Strug. 1986. AIDS and Needle Sharing within the IV-Drug Use Subculture. In *The Social Dimensions of AIDS: Method and Theory,* ed. Douglas A. Feldman and Thomas M. Johnson, pp. 111–125. New York: Praeger.

Falck, Russel, and Harvey A. Siegal. 1991. HIV Risk Reduction for Injection Drug Users and Their Sexual Partners: International Manual. National Institute on Drug Abuse, Community Research Branch, Rockville, Maryland, *in press.*

Falck, Russel, Harvey A. Siegal, Robert G. Carlson, Kathy Baumgartner, and Richard C. Rapp. 1990. The Chit System as a Mechanism for Condom Distribution. Presented at the Second Annual National AIDS Demonstration Research Project Meetings, National Institute on Drug Abuse, Bethesda, Maryland, November, 27–30.

Feldman, Douglas A. 1990. Assessing Viral, Parasitic, and Sociocultural Cofactors Affecting HIV-1 Transmission in Rwanda. In *Culture and AIDS,* ed. Douglas A. Feldman, pp. 45–54. New York: Praeger.

Feldman, Harvey W., and Patrick Biernacki. 1988. The Ethnography of Needle Sharing among Intravenous Drug Users and Implications for Public Policies and Intervention Strategies. In *Needle Sharing among Intravenous Drug Abusers: National and International Perspectives,* ed. Robert J. Battjes and Roy W. Pickens, pp. 28–39. NIDA Research Monograph 80. Rockville, MD: National Institute on Drug Abuse.

Friedland, Gerald. 1989. Parenteral Drug Users. In *The Epidemiology of AIDS: Expression, Occurrence, and Control of Human Immunodeficiency Virus Type 1 Infection*, ed. Richard A. Kaslow and Donald P. Francis, pp. 153–178. New York: Oxford University Press.

Friedman, Samuel R., Don C. Des Jarlais, and Douglas S. Goldsmith. 1989. An Overview of AIDS Prevention Efforts Aimed at Intravenous Drug Users circa 1987. *Journal of Drug Issues* 19:93–112.

Friedman, Samuel R., Don C. Des Jarlais, and Jo L. Sotheran. 1986. AIDS Health Education for Intravenous Drug Users. *Health Education Quarterly* 13:383–393.

Hahn, Robert A., Ida M. Onorato, T. Stephen Jones, and John Dougherty. 1989. Prevalence of HIV Infection among Intravenous Drug Users in the United States. *Journal of the American Medical Association* 18:2677–2684.

Holmberg, Scott D., C. Robert Horsburgh, Jr., John W. Ward, and Harold W. Jaffe. 1989. Biologic Factors in the Sexual Transmission of Human Immunodeficiency Virus. *Journal of Infectious Diseases* 160:116–125.

Kane, Stephanie, and Theresa Mason. 1992. "IV Drug Users" and "Sex Partners": The Limits of Epidemiological Categories and the Ethnography of Risk. In *The Time of AIDS: Social Analysis, Theory, and Method*, ed. Gilbert Herdt and Shirley Lindenbaum, pp. 199–222. Newbury Park, CA: Sage Publications.

Kaslow, Richard A., and Donald P. Francis. 1989. Epidemiology: General Considerations. In *The Epidemiology of AIDS: Expression, Occurrence, and Control of Human Immunodeficiency Virus Type 1 Infection*, ed. Richard A. Kaslow and Donald P. Francis, pp. 87–115. New York: Oxford University Press.

Kleinman, Paula H., Douglas S. Goldsmith, Samuel R. Friedman, William Hopkins, and Don C. Des Jarlais. 1990. Knowledge about and Behaviors Affecting the Spread of AIDS: A Street Survey of Intravenous Drug Users and Their Associates in New York City. *International Journal of the Addictions* 25:345–361.

Koester, Stephen. 1992. Ethnography and High Risk Drug Use. Presented at the Annual Meeting of the College on the Problems of Drug Dependence, Keystone, Colorado, June.

Koester, Stephen, Robert Booth, and Wayne Wiebel. 1990. The Risk of HIV Transmission from Sharing Water, Drug Mixing Containers, and Cotton Filters among IV Drug Users. *International Journal on Drug Policy* 1(6): 28–30.

Krieger, John N., Robert W. Coombs, Ann C. Collier, Susan O. Ross, Kim Chaloupka, Dana K. Cummings, Victor L. Murphy, and Lawrence Corey. 1991. Recovery of Human Immunodeficiency Virus Type I from Semen: Minimal Impact of Stage of Infection and Current Antiviral Chemotherapy. *Journal of Infectious Diseases* 163:386–388.

Leukefeld, Carl G., Robert J. Battjes, and Zili Amsel, eds. 1990. *AIDS and Intravenous Drug Use: Future Directions for Community-based Prevention Research*. NIDA Research Monograph 93. Washington, DC: U.S. Government Printing Office.

Levy, Jay A. 1989. Human Immunodeficiency Viruses and the Pathogenesis of AIDS. *Journal of the American Medical Association* 261:2997–3006.

McCombie, S. C. 1989. Dealing with AIDS: Lessons from Hepatitis B. In *The AIDS Pandemic: A Global Emergency*, ed. Ralph Bolton, pp. 59–65. New York: Gordon and Breach.

McCoy, Clyde B., and Elizabeth Khoury. 1990. Drug Use and the Risk of AIDS. *American Behavioral Scientist* 33:419–431.

McCoy, H. Virginia, Carolyn McKay, Lisa Hermanns, and Shenghan Lai. 1990. Sexual Behavior and the Risk of HIV Infection. *American Behavioral Scientist* 33:432–450.

Miller, Heather G., Charles F. Turner, and Lincoln Moses, eds. 1990. Prevention: The Continuing Challenge. In *AIDS: The Second Decade*. Report of the National Research Council Committee on AIDS Research and the Behavioral, Social, and Statistical Sciences, pp. 81–146. Washington, DC: National Academy Press.

Neaigus, Alan, Meryl Sufian, Samuel R. Friedman, Douglas S. Goldsmith, Bruce Stepherson, Patrice Mota, Jacqueline Pascal, and Don C. Des Jarlais. 1990. Effects of Outreach Intervention on Risk Reduction among Intravenous Drug Users. *AIDS Education and Prevention* 2:253–271.

Neisson-Vernant, C., S. Arfi, D. Mathez, J. Leibowitch, and N. Monplaisir. 1986. Needlestick HIV Seroconversion in a Nurse. *Lancet* 2(8510): 814.

Nelson, K. E., D. Vlahov, S. Cohen, A. Lindsay, L. Soloman, and J. C. Anthony. 1990. Diabetes Is Protective against HIV Infections in IV Drug Users. Presented at the Sixth International Conference on AIDS, San Francisco, June.

Newmeyer, John A. 1988. Why Bleach? Fighting AIDS Contagion among Intravenous Drug Users: The San Francisco Experience. *Journal of Psychoactive Drugs* 20(2): 159–163.

Newmeyer, John A., Harvey W. Feldman, Patrick Biernacki, and John K. Watters. 1989. Preventing AIDS Contagion among Intravenous Drug Users. *Medical Anthropology* 10:167–175.

Nicolosi, Alfredo, Silvia Molinari, Massimo Musicco, Alberto Saracco, Nicoletta Ziliani, and Adriano Lazzarin. 1991. Positive Modification of Injecting Behavior among Intravenous Heroin Users from Milan and Northern Italy, 1987–1989. *British Journal of Addiction* 86:91–102.

O'Donnell, J. A., and J. P. Jones. 1968. Diffusion of the Intravenous Technique among Narcotic Addicts in the United States. *Journal of Health and Social Behavior* 9:120–130.

Oksenhendler, Eric, Martine Harzic, Jeanne-Marie Le Roux, Claire Rabian, and Jean Pierre Clauvel. 1986. HIV Infection with Seroconversion after a Superficial Needlestick Injury to the Finger. *New England Journal of Medicine* 315:582.

Ouellet, Lawrence J., Antonio D. Jimenez, Wendell A. Johnson, and W. Wayne Wiebel. 1991. Shooting Galleries and HIV Disease: Variations in Places for Injecting Illicit Drugs. *Crime and Delinquency* 37:64–85.

Page, J. Bryan. 1990. Shooting Scenarios and Risk of HIV-1 Infection. *American Behavioral Scientist* 33:478–490.

Page, J. Bryan, Dale D. Chitwood, Prince C. Smith, Normie Kane, and Duane C. McBride. 1990. Intravenous Drug Use and HIV Infection in Miami. *Medical Anthropology Quarterly* 4:56–71.

Page, J. Bryan, Prince C. Smith, and Normie Kane. 1991. Shooting Galleries, Their

Proprietors, and Implications for Prevention of AIDS. In *AIDS and Alcohol/ Drug Abuse: Psychosocial Research*, ed. Dennis G. Fisher, pp. 69–85. New York: Harrington Park Press.

Pascal, Chris B. 1988. Intravenous Drug Abuse and AIDS Transmission: Federal and State Laws Regulating Needle Availability. In *Needle Sharing among Intravenous Drug Abusers: National and International Perspectives*, ed. Robert J. Battjes and Roy W. Pickens, pp. 119–136. NIDA Research Monograph 80. Rockville, MD: National Institute on Drug Abuse.

Potterat, J. J. 1987. Does Syphilis Facilitate Sexual Acquistion of HIV? [Letter] *Journal of the American Medical Association* 258:473.

Preble, Edward, and John J. Casey. 1969. Taking Care of Business: The Heroin User's Life on the Street. *International Journal of the Addictions* 4(1): 1–24.

Seligman, Paul J., Robert J. Campbell, Gordon P. Keeler, and Thomas J. Halpin. 1989. Human Immunodeficiency Virus Seropositivity in Intravenous Drug Users in Ohio. *Ohio Medicine* 85:56–59.

Siegal, Harvey A. 1990. Intravenous Drug Abuse and the HIV Epidemic in Two Midwestern Cities: A Preliminary Report. *Journal of Drug Issues* 20(2): 281–290.

Siegal, Harvey A., Robert G. Carlson, Russel Falck, Ling Li, Mary Ann Forney, Richard C. Rapp, Kathy Baumgartner, William Myers, and Morton Nelson. 1991. HIV Infection and Risk Behaviors among Intravenous Drug Users in Low Seroprevalence Areas in the Midwest. *American Journal of Public Health* 81:1642–1644.

Singer, Merrill. 1991. Confronting the AIDS Epidemic among IV Drug Users: Does Ethnic Culture Matter? *AIDS Education and Prevention* 3(3): 258–283.

Singer, Merrill, Ray Irizarry, and Jean J. Schensul. 1991. Needle Access as an AIDS Prevention Strategy for IV Drug Users: A Research Perspective. *Human Organization* 50:142–153.

Trapido, Edward J., Nancy Lewis, and Mary Comerford. 1990. HIV-1-related and Nonrelated Diseases among IV Drug Users and Sexual Partners. *Journal of Drug Issues* 20:245–266.

Turner, Victor. 1974. *Dramas, Fields, and Metaphors: Symbolic Action in Human Society*. Ithaca: Cornell University Press.

van Haastrecht, Harry J. A., Johanna A. R. van den Hoek, Christiane Bardoux, Anne Leentvaar-Kuypers, and Roel A. Coutinho. 1991. The Course of the HIV Epidemic among Intravenous Drug Users in Amsterdam, The Netherlands. *American Journal of Public Health* 81:59–62.

Von Reyn, C. Fordham, and Jonathan M. Mann. 1987. Global Epidemiology. *Western Journal of Medicine* 147:694–701.

Waldorf, Dan, Sheigla Murphy, David Lauderback, Craig Reinarman, and Toby Marotta. 1990. Needle Sharing among Male Prostitutes: Preliminary Findings of the Prospero Project. *Journal of Drug Issues* 20:309–334.

Watters, John K. 1989. Observations on the Importance of Social Context in HIV Transmission among Intravenous Drug Users. *Journal of Drug Issues* 19:9–26.

Weissman, Gloria, and the National AIDS Research Consortium. 1991. AIDS Prevention for Women at Risk: Experience from a National Demonstration Research Program. *Journal of Primary Prevention* 12(1): 49–62.

Wiebel, W. Wayne. 1988. Combining Ethnographic and Epidemiologic Methods in Targeted AIDS Interventions: The Chicago Model. In *Needle Sharing among Intravenous Drug Abusers: National and International Perspectives,* ed. Robert J. Battjes and Roy W. Pickens, pp. 137–150. NIDA Research Monograph 80. Rockville, MD: National Institute on Drug Abuse. Government Printing Office.

Zule, William A., Kenneth N. Vogtsberger, and David P. Desmond. 1990. Needle Risk Behavior in San Antonio: An Ethnographic Perspective. *Research in Progress* (NIDA), December, pp. 38–40. Bethesda, Maryland: NOVA Research.

# 13

# AIDS Risk Behavior among Drug Injectors in New York City: Critical Gaps in Prevention Policy

*Michael C. Clatts, W. R. Davis, Sherry Deren,*
*Douglas S. Goldsmith, and Stephanie Tortu*

It is not known with any degree of precision how many persons use psychoactive narcotic or other drug substances, nor how many of them administer these substances by either subcutaneous or intravenous injection. Some injectors appear to suffer little or no negative effects from the use of narcotic and other drug substances themselves and may even derive certain kinds of benefits from doing so (Clatts, Springer, and Washburn 1990; Springer 1991). Some are even able to control or stop use without formal treatment (cf. Biernacki 1986; Blackwell 1983; Graeven and Graeven 1983). Others, however, are able neither to control their use nor to effectively avail themselves of existing treatment modalities (Hubbard *et al.* 1989) and live with chronic dependency on the experiences afforded by narcotic and drug substances.

Apart from the potentially debilitating effects that this use may pose, however, are the added dangers associated with the illicit manner in which many such substances are often procured and administered. A case in point involves the sharing of injection equipment, commonly known as "works" or "sets," that over the last decade has been increasingly associated with risk for HIV infection (cf. Des Jarlais and Friedman 1987; Kristal 1986).[1] Studies in both the United States and Europe, for example, indicate that the vast majority of cases of HIV infection that derive from heterosexual contact are a consequence of a sex partner who has become infected from shared injection equipment (Drucker 1986; Evans *et al.* 1988). In Europe the sharing of injection equipment is the single most common mode of HIV transmission, and in the United States nearly a third of recently diagnosed cases of AIDS are related to the sharing of drug injection equipment (Centers for Disease Control 1991).

It has also been suggested that drug injectors may be at significantly more risk for developing HIV-spectrum diseases (Des Jarlais, Friedman, and Marmor 1987; Robertson *et al.* 1990; Selwyn *et al.* 1989; Weber *et al.* 1990). First, a number of stimulant drugs, such as cocaine, are typically injected more frequently, with concurrent increases in sharing and reinfection, and may themselves be immunosuppressive. Moreover, at least in the United States, these substances are typically obtained illegally through the street economy and are often adulterated by substances that may also contribute to immune impairment, a factor that may exacerbate dysfunction caused by HIV infection. Additionally, again as a function of the fact that many injected substances are illegal and therefore must be obtained and used surreptitiously, these substances are often administered in a manner that involves the sharing not only of infected needles, but also of related injection equipment including "cookers," cotton, and rinse water (cf. Battjes and Pickens 1988). These factors may also increase the likelihood that a user will be reinfected (cf. Flegg *et al.* 1989), as well as that a user will be exposed to multiple strains of HIV (Hahn *et al.* 1986), both factors that are also believed to accelerate immune dysfunction. Finally, and particularly in areas such as New York City, where the rate of seroprevalence among drug injectors is estimated already to exceed 50 percent (Des Jarlais, Friedman, and Marmor 1987), risk for exposure from sharing "works" is exacerbated not only by the greater likelihood of sharing of infected injection equipment, but also for exposure from unprotected sexual contact with an infected partner (Drucker 1986).

The rate of increase of AIDS cases among some groups initially associated with risk for HIV infection appears to be leveling off, a change that has been widely attributed to reported behavioral changes including increased condom use and a reduction in numbers of sexual partners (cf. Siegel *et al.* 1988). However, parallel changes among those whose risk is associated with the sharing of drug injection equipment has not been as readily forthcoming, at least as such changes can be inferred from seroprevalence studies (cf. Hahn *et al.* 1989). Given the fact that none of the existing AIDS treatments for HIV infection have as yet been demonstrated to have either broad demographic applicability or long-term effectiveness, prevention of the spread of HIV infection remains a critical challenge to public health practice, and the formulation of effective AIDS intervention strategies specific to drug injectors remains a critical problem in public health.

This chapter reviews evidence from a number of studies conducted among drug injectors in New York City. Early studies conducted among drug injectors in the Bronx, Brooklyn, and Manhattan boroughs of New York City in 1986 and 1987 are presented. Findings from a subsequent and more detailed study of knowledge and risk behavior in a sample of out-of-treatment drug injectors in Harlem between 1989 and 1990 are also presented.[2] Our purpose is to identify patterns in knowledge and risk behavior among drug injectors, to explicate disparities between knowledge and continued risk behavior, and to explore the import of these patterns for the formulation of AIDS prevention strategies and policies.

## OVERVIEW OF RISK KNOWLEDGE AND RISK BEHAVIOR AMONG INJECTORS IN NEW YORK CITY

Drug injectors in New York City appear to have had considerable knowledge about AIDS as early as 1984. In a study of fifty-nine individuals enrolled in methadone maintenance programs, for example, all had heard about AIDS, and over half knew that "needle sharing" (see previous chapter for a discussion of this term) was a potential mode of transmission (Friedman, Des Jarlais, and Sotheran 1986). Similarly, in a study conducted by the Street Survey Unit of the New York State Division of Substance Abuse Services in 1987, Hopkins (1988) found considerable awareness of AIDS among drug injectors, but noted that most seemed to perceive risk as primarily pertaining to "homosexuals." Likewise, in a study among drug injectors in jail and in methadone maintenance programs, Selwyn and associates (1985) found that some 97 percent acknowledged that sharing needles could transmit AIDS (see also Selwyn *et al.* 1989).

Data derived from a subsequent series of street surveys conducted in the fall of 1986 in drug-use areas in the Bronx, Brooklyn and Queens boroughs of New York City also suggested high levels of knowledge (see table 13.1) (Kleinman *et al.* 1990).[3] Some 95 percent of those asked about the means of AIDS transmission reported at least one correct answer, 75 percent reported some understanding of a relationship between the sharing of contaminated drug injection equipment and AIDS, and 80 percent reported some understanding of the relationship between sex and AIDS. Thirty-two percent never shared needles, 11 percent always shared needles, and the majority, 57 percent, reported specific kinds of circumstances as mitigating whether or not they shared needles on some occasions (e.g., with spouse only or with a "running partner" only). Almost half never used shooting galleries, 7 percent always used galleries, 4 percent used them only to "cop" (i.e., to purchase drugs), and 42 percent continued to use galleries under some circumstances. Forty-nine percent never used condoms, only 7 percent always used them, and 26 percent used them under some conditions.

A second survey, conducted approximately six months later in the spring of 1987 in drug-use areas in the Bronx, Brooklyn, and Queens, as well as in the area of upper Manhattan known as Harlem, suggested similar levels of knowledge. Of the 125 respondents from the Bronx, Brooklyn, and

Table 13.1
AIDS Knowledge and Practices in New York City

| Time | Location | Sample Size | Ethnicity | Gender | Transmission Knowledge | Gallery Use | Needle Sharing | Condom Use * |
|---|---|---|---|---|---|---|---|---|
| November 1986 | NEW YORK CITY<br><br>(Brooklyn, The Bronx, and Queens) | 137 | B–46%<br>W–15%<br>H–38% | M- 65%<br>F- 35% | 75% Works/AIDS<br>80% Sex/AIDS | 47% Never Use<br>42%Use Circumstantially<br>4% Use Only To Cop<br>7% Always Use | 32% Never Share<br>57% Share Circumstantially<br>11% Always Share | 49% Never Use<br>26% Use Circumstantially<br>7% Always Use |
| June 1987 | NEW YORK CITY<br><br>(Brooklyn, The Bronx, and Queens) | 125 | B–49%<br>W–12%<br>H–39% | M- 67%<br>F- 33% | 85% Works/AIDS<br>74% Sex/AIDS | 52% Never Use<br>34% Use Circumstantially<br>6% Use Only To Cop<br>7% Always Use | 36% Never Share<br>56% Share Circumstantially<br>7% Always Share | 47% Never Use<br>31% Use Circumstantially<br>6% Always Use |
| June 1987 | NEW YORK CITY<br><br>(HARLEM) | 46 | B–55%<br>W–11%<br>H–34% | M- 68%<br>F- 32% | 87% Works/AIDS<br>68% Sex/AIDS | 50% NeverUse<br>28% Use Circumstantially<br>9% Use Only To Cop<br>13% Always Use | 57% Never Share<br>31% Share Circumstantially<br>13% Always Share | 30% Never Use<br>38% Use Circumstantially<br>17% Always Use |
| Apr.'89-Dec.'90 | NEW YORK CITY<br><br>(HARLEM) | 1770 | B–66%<br>W–3.4%<br>H–30.3% | M- 63%<br>F- 37% | 99.7% Works/AIDS<br>99.3% Sex/AIDS | 56.5% Never Use<br>38.7% Use Circumstantially<br>4.8% Always Use | 31.5% Never Share<br>59.5% Share Circumstantially<br>9% Always Share | 46.4% Never Use<br>39.2% Use Circumstantially<br>14.4% Always Use |

B.-Black,not Hispanic
W.-White
H.-Hispanic

* Not all of Sample is Sexually Active

Queens who self-identified as drug injectors, 98 percent reported at least one correct answer regarding knowledge about AIDS. Eighty-five percent reported an association between the sharing of drug injection equipment and AIDS, and 74 percent reported an association between sex and AIDS. Fifty-two percent never used shooting galleries, 34 percent used them circumstantially, 6 percent used them only to cop, and 7 percent always used them. Thirty-six percent reported having always used what they believed to be new needles, 56 percent shared needles under some circumstances, and 7 percent always shared needles. Six percent always used condoms, 31 percent used them circumstantially, and 47 percent never used them.

Of those contacted in Harlem, 96 percent reported at least one correct answer about AIDS. Eighty-seven percent evidenced some understanding of the relationship between AIDS and the sharing of drug injection equipment, and 68 percent reported an association between AIDS and sexual behavior. Fifty-seven percent never shared needles, 31 percent did so under some circumstances, and 13 percent always shared needles. Fifty percent never used shooting galleries, 28 percent did so under some circumstances, 9 percent used them only to cop, and 13 percent always used them. Thirty percent never used condoms, 38 percent used them under some conditions, and only 17 percent always used them.[4]

While the kinds of conclusions that may be drawn from these initial studies are limited, they do suggest that there was a substantial understanding of the relationship between needle use and risk for AIDS among drug injectors in New York City. Admittedly, this association was sometimes quite vague. Some respondents associated risk for infection with the drugs themselves rather than with injection equipment, or with needles used during blood transfusions rather than with sharing drug injection equipment. Responses also indicated that risk from sharing of needles or blood products during transfusions, for example, was often conceptualized within socially derived boundaries, such that sharing needles was only considered dangerous when it involved persons thought to belong to other risk categories (e.g., gay men). In general, responses in the street surveys suggested that most of those contacted did not believe themselves to be personally at risk from needle sharing. Similarly, although the survey data showed a relatively high level of awareness of the relationship between AIDS and sexual activity, many of the respondents associated risk for AIDS from sex with certain kinds of persons (e.g., "gays"), regardless of any commonality between the particular sexual acts involved. Again, many respondents in the street survey study did not believe that they were personally at risk from unprotected sexual behavior.

## THE HARLEM STUDY

Given the limited size of these early studies, these data perhaps pose more questions than they resolve. As noted, they were derived from responses recorded in relatively "loose" contexts, with concurrent limitations in detail and sample selection. Moreover, and in and of themselves, they tell us little about the meaning that risk behaviors have in the everyday lives of drug injectors, the social and economic correlates of risk behavior, or the ways in which these correlates constrain consistent risk reduction. What is clear, however, is that in and of itself knowledge does not result in sustained risk reduction, a fact that is well substantiated in other literature on health behavior (cf. Fisher 1988). The issue, at least regarding AIDS prevention policy, therefore, is to identify those factors that impinge upon effective transformation of knowledge to action.

Here the longitudinal findings from a larger study in Harlem, the Harlem AIDS Project (HAP), may be of more analytic saliency.[5] Between April 1989 and December 1990 the HAP recruited 1,770 individuals, including 1,470 drug injectors and 300 sexual partners of drug injectors, from West, Central, and East Harlem (see table 13.1). Virtually all reported some understanding of the relationship between the sharing of "works" and AIDS, and almost all acknowledged that unprotected sex was a risk factor for AIDS. Despite these high levels of knowledge, however, both kinds of risk behavior persisted among most individuals in the sample. If we combine those injectors who sometimes (38.7 percent) or always (4.8 percent) used a shooting gallery, nearly half of the sample continued to do so. If we combine those who always shared needles (9 percent) and those who did so under some circumstances (59.5 percent), it is clear that the majority of the sample also continued to share injection equipment. Finally, nearly half of the total sample (46.4 percent) never used condoms, and much of the other half of the sample did so only circumstantially (39.2 percent). Thus while the changes in behavior that were indicated in these data were in the direction of increased risk reduction, a considerable amount of both injection and sex risk behavior continued to occur.

These patterns are also reflected in information gathered in data derived from qualitative ethnographic interviews (e.g., life-history and illness narratives), as well as from field observation in contexts in which high-risk behavior occurs (e.g., shooting galleries and crack houses). In particular, changes observed and noted in ethnographic research suggest that to a very large extent this decision making is situational and contextually defined. Specific kinds of conditions were often cited as overriding factors in decision-making processes relating to risk reduction, often in direct contradiction to stated knowledge and concern about the nature of risk.[6]

## RISK FROM NEEDLE SHARING

Although an increasing number of drug injectors contacted in informal street ethnography report that they view shooting galleries as undesirable places in which to shoot, the sharing of injection equipment in a variety of

contexts that are defined as explicitly social continues. In ethnographic interviews drug injectors report that they now prefer to shoot up in someone's
home, where the individuals involved are described as "known." Jimmy,
an African-American male who has used heroin for nearly thirty years, only
shoots with a group of long-term "running partners." They continue to
gather, as they have for nearly two decades, in the apartment of one member of the group to listen to jazz music and "share a bag of dope." They
have "always" shared needles, and although Jimmy knows that there is risk
involved in doing so, he specifically articulated the fact that he has known
all the members of the group for many years and the fact that none of
them have ever had any other needle-related infections (e.g., hepatitis) as
factors in his decision to continue sharing. Jimmy explained this practice
as originating from the fact that needles were and are sometimes difficult
to acquire. In addition to periodic fluctuations in the supply of needles, he
emphasized that carrying needles, which is illegal in New York City, represented an added danger for arrest.

It is noteworthy, moreover, that in the descriptions of the social importance of sharing needles often were embedded the ritualized meanings associated with the sharing of other kinds of socially constituted space, often
overlapping in context and meaning with other kinds of risk behavior. This
was particularly true of individuals who claimed to share needles only with
their primary sex partners. Natalie, a Hispanic female, for example, described a stormy relationship with her husband, including several occasions
when he had become violent and beaten her. Equally vivid, however, was
her description of subsequent reconciliations in which he would inject with
her rather than with his regular "running buddies." These events stood out
in the narrative as those that she identified as among the most important
in her experiences in her life. In particular, it is noteworthy that the sharing
of injection equipment, at least on her part, came to signify the renewed
bond between them, a pattern that was also echoed among other women.

These interpersonal dynamics notwithstanding, perhaps more representative of the kinds of circumstances that were reported as influencing
whether or not someone shares "works," were those factors that involved
some kind of practical necessity to share injection equipment. This was
particularly true of explanations of sharing "works" in shooting galleries.
"Feeling sick," a generalized experience of pain and acute anxiety that is
associated with heroin withdrawal, or for some reason not being able to
go home to shoot, are the two circumstances most often cited as reasons
for using a shooting gallery.

"Not being able to go home" is sometimes explained in terms of the time
it takes to "cop" and then travel home to shoot when one is feeling "sick,"
or the dangers of assault or arrest from carrying drugs on the streets. Others
report having to conceal their drug use from individuals within their households. However, the explanation "not being able to go home to inject" is

also sometimes a literal explanation as well. Approximately one-fifth of the drug injectors in the final HAP sample reported living on the streets or in a homeless shelter, a circumstance that was strongly associated with risk behavior.[7] Higher frequencies of drug use exist among homeless injectors, including more frequent use of crack, injected heroin, alcohol, and "speedballs" (heroin and cocaine mixed). In ethnographic interviews among homeless drug injectors, the use of multiple narcotic substances was also consistently described in direct association with the experience of homelessness, including frequent hunger and chronic feelings of despair and alienation. Life-history narratives are filled with extended descriptions of self-doubt and self-hate and are rife with pained images of despair and self-destruction. These emotions are often "medicated" through the use of stimulant drugs, especially freebase cocaine and speed. The use of speedballs seems to have particular importance among the homeless and, at least in street folklore, is also said to be a way of stretching the effects of a low dosage of heroin.

Moreover, homeless drug injectors in this study were also shown to be more likely to use a shooting gallery, more likely to shoot at a dealer's house, and more likely to shoot in a park, alley, or abandoned building than nonhomeless drug injectors, all contexts that are strongly associated with sharing injection equipment.[8] Jerry, for example, a white male in his early forties who has run in the street economy of Harlem since his early teens, is homeless, making his way by whatever he "boosts" (steals) from supermarkets and drug stores and can later sell on the streets. He lives in a "coke gallery," where he injects both cocaine and amphetamines. Often he cannot afford to purchase new "works" on the streets and consequently must rent "house works," often shooting with one or more persons within a wide, fluid, social street network of individuals who occupy similar positions in the street economy. In addition, it is noteworthy that in a pattern typical of injectors who are dependent upon stimulant drugs such as cocaine, he injects much more often than does the typical user of heroin, a fact that increases the number of times that he is likely to share, and consequently his risk for HIV infection (cf. Des Jarlais and Friedman 1988).

## RISK FROM UNPROTECTED SEX

Responses obtained in both the earlier street survey data and the Harlem study indicate the interdependence of risks associated with needle sharing and those associated with high-risk sexual behavior. Danger is frequently represented as pertaining to certain kinds of persons (e.g., "gays" and "crackheads"), and respondents often claim that they are not personally at risk because of socially derived knowledge of the person with whom they are engaging in risk behaviors. The length of time that a person has been known and the fact that they have engaged in risk behavior (both needle sharing and unprotected sex) on previous occasions without apparent harm are frequently cited examples. However, foremost in these discussions were the difficulties encountered in attempting to introduce safer sex practices (e.g., the use of condoms) into ongoing relationships without seeming to undermine the complex interpersonal expectations upon which those relationships were founded. Indeed, and again reminiscent of the social meanings that are sometimes associated with needle sharing between sexual partners, some respondents have described engaging in risk behaviors, particularly sex without a condom, as one way in which commitment to a relationship is signified (Worth 1989).

Ethnographic material obtained during life-history interviews also suggests that reported increases in the use of a number of noninjected drugs, particularly crack and alcohol, is a direct response to emergent concerns about risk for AIDS now associated with sharing needles (cf. Abramowitz et al. 1989; Buffum 1988; Clatts et al. 1990; Landry and Smith 1988; Worth 1989). A wide range of drugs are available in "crack houses," or what are sometimes known in New York City as "freak houses" or "get off houses." Snorting cocaine and smoking crack cocaine, both in conjunction with heroin ("chasin' the dragon"), alcohol ("to smooth it out"), or angel dust ("space base"), are also frequent occurrences in these settings. In addition to the fact that some of these places function as places of temporary refuge for many homeless drug injectors, as well as a place in which to acquire and use drugs in general, they are also frequently a site in which drugs are exchanged for sex. It is noteworthy, for example, that of the 971 individuals in the HAP sample who had multiple sex partners, nearly 40 percent reported having exchanged sex for money, and nearly 35 percent reported exchanging sex for drugs. Although the use of crack is not itself a vector for HIV transmission, chronic dependence on a drug like crack is certainly a risk to general health and may also contribute to impairing or constraining judgment regarding sexual risk behavior (cf. Clatts, Davis, Deren, and Tortu 1991; Friedman et al. 1988; Kronliczak 1990).

## DISCUSSION

A substantial number of questions remain unresolved in attempting to compare and interpret the data presented here. First, as previously noted, the initial survey data were based on self-reports from informal, somewhat casual conversations. In contrast, the data gathered in the context of the HAP study, while also based on self-reports, were obtained in the course of highly structured interviews conducted by trained interviewers in a private office at a research site.[9] Thus the data are not completely comparable. Second, it is noteworthy that the initial street surveys included a much larger percentage of individuals whom street survey workers identified as Hispanic, while the subsequent study initially consisted largely of individuals who self-identified as African-American.[10] Though the ratio of African-Americans to Hispanics in the final HAP sample appears comparable to the ratios in the earlier studies, the issues of accuracy and comparability remain, as do limitations in comparing information provided in the course of street conversation with that provided in highly structured interviews.

With these methodological sampling differences and consequent inferential limitations in mind, and given the relatively small sample size of the street survey data, it would be difficult to infer definitive conclusions with regard to either general knowledge about AIDS or risk behavior. What is perhaps most notable about the data taken as a whole, however, is the fact that a considerable number of individuals continue to engage in high-risk behavior, apparently with considerable frequency and despite high levels of knowledge about both AIDS risk behavior and AIDS risk reduction. That is, despite considerable knowledge about AIDS in the Harlem community, documented over a four-year span of time, the data suggest that a substantial number of drug injectors continue to frequently engage in a number of high-risk behaviors, or, conversely, that they engage in protective or low-risk behaviors inconsistently or only circumstantially.

As noted previously, the risk behaviors that have been implicated in the spread of HIV infection cannot be understood apart from the social, cultural, economic, and political institutions and contexts in which they are embedded. That is, behavioral processes are configured not only as a function of individual knowledge and will, but also by the larger structural circumstances that may serve to constrain individual action. While continued AIDS education is of great importance in this community, the findings presented here indicate that perhaps paramount among the factors that undermine risk reduction are structural constraints that are embedded in the social, economic, and political institutions that prevail in this community (see also Marion and Amann 1989).

Earlier in this chapter we noted that the kinds of behavior changes that have been attributed to other risk communities, such as gay men, have generally not emerged on a parallel scale among drug injectors, at least in New York City. While there are clear differences both in the risk behaviors themselves and in the sociocultural meanings that attend them, it is noteworthy that there are also marked economic differences between these two "risk groups."[11] For example, the fact that a substantial number of individuals are dependent upon street prostitution, a circumstance that is strongly associated with both high-risk sex and chronic drug dependency, cannot be adequately understood outside the context of the dearth of educational and employment opportunities that exists in this community. Similarly, risk behavior among the homeless cannot be understood apart from the social and economic factors that function both to create and to maintain a substantial population who do not have access to employment, housing, and health care resources (cf. Benker, Boone, and Dehavenon

1990; Clatts 1993). Nor can the form and function of the use of a number of street drugs among them, as well as chronic drug dependency, be adequately understood apart from the demoralizing and debilitating effects of homelessness itself (Clatts, Beardsley, Deren, and Tortu 1991). Moreover, and in addition to vastly inadequate primary health care and prevention resources in this community (McCord and Freeman 1990:173–177), there are also vastly inadequate resources for both drug treatment (cf. Des Jarlais and Friedman 1991) and research on alternative treatment modalities.[12]

The scope of this chapter does not permit a full examination of the health policy implications of these multiple and admittedly very complex issues. The data do, however, support the conclusion that while knowledge is a necessary condition for risk reduction, it often is not a sufficient one. These data also suggest that there is a lack of fit between AIDS prevention policies that target reduction in "supply" for drugs and those policies that are focused on reduction of unsafe drug-administration practices.

As Newcombe (1990), among many others, has indicated, risk for injection-related harm is as much a function of laws, strictures, de facto treatment of drug users, and a supply-side approach to the use of controlled substances as it is a product of the use of drugs themselves. Supply strategies do not need to be considered antithetical to those that focus on demand. Indeed, programs providing treatment to reduce drug injection and programs providing means for safer injection practices, such as needle-exchange projects, can and should be seen as complementary rather than contradictory (cf. Des Jarlais et al. 1989). However, such initiatives are often represented as contradictory and in practice are made incompatible when, as in New York City, health care policies and health care resources are not adequately focused on critical AIDS intervention goals, particularly reduction in needle sharing. For example, the inordinate level of resources that have been put into supply reduction have had little if any real effect on demand, at least among chronic users in this community (cf. Clatts, Davis, Deren, and Tortu 1990; Hamid 1990, 1991; Johnson et al. 1989)—this at a time when many in this community suffer from inadequate housing, health care, and educational resources.

Furthermore, the political discourse in which current supply strategies have been forged, one that both criminalizes drug use and stigmatizes the drug user, has had a number of negative effects on AIDS prevention policy and prevention practice (Rivera-Beckman, Friedman, and Clatts 1990; Sorge 1991). For example, many street-based AIDS education programs have become almost exclusively focused on HIV testing and surveillance and have been characterized by a style that has served to alienate those most in need of AIDS prevention services and resources (cf. Rivera-Beckman, Friedman, and Clatts 1990). Similarly, the debate in New York City over bleach distribution and needle exchange has been so tangled in complex racial and class power conflicts that it has thus far virtually immobilized the formulation of a rational health policy.

For example, in November 1989 the number of persons in New York City diagnosed with AIDS whose primary risk factor was drug injection was 1,163, accounting for 42 percent of all cases. In 1990, the year following the closing of a very modest and limited needle-exchange program, the number of those whose primary risk factor was associated with drug injection more than doubled to a total of 2,499, increasing to approximately 46 percent of all cases.[13] While final figures are not yet available, it is anticipated that similar patterns of increase among drug injectors, their sexual partners, and their children will emerge.[14] In a city where over half the drug injectors are estimated to be HIV infected, these figures serve to illustrate both the seriousness of the situation and the contradictory character of the social and political discourse that has underpinned AIDS prevention policy and decision making.

## SUMMARY AND CONCLUSIONS

This chapter has had two primary goals. The first is to report evidence from a variety of research efforts that have been initiated among drug injectors in New York City since 1989. In particular, we have examined knowledge about AIDS and the persistence of a number of risk behaviors, notably needle sharing, the use of shooting galleries where needle sharing has often been known to occur, and unprotected sex, despite a relatively high level of knowledge about the risks for HIV infection. The second goal, an outgrowth of the first, is to show the way in which data gathered by utilizing diverse research strategies can be effectively integrated, how they can be used to interpret community responses to AIDS, and how they can be brought to bear in discussion of prevention policy.

Two broad conclusions respective to AIDS prevention policy among drug injectors can be drawn from this discussion: in and of itself, knowledge about risk does not result in behavioral change among a substantial portion of those involved in drug injection. As indicated elsewhere in the health literature, decision-making processes relating to health often involve management of competing "goals" extant within the larger social and economic fabric of the community in which an individual lives. The ethnographic interviews indicate that the need to assuage feelings of "sickness" associated with drug withdrawal, for example, significantly constrains decision-making processes related to needle sharing. Chronic use of crack and other stimulant drugs also appears to be directly related to the need to "medicate" acute feelings of panic, fear, and depression. Similarly, decision making relating to the use of condoms during sexual intercourse appears to be constrained by a host of social and economic factors whose force and immediacy compete with concerns about potential risk for HIV infection.

The finding that high-risk behaviors in the community are circumstantially governed by such factors as the onset of withdrawal pains and chronic feelings of depression has a number of important implications for intervention. One such implication is that consistent behavioral change in regard to the sharing of drug-use equipment is likely to be contingent not simply upon the possession of knowledge about the risks inherent in these behaviors, but also upon the availability of alternatives with which to respond to the urgency that everyday experiences of dependency impose. Minimally, these alternatives must include the availability of sterile injection equipment, but they must also include opportunities for drug treatment. It is noteworthy, however, that although some drug users benefit from treatment, there is a sizeable group who never enter treatment (cf. Biernacki 1986). Many others are unable to complete the program or relapse after treatment. It has been estimated in some European studies, for example, that perhaps no more than 10 to 25 percent of drug users have a long-term benefit from treatment (Burning 1991; see also Baekeland and Lundwall 1975; Hubbard *et al.* 1989). Thus successful AIDS prevention among out-of-treatment injectors necessarily involves identifying and making available safer injection alternatives.

Moreover, the finding that risks associated with needle sharing are defined by indigenous perceptions of safety (e.g., shooting at home) and by conceptualizations of social intimacy (e.g., shooting with someone who is "known," such as a regular sexual partner), suggests that behavioral change is likely to be highly dependent upon an individual's personal skills. These skills include not simply the ability to recognize personal risk, but also the perception that one is able to introduce behavioral changes within socially defined relationships that will not threaten the expectations of appropriate social closeness upon which those relationships have been founded. AIDS prevention programs that do not articulate risk-reduction messages within the larger structure of social and economic choices in which individual decision making occurs are unlikely to make a substantial and lasting impact on behavioral change.

Finally, we have explored the impact of ambiguous and often contradictory AIDS prevention policies on the spread of HIV infection among drug injectors in New York City. Several studies have indicated that drug injectors are receptive to risk-reduction strategies, especially those that are specific to changes in shooting behavior (cf. Jackson, Rothkiewitz, and Wells 1988; Jain 1988; Lowenstein 1988). However, particularly as these strategies relate to resource allocation in general, and to needle exchange in particular, we have raised concerns about the way in which the public health goal of preventing the spread of HIV infection appears to have been subverted by competing political interests and an anti–drug-user public health discourse.

## NOTES

We would like to acknowledge the work of D. Des Jarlais, S. Friedman, and P. Kleinman of NDRI, and W. Hopkins of the New York State Division of Substance Abuse Services and his street unit, in the development and administration of the street survey data that are reviewed in this chapter. The research presented from the Harlem AIDS Project was supported by grant DA05746 from the National Institute on Drug Abuse. The views expressed in this chapter do not necessarily represent those of Narcotic and Drug Research, Inc., the New York State Division of Substance Abuse Services, or the National Institute on Drug Abuse.

1. A number of street terms are used in this chapter. In New York City the term *works* (in some places also known as *sets* or *rigs*) refers to an array of injection-related equipment, including a *pin* (hypodermic needle and syringe), a *cooker* (a small container, often a bottle cap, used to dissolve and heat heroin), and *cotton* (a piece of cotton used to strain impurities from dissolved heroin). A *shooting gallery* is a semipublic place, such as an abandoned building, in which drugs are purchased and injection activity occurs. The counterpart of a gallery for the use of crack is called a *crack house*. To *cop* or *copping* refers to some manner of acquiring drugs, usually heroin. *Feeling sick* is used in particular linguistic contexts to refer to physical pain associated with heroin withdrawal. *Running* is a term that generally refers to the life of heroin injection (cf. Agar 1973). A *running partner*, sometimes also referred to as a *running buddy*, is an individual with whom one regularly injects, usually including common purchase of drugs and use of common injection equipment.

2. There are a number of limitations in the comparability of these various sources of data, particularly the early street-based studies. These limitations are readily acknowledged in the course of their presentation. However, we believe that the material does serve to prepare us to ask some rather specific questions of the data gathered in the subsequent Harlem study, questions that are important policy issues relating to AIDS prevention among drug injectors.

3. The survey data sets involved the same interview staff, working on roughly the same or immediately contiguous blocks or streetcorners. Since no identifying information was recorded in either survey, it is not known how many of those initially contacted also participated in the subsequent survey. Moreover, it was not possible in the context of these interviews to establish whether or not all of these respondents resided in Harlem. Since Harlem functions as a center for the New York metropolitan area where drugs are sold, it is likely that at least some of those contacted resided outside the Harlem community.

4. While important as initial assessments of knowledge about AIDS among drug injectors, the scope of these earlier studies provides the basis for only a very limited analysis of levels of knowledge and risk behavior. These studies were conducted in an informal manner, and respondents did not know that information contained in their conversation was part of a research study. Since specific areas of inquiry relating to knowledge about AIDS, condom use, and needle sharing were explored during casual conversation, it was sometimes difficult to explore particular issues in depth. Furthermore, although the interviews were conducted by trained, experienced personnel, the setting and nature of the study site itself placed some

limitations on the research process. Conversations were frequently interrupted and probably reflected respondents' most salient reactions to any particular issue, rather than their complete knowledge and understanding (Kleinman et al. 1990). Finally, it is noteworthy that responses were recorded after interviewers were able to find a discrete place on the streets to record notes about the content of the interview and often reflect the interviewers' "gloss" on the substance of the exchange.

5. All participants in the HAP study were out-of-treatment drug injectors or a sexual partner of a drug injector. Each was asked to participate in structured interviews that included a number of specific questions regarding their knowledge about AIDS (i.e., means of HIV transmission and prevention), as well as about specific kinds and frequencies of drug use and high-risk sexual behavior. Participants were subsequently offered the opportunity to participate in a series of AIDS education group sessions and were reinterviewed at six-month and one-year intervals in an effort to examine the extent to which the information provided and the risk-reduction skills taught in the group sessions had resulted in behavioral change. This study also included a formal ethnographic component that involved both gathering life-history narratives using open-ended questions and "participant observation" of high-risk activities (e.g., shooting galleries and crack houses) in the Harlem community. The purpose of the ethnographic research was to acquire some understanding of the larger social fabric of the community, to document participants' responses to, and experience of, the intervention program, and to document changes in risk behavior among drug injectors in the community. Life-history interviews generally lasted approximately three hours and methodologically were conducted in a loose, open-ended format suited to the goal of acquiring an understanding of the drug injectors' own interpretations of risk. For more general discussions of the use of ethnography in AIDS prevention research, see Adler (1990) and Feldman and Aldrich (1990).

6. For further discussion, see Clatts (1993) and Clatts, Davis, Deren, and Tortu (1990). Similar findings have been reported in parallel studies conducted elsewhere. See, for example, Goldsmith and Friedman (1991) and Newmeyer et al. (1989).

7. There were no statistically significant differences relating to these aspects of knowledge about risk behavior between homeless and nonhomeless drug injectors in this sample. For further discussion of risk behavior among homeless drug injectors, see Clatts (1991); Goldsmith and Friedman (1991); and Popkin et al. (1991).

8. Homelessness increases the likelihood that a drug injector will share "works" for two reasons. First, homeless drug injectors rarely have enough money to buy their own drugs, or to buy them in large quantities. Second, they do not have a reliable or secure place in which they can store drugs. Consequently, they tend to "cop" a single dose at a time, and to inject immediately, often using "house works" since it is illegal and therefore dangerous to carry their own on the streets. Because of both constraints, they may "split a bag" with someone else, a circumstance that is likely to promote needle sharing. Indeed, the emergence of a market in the early 1980s for cocaine hydrochloride powder for conversion into freebase (crack) for smoking was directly tied to circumstances in the underground drug economy that favored marketing a readily usable noninjected substance that could be easily sold in small, easily concealed, one-time doses (cf. Hamid 1991). Thus, in addition to the substantial experiential functions that this particular drug serves, it also fits a

particular economic and statutory niche. For more extensive discussion of the data on the homeless in this sample, see Clatts, Beardsley, Deren, and Tortu (1991).

9. While these more structured contexts provide a more suitable context for conducting certain kinds of survey research, they also have a number of methodological and interpretive limitations. For an extended discussion of these issues, see Amsel *et al.* (1976); Kleyn and Day (1990); Maddux and Desmond (1975); Page and Lai (1990); Stephens (1972); van Meter (1990); Watters and Cheng (1991); and Wiebel (1989, 1991).

10. Harlem is a multiethnic community that includes large numbers of individuals of Caribbean island and Central American birth or descent, as well as African-Americans. Ethnic affiliation among some members of these groups is often quite fluid, and ethnic membership is subject to situational negotiation (cf. Brettel 1977; DeVos 1975). The latter circumstance presents a serious obstacle to attempts to derive any absolute conclusions about ethnic groups in the community, particularly as these relate to behaviors implicated in HIV infection. For specific discussion of this issue in relation to AIDS prevention among Hispanics, see Deren *et al.* (1991).

11. We acknowledge the difficulty of using the term *risk groups*. In New York City, for example, there is overlap between men who have sex with men and men who inject drugs; hence there are limitations in treating these groups as if they existed independent of one another. We use the term here heuristically and for the limited purposes of certain parts of our discussion. In general, however, we caution against imputing any absolute empirical distinction between the referents (cf. Carrier and Bolton 1991; Clatts and Mutchler 1989:113; Inhorn and Brown 1990).

12. It is noteworthy that although the HAP sample was explicitly drawn from out-of-treatment drug injectors, much of the sample had been in treatment at some time in their lives, many on several occasions. In ethnographic interviews many of these individuals reported the perception that it was not possible for them to live without drugs and revealed the expectation that they would always be drug dependent.

13. As of 1994, there have been five programs that have been exempted from the New York City law that makes needle exchange illegal. However, it remains unclear if, as in the previous trial exchange program, politics will determine the structure of the program to such an extent as to undermine its potential effectiveness, and in the process thereby virtually insure its own self-destruction (cf. Sorge 1991). For more general discussions of the impact of social and political discourse on both AIDS prevention and AIDS research, see Clatts and Mutchler (1989) and Lessor and Jurich (1986).

14. The "window" period between initial infection and seroconversion is currently believed to be as much as six months. More poorly defined, however, is the time between seroconversion and the onset of AIDS-spectrum diseases that may or may not result in actual diagnosis. Consequently, it is not possible to determine the potential role that the closing of the program may have had on the subsequent increases in seroprevalence and AIDS cases among drug injectors.

## REFERENCES

Abramowitz, A., J. Guydish, W. Woods, and W. Clark. 1989. Increasing Crack Use among Drug Users in an AIDS Epicenter: San Francisco. Poster presentation at the V International AIDS Conference, Montreal.

Adler, P. 1990. Ethnographic Research on Hidden Populations: Penetrating the Drug World. In *The Collection and Interpretation of Data from Hidden Populations*. NIDA Research Monograph 90, pp. 96–112.

Agar, M. 1973. *Ripping and Running: A Formal Ethnography of Urban Heroin Addicts*. New York: Seminar Press.

Amsel, Z., W. Mandell, L. Matthias, C. Mason, and I. Hocherman. 1976. Reliability and Validity of Self-reported Illegal Activities and Drug Use Collected from Narcotic Addicts. *International Journal of the Addictions* 11:325–336.

Baekeland, F., and L. Lundwall. 1975. Dropping out of Treatment: A Critical Review. *Psychological Bulletin* 82(5): 738–783.

Battjes, R., and R. Pickens, eds. 1988. *Needle Sharing among Intravenous Drug Abusers: National and International Perspectives*. NIDA Research Monograph 80. Rockville, MD: National Institute on Drug Abuse.

Benker, K., M. Boone, and A. Dehavenon. 1990. *The Tyranny of Indifference: A Study of Hunger, Homelessness, Poor Health, and Family Dismemberment in 1,325 New York City Households with Children, 1989–1990*. New York: Action Research Project on Hunger, Homelessness, and Family Health.

Biernacki, P. 1986. *Pathways from Heroin Addiction: Recovery without Treatment*. Philadelphia: Temple University Press.

Blackwell, J. 1983. Drifting, Controlling, and Overcoming: Opiate Users Who Avoid Becoming Chronically Dependent. *Journal of Drug Issues* No. 13 (Spring): 219–235.

Brettel, C. 1977. Ethnicity and Entrepreneurs: Portuguese Immigrants in a Canadian City. In *Ethnic Encounters: Identities and Contexts*, ed. G. Hicks and P. Leis. North Scituate, MA: Duxbury Press.

Buffum, J. 1988. Substance Abuse and High-Risk Sexual Behavior: Drugs and Sex— The Dark Side. *Journal of Psychoactive Drugs* 20(2): 165–167.

Burning, E. 1991. Harm Reduction Is Mainstream Thinking. Paper presented at the Second International Conference on the Reduction of Drug-related Harm, Barcelona, Spain, March.

Carrier, J., and R. Bolton. 1991. Anthropological Perspectives on Sexuality and HIV Prevention. *Annual Review of Sex Research*.

Centers for Disease Control. 1991. *HIV/AIDS Surveillance: Year-End Edition: U.S. AIDS cases Reported through December 1990*. Atlanta: CDC.

Clatts, M. 1991. Ethnography and AIDS Intervention in New York City: Life History as an Ethnographic Strategy. In *Community-based AIDS Prevention: Studies of Intravenous Drug Users and Their Sexual Partners*. Rockville, MD: National Institute on Drug Abuse.

———. 1993. Poverty, Drug Use, and AIDS: Converging Lines in the Life Stories of Women in Harlem. In *Wings of Gauze: Gender and the Experience of Illness*, ed. B. Blair and S. Cayleff. pp. 328–339. Detroit: Wayne State University Press.

Clatts, M. C., M. Beardsley, S. Deren, and S. Tortu. 1991. Economies of Scale and the Homeless Drug Injector: Contradictions in AIDS Prevention Practice. Paper presented at the Third Annual AIDS Demonstration Conference, Bethesda, Maryland.

Clatts, M. C., R. Davis, S. Deren, and S. Tortu. 1991. NIDA Community based AIDS Prevention Among Intravenous Drug Users and Their Sexual Partners. Rockville, Maryland: NIDA.

Clatts, M. C., S. Deren, and S. Tortu. 1991. What's in a Name? AIDS and the Social Construction of Risk in the Moral Imagination of Drug Users in Harlem. *Anthropologie et Societes* 15(2–3).

Clatts, M. C., and K. M. Mutchler. 1989. AIDS and the Dangerous Other: Metaphors of Sex and Deviance in the Representation of Disease. *Medical Anthropology* 10(2–3):105–114.

Clatts, M. C., E. Springer, and M. Washburn. 1990. Outreach to Homeless Youth in NYC: Implications for Planning and Practice in Social Services. Paper presented at the meetings of the American Public Health Association, New York, N.Y.

Des Jarlais, D. 1989. AIDS Prevention Programs for Intravenous Drug Users: Diversity and Evolution. *International Review of Psychiatry* 1:101–108.

Des Jarlais, D., and S. R. Friedman. 1987. HIV Infection among Intravenous Drug Users: Epidemiology and Risk Reduction. *AIDS* 1(2):67–76.

———. 1988. HIV Infection among Persons Who Inject Illicit Drugs: Problems and Prospects. *Journal of Acquired Immune Deficiency Syndromes* 1:267–273.

———. 1991. *Waiting Lists for Drug Abuse Treatment*. Washington, DC: National Academy of Sciences.

Des Jarlais, D., S. R. Friedman, and M. Marmor. 1987. Development of AIDS, HIV Seroconversion, and Potential Co-factors for T4 Cell Loss in a Cohort of Intravenous Drug Users. *AIDS* 1:105–111.

Des Jarlais, D., S. Friedman, D. Novick, and J. Sotheran. 1989. HIV-1 Infection among Intravenous Drug Users in Manhattan, New York City, from 1977 through 1987. *Journal of the American Medical Association* 261:(7) 1008–1012.

DeVos, G. 1975. Ethnicity: Vessel of Meaning and Emblem of Contrast. In *Ethnic Identity: Cultural Continuities and Change,* ed. G. DeVos and L. Romanucci-Ross. Palo Alto, CA: Mayfield.

Drucker, E. 1986. AIDS and Addiction in New York City. *American Journal of Drug and Alcohol Abuse* 12(1–2):165–181.

Evans, B., S. McCormack, R. Bond, K. MacRae, and R. Thorp. 1988. Human Immunodeficiency Virus Infection, Hepatitis B Virus Infection, and Sexual Behaviour of Women Attending a Genitourinary Medicine Clinic. *British Medical Journal* 296:473–475.

Feldman, H., and M. Aldrich. 1990. The Role of Ethnography in Substance Abuse Research and Public Policy: Historical Precedent and Future Prospects. In *The Collection and Interpretation of Data from Hidden Populations,* NIDA Research Monograph 90, pp. 12–30.

Fisher, J. D. 1988. Possible Effects of Reference Group–based Social Influence on AIDS-Risk Behavior and AIDS Prevention. *American Psychologist* 43(11): 914–920.

Flegg, P., M. Jones, L. MacCallum, A. Bird, J. Whitelaw, and R. Brettle. 1989. Continued Injecting Drug Use as a Cofactor for Progression of HIV. Poster presentation at V International Conference on AIDS, Montreal.

Friedman, S. R., D. Des Jarlais and J. Sotheran, 1986. AIDS Health Education for Intravenous Drug Users. *Health Education Quarterly* 13(4): 383–393.

Friedman, S., C. Dozier, C. Sterk, T. Williams, J. Sotheran, and D. Des Jarlais. 1988. Crack Use Puts Drug Smoking Women at Risk for Heterosexual

Transmission of HIV from Intravenous Drug Users. Paper presented at the IV International AIDS Conference, Stockholm, Sweden.

Goldsmith, D., and S. R. Friedman. 1991. Drugs, Sex, AIDS, and Street Survival: The Voices of Five Women. *Anthropologie et Societes* 15(2–3):13–36.

Graeven, D., and K. Graeven. 1983. Treated and Untreated Addicts: Factors Associated with Participation in Treatment and Cessation of Heroin Use. *Journal of Drug Issues* (Spring):13:207–208.

Hahn, B., G. Shaw, and M. Taylor, et al. 1986. Genetic Variation in HTLV-III/LAV over Time in Patients with AIDS or at Risk for AIDS. *Science* 232: 1548–1553.

Hahn, R., I. Onorato, T. Jones, and J. Dougherty. 1989. Prevalence of HIV Infection among Intravenous Drug Users in the United States. *Journal of the American Medical Association* 18:2677–2684.

Hamid, A. 1990. The Political Economy of Crack-related Violence. *Contemporary Drug Problems* 3:31–77.

———. 1991. From Ganja to Crack: Caribbean Participation in the Underground Economy of Brooklyn. *International Journal of the Addictions* 26(8):31–78.

Hopkins, W. 1988. Needle Sharing and Street Behavior in Response to AIDS in New York City. In *Needle Sharing among Intravenous Drug Abusers: National and International Perspectives,* ed. R. Battjes and R. Pickens. NIDA Research Monograph 80. Rockville, MD: National Institute on Drug Abuse.

Hubbard, R. L., M. Marsden, J. Rachal, H. Harwood, E. Cavanaugh, and H. Ginzburg. 1989. *Drug Abuse Treatment: A National Study of Effectiveness.* Chapel Hill: University of North Carolina Press.

Inhorn, M. C. and P. Brown. 1990. The Anthropology of Infectious Disease. *Annual Review of Anthropology* 19:87–117.

Jackson, J., L. Rothkiewitz, and D. Wells. 1988. IVDU AIDS Knowledge and Behavioral Change. Poster paper presented at the IV International Conference on AIDS, Stockholm, Sweden.

Jain, S. 1988. IV Drug Users and AIDS: Changing Attitudes and Behavior. Poster presented at the IV International Conference on AIDS, Stockholm, Sweden.

Johnson, B., T. Williams, K. Dei, and H. Sanabria. 1989. Drug Abuse and the Inner City: Impact of Hard Drug Use and Sales on Low Income Communities. In *Crime and Justice: A Review of Research* Chicago: University of Chicago Press.

Kleinman, P., D. Goldsmith, S. R. Friedman, W. Hopkins, and D. Des Jarlais. 1990. Knowledge about and Behaviors Affecting the Spread of AIDS: A Street Survey of Intravenous Drug Users and Their Associates in New York City. *International Journal of the Addictions* 25(4): 345–361.

Kleyn, J., and L. Day. 1990. Sex, Drugs, and Truth: New Findings on the Reliability of Intravenous Drug Users' Self-Reports. Paper presented at the 1990 Annual Meetings of the American Society of Criminology.

Kristal, A. R. 1986. The Impact of the Acquired Immune Deficiency Syndrome on Patterns of Premature Death in New York City. *Journal of the American Medical Association* 255:2306–2310.

Kronliczak, A. 1990. Update on High-Risk Behaviors among Female Sexual Partners of Injection Drug Users. *NADR Network* [Special issue]. Bethesda, MD: National Institute on Drug Abuse.

Landry, M., and D. Smith. 1988. AIDS and Chemical Dependency: An Overview. *Journal of Psychoactive Drugs* 20(2): 141–147.

Lessor, R., and K. Jurich. 1986. Ideology and Politics in the Control of Contagion: The Social Organization of AIDS Care. In *The Social Dimensions of AIDS,* ed. D. Feldman and T. Johnson, pp. 245–259. New York: Praeger.

Lowenstein, W. A. 1988. Changes of Behavior in French IV Drug Addicts. Poster presented at the IV International Conference on AIDS, Stockholm, Sweden.

Maddux, J., and D. Desmond. 1975. Reliability and Validity of Information from Chronic Heroin Users. *Journal of Psychiatric Research* 12:87–95.

Marion, I., and K. Amann. 1989. Determinants of Needle Sharing among Intravenous Drug Users. *American Journal of Public Health* 79:459–462.

McCord, C., and H. Freeman. 1990. Excess Mortality in Harlem. *New England Journal of Medicine* 322(3): 173–177.

Newcombe, R. 1990. The Reduction of Drug-related Harm: A Conceptual Framework for Theory, Practice, and Research. Paper presented at the First International Conference on the Reduction of Drug-Related Harm, University of Liverpool, Liverpool, England, April 9–12.

Newmeyer, J., H. Feldman, P. Biernacki, and J. Watters. 1989. Preventing AIDS Contagion among Intravenous Drug Users. *Medical Anthropology* 10:167–175.

Page, J. B., and S. Lai. 1990. Longitudinal Study of Street Recruited Intravenous Drug Users. Paper presented at the Annual Meeting of the American Anthropological Association, New Orleans, Louisiana, November 28.

Page, J. B., and P. Smith. 1990. Venous Envy: The Importance of Having Functional Veins. *Journal of Drug Issues* 20(2): 291–308.

Popkin, S., W. Johnson, M. C. Clatts, W. Wiebel, and S. Deren. 1991. Homeless and Risk Behaviors among IVDUS in Chicago and New York. Poster presented at the VII International AIDS Conference, Florence, Italy.

Rivera-Beckman, J., S. R. Friedman, and M. C. Clatts. 1990. Inside-outside: Social Processes in Street Outreach. Paper presented at the Second Annual AIDS Demonstration and Research Conference, National Institute on Drug Abuse, Bethesda, Maryland.

Robertson, J. R., C. Skidmore, J. Roberts, and R. Elton. 1990. Progression to AIDS in Intravenous Drug Injectors, Co-factors, and Survival. Poster VI International Conference on AIDS, San Francisco.

Selwyn, P. A., C. P. Cox, C. Feiner, C. Lipshutz, and R. Cohen. 1985. Knowledge about AIDS and High-Risk Behavior among Intravenous Drug Abusers in New York City. Paper presented at the Annual Meeting of the American Public Health Association, Washington, D.C., November 18.

Selwyn P. A., D. Hartel, W. Wasserman, and E. Drucker. 1989. Impact of the AIDS Epidemic on Morbidity and Mortality among Intravenous Drug Users in a New York City Methadone Maintenance Program. *American Journal of Public Health* 79(10): 1358–1362.

Siegel, K., L. Bauman, G. Christ, and S. Krown. 1988. Patterns of Change in Sexual Behavior among Gay Men in New York City. *Archives of Sexual Behavior* 17(6): 481–497.

Sorge, R. 1991. Drug Policy in the Age of AIDS: The Philosophy of "Harm Reduction." *National Alliance of Methadone Advocates Educational Series*, no. 2 (reprinted from *Health PAC Bulletin* 1990, 20(3): 4–10).

Springer, E. 1991. Effective AIDS Prevention with Active Drug Users: The Harm Reduction Model. *Journal of Chemical Dependency Treatment* 4(2): 141–157.

Stephens, R. 1972. The Truthfulness of Addict Respondents in Research Projects. *International Journal of the Addictions* 7:549–558.

van Meter, K. 1990. Methodological and Design issues: Techniques for Assessing the Representatives of Snowball Samples. In *The Collection and Interpretation of Data from Hidden Populations*. NIDA Research Monograph 90, pp. 31–43.

Watters, J., and Y. Cheng. 1991. Toward Comprehensive Studies of HIV in Intravenous Drug Users: Issues in Treatment-based and Street-based Samples. In *Longitudinal Studies of HIV Infection in Intravenous Drug Users*. NIDA Research Monograph 109, pp. 63–73.

Weber, R., B. Lederberber, M. Opravil, and R. Luthy. 1990. Cessation of Intravenous Drug Use Reduces Progression of HIV Infection in HIV+ Drug Users. Poster VI International Conference on AIDS, San Francisco.

Wiebel, W. 1989. Identifying and Gaining Access to Hidden Populations. In *The Collection and Interpretation of Data from Hidden Populations*. NIDA Research Monograph 98, pp. 4–11.

———. 1991. Sampling Issues for Natural History Studies Including Intravenous Drug Abusers. In *Longitudinal Studies of HIV Infection in Intravenous Drug Users*. NIDA Research Monograph 109, pp. 51–62.

Worth, D. 1989. Sexual Decision-making and AIDS: Why Condom Promotion among Vulnerable Women Is Likely to Fail. *Studies in Family Planning*. 20(6):297–307.

# 14

# Conclusion

*Douglas A. Feldman*

Developing a coherent, unified global AIDS policy that is appropriate and applicable in the totality of diverse cultures and social settings is a formidable task indeed. Some have argued that different cultures should be judged by different standards and have maintained that in some societies where group cohesion is more highly regarded than individual needs, it would be wrong for the rights of the individual to interfere with the good of the whole (Herskovits 1973; cf. Edgerton 1992). Cuba is a good example of this.

In 1986, rather than embarking on a program emphasizing AIDS education and HIV risk reduction, the government of Cuba began to devote its resources to mandatory HIV testing of every citizen on the island and forced mass quarantine for life of all persons testing HIV positive. Pregnant women found to be HIV positive are required to undergo an abortion, even though it is known that most of the children would not become HIV infected. Today, most of the degrading conditions found in the original quarantine camps have been eliminated, and the quality of life provided has significantly improved. Those patients designated as "trustworthy," usually heterosexual men who served in the Cuban army in Angola, are granted considerable freedom of movement outside the sanatoria. But those who are deemed "untrustworthy," more often women or gay men, are rarely or never permitted to leave the sanatoria. Those who attempt to escape or commit other major infractions are sent to the local prison for months at a time.

It is difficult to know how effective this approach is in controlling the spread of AIDS in Cuba since independent confirmation of Cuban government data is not permitted. But if we assume that the claims of the Cuban government that it has successfully limited the spread of HIV throughout its island are correct, it is important that we focus upon the high cost in lost human dignity and freedom in carrying out this Stalinist policy (Feldman 1993; Kane 1994).

The Cuban approach to HIV control is by no means unique. Bulgaria began a similar policy of HIV quarantine, but abandoned it because it was too costly. The Kenyan government threatened HIV quarantine camps, but failed to carry this out. Observers of South Asia believe that some nations there (e.g., Myanmar and Singapore) are prepared to develop a similar approach. Douglas (1966) informed us that societies consider polluting phenomena dangerous, and those with what are perceived as polluting diseases will be ostracized and stigmatized. Like leprosy throughout human history and cholera especially in the early nineteenth century, the dehumanizing reaction to persons with HIV and AIDS has too often been to cast them out or to isolate them from the rest of society. We have seen this repeatedly in the United States, where Ryan White was forced out of his school and community because he was HIV positive. The Ray family in Arcadia, Florida, had their house burned to the ground. A facility for babies with AIDS in Queens, New York, was similarly set ablaze. Countless persons with AIDS have lost their jobs, their apartments or homes, and their insurance or have been denied basic health and other services as a direct result of AIDS-related discrimination. There is no viable excuse for such discrimination, and a sound AIDS policy, applicable in all nations and among all cultures, needs to condemn every form of coercion and ostracism, including quarantine camps (no matter how pleasant the surroundings), grand-scale mandatory HIV testing, denial of services, or other forms of rejection and discrimination against persons with HIV and AIDS.

As we have learned from several chapters in this volume, the problem has less often been one of blatant discrimination and denial of services, and more often one of neglect, corruption, incompetence, and a general lack of services. In most developing countries this has been compounded by grossly inadequate funding to begin to meaningfully address the health and social crisis. There is an urgent need for donor nations and agencies to reassess their levels of financial commitment in attacking the HIV pandemic on a global level.

Every major corporation doing business in Third World nations needs to reassess its corporate donor policy for HIV-related funding, to strengthen or initiate its comprehensive program for prevention of AIDS in the workplace, and to develop compassionate policies and services designed to assist its employees with AIDS and their families or loved ones. Every religious organization needs to reevaluate its role in the struggle against AIDS. Religious organizations should ask themselves whether they have been using the AIDS epidemic as a mechanism for promoting antisexual values and exploiting persons with HIV to make a "moral" statement, or whether they are educating their congregations about HIV and providing caring help to persons living with AIDS.

Every political leader needs to rethink HIV-related policy issues for his or her nation. Are these policies repressive or neglectful, or are they supportive of persons with AIDS and proactive in developing HIV prevention on a national, communitywide, and interpersonal level? What is being done to eliminate the incompetence and corruption afflicting so many nations in the delivery of AIDS-related services and HIV prevention programs?

No other phenomenon more dramatically reveals the urgent need for a restructuring of the political economy of Third World nations than does AIDS. It is difficult to develop sound, well-funded AIDS prevention and social services programs in a nation where the health and social services facilities are wholly inadequate, understaffed, poorly equipped, and underfinanced, and the per capita expenditure in health is only a few dollars per year. It is difficult to discourage teenage girls from exchanging sex for money in a nation where there is no other way for them to obtain muchneeded pocket change. It is difficult for a married woman to demand that her husband use condoms, even when she knows that he is having extramarital relations, in a nation where decisions about sexual behavior are reserved for the man.

The wide gap between the few who are rich and the many who are poor, the desperate poverty of much of the populace, rapid population growth, and the low status of women are omnipresent realities in most Third World nations. Changes in the Third World should entail prioritizing health, education, and social needs, expanding market-driven economies with strong but efficient government regulation, augmenting taxation of the wealthy and major corporations, strongly promoting zero population growth, decreasing corruption and incompetence in government, altering social institutions that perpetuate sexual inequality and homophobia, promoting job-skill training and employment, maintaining internal security and decreasing rising urban crime, deemphasizing military power and armaments, eliminating two-tiered systems of monetary valuation, and developing programs that erode extraordinary income inequality.

But while changing the global political economy is a necessity and a long-term goal, the AIDS crisis is immediate and requires short-term solutions within the current political and economic framework. If we wait for the world to get better before we do something about AIDS, it will be too late.

A short-term strategy for global AIDS prevention and control, at least until an effective vaccine becomes universally available, is to strive for the following:

1. *HIV Education and Risk Reduction.* Sexual behavior can be changed. People in all cultures can be taught to regularly and properly use condoms and engage in other forms of safer sex. Norms need to be altered on the community level so that it is no longer acceptable to practice unsafe sex outside of a faithful monogamous or closed polygynous or polyandrous

marriage. Attitudes need to be changed on the interpersonal level so that persons have the self-esteem, the skills, and the capacity to initiate a negotiation for safer sex.

Education and peer-led risk-reduction workshops need to be culturally appropriate and directed especially toward youth (in and out of school), sexually active adult men and women, the military, and corporate employees. The media need to become fully involved in promoting explicit messages about AIDS. Traditional healers need to be enlisted in the fight against AIDS, since in many developing nations they are the primary health providers.

2. *AIDS Programs and Services.* HIV-spectrum disease often takes a devastating toll on persons and families suffering from this ongoing affliction. Previously healthy, productive individuals suddenly find themselves unable to work or to provide for their families. AIDS orphans currently number in the millions. Home-based care, meals-on-wheels, visiting nurses, AIDS buddies, psychosocial counseling, HIV support groups, social activities for persons with HIV, and family support (including financial support) are some of the programs needed in every nation through well-funded AIDS service organizations.

3. *Human Rights and HIV Legislation.* If you want to learn what is wrong with a given society, look at how it handles the question of AIDS. Nations under the sway of religious fundamentalism, fascism, or totalitarianism are quick to employ the emergence of HIV as a mechanism to further political repression. Legislation, enforcement, and changing attitudes are needed to protect the human rights of persons living with HIV. There is no acceptable rationale for discriminating against a person based upon his or her HIV serostatus.

4. *Research.* While HIV-related basic biomedical, clinical, and epidemiologic research have been fairly well funded, social and behavioral research have not. There is a need for good qualitative and quantitative research studies in AIDS program evaluation, HIV prevention, human sexuality, the social consequences of AIDS, social and health services for persons with AIDS, and both rapid assessment and long-term ethnographies by trained social scientists on the cultures of at-risk communities and other groups.

The time has come for a renewed commitment against AIDS and HIV infection. We must assemble all of our resources, both human and financial, to wage unconditional war against this pandemic. We have made mistakes in the past, but we must learn from these mistakes. The challenge is now ours. We can succeed.

## REFERENCES

Douglas, Mary. 1966. *Purity and Danger: An Analysis of the Concepts of Pollution and Taboo.* London: Routledge and Kegan Paul.

Edgerton, Robert B. 1992. *Sick Societies: Challenging the Myth of Primitive Harmony.* New York: Free Press.

Feldman, Douglas A. 1993. "Sacrificing Basic Civil Liberties," *Anthropology Newsletter,* p. 2, December.

Herskovits, Melville J. 1973. *Cultural Relativism: Perspectives in Cultural Pluralism.* New York: Vantage Books.

Kane, Stephanie. 1994. "AIDS Quarantine: Human Rights and Anthropology," *Anthropology Newsletter,* p. 48, February.

# Index

# About the Editor and Contributors

ROBERT G. CARLSON is director of ethnography on the Dayton/Columbus AIDS Prevention Research Project based in the Substance Abuse Intervention Programs, Wright State University School of Medicine. His interests include medical anthropology, psychoactive drugs, AIDS, political economy, and structural and symbolic analysis.

CINDIE CARROLL-PANKHURST is a doctoral candidate in epidemiology, Department of Epidemiology and Biostatistics, School of Medicine, Case Western Reserve University. Her interests include maternal mortality and reproductive health in developing countries.

MICHAEL C. CLATTS is a medical anthropologist whose principal area of interest is the study of social change, particularly the use of qualitative research methodologies in the formulation, implementation, and evaluation of technology-transfer strategies. He is currently conducting AIDS intervention research among both the adult drug injector and homeless youth populations in New York City.

W. R. DAVIS has worked on a wide variety of studies in the social sciences, but since 1987 has been involved primarily in drug-use and AIDS research at Narcotic and Drug Research Inc. (NDRI) in New York City.

SHERRY DEREN is currently director of the Institute for AIDS Research at NDRI. She is also principal investigator on NIDA- and CDC-funded AIDS prevention projects. Her other areas of interest have included children of substance abusers and program evaluation.

RUSSEL S. FALCK is project director of the AIDS Prevention Research Project and health education director for Substance Abuse Intervention Programs at Wright State University School of Medicine, Dayton, Ohio.

DOUGLAS A. FELDMAN is a medical anthropologist and President of D. A. Feldman & Associates, a behavioral and program evaluation research organization in Hollywood, Florida. He teaches "AIDS as a Public Health Issue" at the University of Miami School of Medicine. He is the coeditor of *The Social Dimensions of AIDS: Method and Theory* (Praeger, 1986), the editor of *Culture and AIDS* (Praeger, 1990), and the former editor of the *AIDS and Anthropology Bulletin*. He has conducted AIDS behavioral research in the United States, Zambia, Rwanda, Uganda, Senegal, and Thailand.

VINCENT E. GIL is professor of anthropology and human sexuality at Southern California College and conducts research on sexual culture and the epidemiology of AIDS. His research areas include the Caribbean and the People's Republic of China.

DOUGLAS S. GOLDSMITH, an ethnographer with NDRI since 1980, has participated in interdisciplinary research on street drug usage, treatment program behaviors, and AIDS-related beliefs. A volunteer advocate for people with AIDS since 1984, in the street, hospitals, and prisons, he was a member of the AIDS Task Force of the American Anthropological Association.

PAMELA HARTIGAN is responsible for promoting, facilitating, and coordinating activities of the Pan American Health Organization (PAHO/WHO) with NGOs working in health and development in Latin America and the Caribbean.

NORRIS G. LANG is associate professor and chair of the Department of Anthropology at the University of Houston, Central Campus, and associate clinical practitioner at the New Counseling Center in Houston.

JANET W. MCGRATH is associate professor of anthropology, Case Western Reserve University. Her research interests include the biological and social impact of AIDS and other diseases. She served on the American Anthropological Association's AIDS Task Force and is the chair of the AIDS and Anthropology Research Group.

M. E. MELODY is a professor of political science at Barry University in Miami Shores, Florida. He has also served for more than seven years as a volunteer "buddy," and then a director of Health Crisis Network, Inc., Miami's major AIDS-related organization.

REBECCA MUKASA is a research assistant in the Department of Sociology, Makerere University, Kampala, Uganda. She has been involved in AIDS research since 1990.

SYLVIA NAKAYIWA is a research assistant in the Department of Sociology, Makerere University, Kampala, Uganda. Currently she is a graduate student in demography and populations studies at the Institute of Statistics and Applied Economics, Makerere University.

LUCY NAKYOBE is a research assistant in the Department of Sociology, Makerere University, Kampala, Uganda. She has been involved in AIDS research since 1990.

BARBARA NAMANDE is a research assistant in the Department of Sociology, Makerere University, Kampala, Uganda. Currently she is a graduate student in sociology at Queens University, Ontario, Canada.

RICHARD G. PARKER is professor of medical anthropology and human sexuality in the Institute of Social Medicine at the State University of Rio de Janeiro and is a director of the Brazilian Interdisciplinary AIDS Association. He is the author of *Bodies, Pleasures, and Passions: Sexual Culture in Contemporary Brazil* and coauthor with Herbert Daniel of *AIDS: A Terceira Epidemia* and *Sexuality, Politics, and AIDS in Brazil.*

ROBERT W. PORTER is a social anthropologist with Porter/Novelli, a marketing communications firm in Washington, D.C. He serves on technical advisory groups for the World Bank, the National Research Council, and Princeton University.

MICHAEL D. QUAM is professor of anthropology and public health at Sangamon State University in Springfield, Illinois. He is the author and coauthor of a number of papers and articles on AIDS policy in the United States.

DANA RAPHAEL, a medical anthropologist, is director of the Human Lactation Center, Ltd., Westport, Connecticut. Her publications include *Only Mothers Know: Patterns of Infant Feeding in a Hungry World* (Greenwood Press) and *The Tender Gift: Breastfeeding.*

CHARLES B. RWABUKWALI is a senior lecturer in the Department of Sociology, Makerere University, Kampala, Uganda. His research interests are in health resources utilization, social aspects of AIDS, and patterns of fertility regulation. He is a doctoral student in medical anthropology at Case Western Reserve University, Cleveland, Ohio.

DEBRA A. SCHUMANN is a research associate in the Department of Population Dynamics, Johns Hopkins University School of Hygiene and Public Health, and population advisor, Office of Women in Development, United States Agency for International Development. Her research interests include behavioral research on AIDS and other infectious diseases.

HARVEY A. SIEGAL is director of Substance Abuse Intervention Programs, Wright State University School of Medicine, and principal investigator of the AIDS Prevention Research Project, Wright State University School of Medicine, Dayton, Ohio.

STEPHANIE TORTU is a co-investigator on an AIDS-related research project in East Harlem and a faculty member of New York University. She has authored scientific publications, presented at national conferences, and conducted various training workshops.

VIRGINIA VAN DER VLIET is a lecturer at the University of Western Cape. Her research interests are contemporary African family life, demography, and the growing South African AIDS epidemic.

ISBN 0-89789-282-8

EAN

9 780897 892827

HARDCOVER BAR CODE